JANE BRODY'S
NUTRITION BOOK

"A marvelous combination of sound science and common sense.
. . . The best home reference on nutrition I have seen."
>—G. Timothy Johnson
editor, Harvard Medical
School Health Letter

"I heartily recommend it for every home library."
>—Jean Mayer, former
chairman, White House
Conference on Food,
Nutrition and Health

"For all of those people who have looked for a single source of
reliable information on nutrition . . . Jane Brody's book may be the
answer."
>—*The Washington Post*

"Unsurpassed as a guide for individual action."
>—*Kirkus Reviews*

"The very best book of its kind ever written."

h

"As helpful to anxious eaters as
anxious parents."

D1042615

Revised and Updated

JANE BRODY'S NUTRITION BOOK

*A Lifetime Guide to
Good Eating for Better Health
and Weight Control by the
Personal Health Columnist of*
The New York Times

BANTAM BOOKS
TORONTO · NEW YORK · LONDON · SYDNEY · AUCKLAND

JANE BRODY'S NUTRITION BOOK

A Bantam Book / published by arrangement with
W. W. Norton & Co., Inc.

PRINTING HISTORY

Norton edition published March 1981
A Featured Alternate selection of Book-of-the-Month Club, August 1981, Main selection of Cooking and Crafts Club, An Alternate selection of Young Parents Book Club, March 1982, and a Special selection of Macmillan Book Clubs (to all clubs), February 1982.

Serialized in The New York Times *Special Features Syndicate, April 1981;* Book Digest, *August 1981;* Reader's Digest Condensed Books, *September 1981;* Reader's Digest Families Magazine, *December 1981 and May 1981;* Runner's World Magazine, *September, October and November 1981;* House and Garden Magazine, *September 1981;* Redbook Magazine, *October 1981;* Working Mother Magazine, *January 1982;* Saturday Evening Post, *July 1981 and September 1981;* Cosmopolitan *magazine, November 1981;* Weight Watcher's *magazine, October 1981;* Lady's Circle *magazine, October 1981;* Event, *Summer 1981 issue;* Shape Magazine, *January/February 1981;* Health Quarterly *magazine, September/October 1981 and January/February 1982;* Your Good Health *magazine;* Beauty Digest, *May 1982;* Women Sports *magazine, March 1982* and Cosmopolitan's Beauty Digest, *Spring/Summer 1982.*

Excerpted in Woman's Day, Self *and* Family Circle.

Bantam edition / December 1982
Bantam Revised Edition / February 1987
3 printings through March 1988

The "Ape Shake" recipe that appears on page 371 is reprinted from Love at First Bite by Jane Cooper. Copyright © 1977 by Jane Cooper. Reprinted by permission of Alfred A. Knopf, Inc. The height and weight table on page 287 was developed by Pacific Mutual Life Insurance Company, Newport Beach, California, from a study by the Association of Life Insurance Medical Directors and the Society of Actuaries. "What to Drink, When, and Why," which appears on page 423, is reprinted with the permission of The Runner and of Dr. David Costill, William Fink, and Hal Higdon. The following recipes are ©, reprinted with the permission of the American Heart Association: "Cinnamon Toasties," page 91; "Beef Bourguignon," page 213; "Chicken Cacciatore," page 213; "Tomato Crown Fish," page 214; "Potato Salad," page 214, The fats and oils table on page 85 and "How to Season Your Food without Salt" on page 212 are also ©, reprinted with the permission of the American Heart Association. The "Company Beans with Rice" recipe on page 44 is reprinted with the permission of Environmental Nutrition. The illustration of the wheat kernel, which appears on page 107, is reprinted with the permission of the Kansas Wheat Commission. The recipes for "Fluffy Yogurt Gelatin" and "Strawberry-Pineapple Frozen Yogurt," which appear on page 40, are reprinted from Eater's Almanac with the permission of Giant Foods, Inc., and the National Heart, Lung, and Blood Institute. "How Much Sodium Is in Processed Foods?," page 208, is adapted from Consumer Reports, March, 1979, issue, and reprinted with permission of Consumer Reports. "Dining Out the Low-Fat Way," page 89; the menu plan that appears on page 320; and "One Day's Sample Menu during Pregnancy," which appears on page 340, are all reprinted with permission from Nutrition and Health. "How Alcohol Affects You," which appears on page 259, is reprint from How Drinking Can Be Good for You by Morris E. Chafetz, © 1976 by Morris E. Chafetz, with the permission of Stein & Day Publishers.

All rights reserved.
Copyright © 1981, 1987 by Jane E. Brody.
Cover photograph © 1987 by Tom Victor.
No part of this book may be reproduced or transmitted
in any form or by any means, electronic or mechanical,
including photocopying, recording, or by any information
storage and retrieval system, without permission in
writing from the publisher.
For information address: W. W. Norton & Co., Inc.,
500 Fifth Avenue, New York, N.Y. 10110.

Library of Congress Cataloging-in-Publication Data
Brody, Jane E.
Jane Brody's Nutrition Book.
Includes index.
1. Nutrition.   2. Diet   I. Title.   II. Title:
Nutrition book. [DNLM: 1. Nutrition—popular works.
QU 145 B8645n]
TX353.B76   1987   613.2   86-26599
ISBN 0-553-34332-7

Published simultaneously in the United States and Canada

Bantam Books are published by Bantam Books, a division of Bantam Doubleday Dell Publishing Group, Inc. Its trademark, consisting of the words "Bantam Books" and the portrayal of a rooster, is Registered in U.S. Patent and Trademark Office and in other countries. Marca Registrada. Bantam Books, 666 Fifth Avenue, New York, New York 10103.

PRINTED IN THE UNITED STATES OF AMERICA

FG   12 11 10 9 8 7 6

CONTENTS

PART ONE

What to Eat

PART TWO
———
The Noncaloric Nutrients

PART THREE

What to Drink

PART FOUR
─────

What to Do about Your Weight

PART FIVE

Food for Special Lives

PART SIX

What's in Your Food

RECIPES

TABLES

CHARTS

ACKNOWLEDGMENTS

WRITING A BOOK is a family affair, and this one was no exception. It could never have happened without the cooperation, encouragement, and assistance of my family: my beloved husband, Richard Engquist, who read and typed the entire manuscript (and in the process further transformed the family diet) and who for a year and a half took on far more than his share of household responsibilities; and our sons, Lorin and Erik, who stayed out of my hair as much as 10 year olds can and who, with good-natured indulgence if not always outright enthusiasm, played guinea pig for years of cooking experiments.

I also want to thank my parents, mother-in-law and other relatives, my devoted friends, and my editors at the *New York Times* for giving me much-needed mental space and time in which to work. Special thanks go to my dear friend JoAnn Friedman, president of Health Marketing Systems, Inc., who, in addition to directing me to invaluable sources of information, was always ready to reapply the glue whenever I threatened to fall apart at the seams.

I am indebted to the countless researchers who have given so generously of their time and knowledge through the years, helping me to acquire a sound understanding of the intricacies of human nutrition and an appreciation for the need to act now to improve our diets. I am particularly grateful to Dr. Myron Winick, director of the Institute of Human Nutrition at Columbia University College of Physicians and Surgeons, who reviewed the entire manuscript for technical accuracy. My thanks, too, to Dr. Jules Hirsch, obesity specialist at the Rockefeller University; Dr. Henry Blackburn, preventive-medicine specialist at the University of Minnesota; and Dr. David Kritchevsky, fiber expert at the Wistar Institute, all of whom reviewed portions of the manuscript in their areas of expertise.

Without the patient, perceptive, and intelligent editing of Edwin Barber and Mary Cunnane at W. W. Norton & Company this book would have been a third heavier. Thank you, Ed and Mary, for always being upbeat about your comments and criticisms and flexible about changes. Thanks to Marjorie J. Flock for her hard work on the many design problems that the manuscript presented. Thanks, too, to Carol Flechner, who copy-edited the manuscript with extraordinary care and sensitivity. And thanks to everyone at Norton who from the outset supplied continuous enthusiasm and support for the project.

JANE
BRODY'S
NUTRITION
BOOK

TO THE READER

NUTRITION is a subject in constant flux. The recent explosion of consumer interest in the nutritive as well as the culinary aspects of food has prompted a dramatic increase in professional attention to what people should be eating to maintain good health and a normal body weight. As new information emerges from responsible research laboratories here and abroad, the "facts" about human nutrition are necessarily modified. In the five years since I wrote *Jane Brody's Nutrition Book,* there's been a slew of new findings of major health significance: about fats, fiber, calcium, coffee, sweeteners, alcohol, as well as other aspects of food and drink. At the same time, food products and how they are sold have changed too.

The book you are now reading has been updated to reflect the new findings as well as the changes in the marketplace and in the thinking of qualified professionals in the field of nutrition. The information herein represents the best available research in human nutrition as of the mid-1980s. From time to time, new findings will continue to change our understanding of this long-neglected subject and the nutritional guidance derived from it, and when this happens, I will make further changes in this book. For now, however, we all have to eat. We cannot wait for the "last word" on nutrition before we decide how to structure our diets. We know enough now about healthful eating to make reasonable recommendations for most people, who quite naturally want to enjoy their food for as many healthful years as possible.

This book is a guide to good nutrition throughout your life. Although the emphasis is on eating to preserve health, it does not contain dietary prescriptions for specific medical problems. *Do not use any of the advice herein for self-treatment without your physician's knowledge and okay. Even if you are perfectly healthy, a radical, abrupt change in your diet is unwise without first consulting your physician.*

A certain amount of redundancy has been built into the book. Since many topics in nutrition are closely interrelated and since many readers are likely to refer to individual chapters from time to time, particular points have been made wherever they happen to be relevant. And in many cases, the reader is referred to other chapters for expanded discussions of certain points. For example, while animal fats are discussed primarily in the chapter on fats and cholesterol, they are also mentioned in the chapters on protein and vegetarian diets.

The chapters in this book have been read for technical accuracy by area specialists (see acknowledgments). These specialists are highly regarded not only for their expertise, but also for their unbiased approach to research.

Throughout the book, unless otherwise attributed, all opinions expressed are those of the author, who is beholden to no special interest group or industry. I have based my conclusions on an extensive and detailed study of the findings of scientifically sound nutrition research.

Unless you have a chronic illness like diabetes or are genetically prone to heart disease, you need not become an extremist or an ascetic, nor do you have to give up everything you love forever, to live healthfully and enjoyably. Through the principles of moderation, you can enjoy good health and a good life. You need only decide it's something you want to do.

The philosophy of this book is one of understanding and logic. On the basis of personal experience, observation of others, and conversations with experts, I believe that people are most likely to loosen their hold on old habits and make constructive changes in their lives when they understand and appreciate the rationale for those changes and are given some guidance as to how to go about them. This, at least, is how it worked for me and my family. Keep reading and see if you agree.

JANE E. BRODY

PART ONE

What to Eat

1 ⚬ THE NEW NUTRITION: YOU ARE WHAT YOU EAT

W HETHER you are hell-bent on living to 100 or you'd settle for a mere threescore and ten, no doubt you'd like to look well and feel well all your life. Whether nature gave you large bones or small ones, you probably want to be trim without suffering the rigors and deprivations of one "diet" after another, 90 percent of which are doomed to fail anyhow.

Your success in reaching these goals depends very much on what and how and how much you eat. Your daily diet can influence your risk of developing an imposing list of life-shortening and typically American diseases, including heart disease, cancer, stroke, diabetes, and high blood pressure, not to mention the less threatening but painful problems of tooth decay, bone fractures, and—America's leading ailment—obesity.

If indeed you are what you eat, what can you do about it? Nutrition studies have shown that for the vast majority of Americans a healthful diet depends not so much on consuming any particular nutrient or group of nutrients, but rather on the overall structure of the diet —the total balance of foods we eat. Currently, our balance is greatly distorted: Americans eat too much fat, too much sugar, too many calories, and even too much protein.

We are a people ignorant of good nutrition. And the reasons why are as close as the local supermarket, where shelves are lined with thousands of smartly packaged food products that have little nutritive value or are so highly processed that they bear small resemblance to the original farm product. More than half the foods we eat are processed and packaged. Fifty percent of these manufactured food items didn't exist a decade ago. Experts estimate that ten years from now, 80 percent of the food items sold in supermarkets will be less than a decade old. As many as 500 new products may be introduced in a given year.

How can consumers faced with this array of new and unfamiliar foods know if they're getting their nutritional money's worth? Too often, they can't. The food industry spends more than $2 billion a year advertising its wares, mostly pushing the nutritionally deficient ones—snacks, candy, and soft drinks laden with fat, sugar, and calories. Rarely are there equally enticing ads for whole grains, fresh fruits, or vegetables.

Many people who've become disillusioned with what industry has done to foods have opted for so-called natural and organic products, and often end up paying through the nose for nutrition that is no better than what the supermarket offers. Others have abandoned the "standard American diet" for the vegetarian regimens of our evolutionary forebears, and some shortchange their bodies on essential nutrients because they don't know enough to construct a nutritionally sound vegetarian diet. Still others sprinkle fiber like holy water on everything they eat, but lack any appreciation for what the different kinds of fiber can and cannot do for the body. And tens of millions are beset with dietmania, often choosing hazardous schemes in their eternal search for a way to eat themselves to slimdom.

In general, a public ignorant of sound nutritional facts is at the mercy not only of nutritionally immoral food companies but also of a growing army of food faddists, diet mongers, vitamin hawkers, and self-styled nutritionists. As a result, many of the choices people make in an effort to improve their nutritional well-being are based on sweeping generalities, half-baked data, ignorance, prejudice, and superstition.

At a Christmas buffet, I watched a young man pick apart an eggplant casserole to be sure it contained no meat. He said that he doesn't eat meat or chicken because "they are contaminated with dangerous chemicals." But he had no qualms about eating fish. He admitted that many fish are harvested from waters laced with chemical poisons, but he said "at least they got there naturally—someone didn't deliberately add them to the fish."

A friend never drinks coffee because she says it keeps her awake at night. But she thinks nothing of downing two or three cups of tea after dinner, which contain more caffeine than a cup of coffee.

Another friend refuses to eat the rice at Chinese restaurants because it isn't brown rice.

At dinner in an elegant New York restaurant, a companion asked the waiter for Sweet 'N Low for her coffee, which accompanied her 600-calorie dessert of raspberry pie a la mode. As she emptied the pink packet of no-calorie saccharin into her cup to replace the 18 calories in a teaspoon of sugar, she said to me apologetically, "I know this probably causes cancer, but . . ."

I was waiting for a drink at the office fountain while the young man ahead of me swallowed no less than six pills and tablets, one after the other. Concerned, I asked him if he was all right. "Sure," he said, "these are . . ." and he rattled off a laundry list of vitamins, minerals, and quasi nutrients, which he said he takes three times a day. "They're good for you," he assured me.

In the face of nutritional ignorance, myths and downright quackery have gained a strong foothold. People lambaste "chemicals" in our foods and overlook the fact that major nutrients like fat and sugar are actually doing the most damage. Millions search for the elixir of youth in bottles of vitamins and minerals, cakes of yeast, or jars of wheat germ. The current interest in micronutrients—vitamins, minerals, and trace elements—has prompted many to conclude that haphazard eating habits and unbalanced menus can be compensated for by swallowing a pill or potion of concentrated nutrients. This is not true. It's comparable to giving a Lincoln Continental an occasional shot of premium gasoline to make up for the low-octane fuel you fill it with most of the time. Your body is a machine; it will run as well as its fuel allows.

This book is designed to steer you between the profit-motivated food companies and faddism. It is meant to help you understand the why and wherefore of good nutrition and to put them into practice if you decide to. It is necessarily based on less-than-complete information. Nutrition research has long sucked the hind teat of the nation's multibillion-dollar biomedical research cow, and even now is not receiving the research support it deserves. But if you put together all that we do know, you'll have plenty of guidance to make sensible and healthful adjustments in your diet.

It's important to realize that good nutrition is not necessarily incompatible with pleasurable dining. Food has long been—and should continue to be—a great source of enjoyment for people. You needn't give up everything you now love to eat in order to protect your health. But you do have to learn to practice discretion and moderation in your food choices. A Harris poll taken in 1978–1979 revealed that two in three Americans think they'd be healthier if they changed their diets, but they continue to eat the way they always have because they enjoy it and lack the will power to change.

The Good Word about Good Nutrition

Most of us grew up thinking nutrition was a great bore. We learned the Basic Seven food groups (which became the Basic Four in the mid-1950s) and how many servings per day we were supposed to eat of each to pack in enough protein, vitamins, and minerals to grow on. Maybe a brightly illustrated chart accompanied the lesson, which advised eating two servings a day of meat or a meat equivalent, two to four servings of milk and dairy products, four or more servings of fruits and vegetables, and four or more servings of bread, grains, and cereals. But most of us went on eating precisely as we had before, and after passing the quiz, even forgot the groupings, not to mention the recommended number of servings.

Until recently, nutrition was a dead word. It didn't "sell." It was equated in the public mind with having to eat foods we disliked and giving up those we loved for the sake of some textbook formula for good health. Except for a small audience of "health nuts" who frequented "health food" stores scattered about the country's major metropolitan areas, nutrition simply turned people off. Even the late health-food guru Adelle Davis didn't use the word nutrition in her book titles!

Then in the 1970s, nutrition came out of the closet. The first wedge in the door was a negative one—tales of harmful food substances that might be poisoning us all. Farm produce was said to be riddled with pesticide residues, meat and poultry laced with potent hormones and antibiotics, fish polluted with toxic industrial chemicals, and processed foods filled with long strings of unpronounceable chemicals to make them resemble foods that they were not. What are these chemical concoctions you shake and bake and whip and chill, the instant breakfasts and hamburger helpers, the meals in a box and frozen dinners? And are they good for you?

The emerging crisis in confidence in the safety and healthfulness of the American food supply was nurtured by an increasingly aggressive health-food movement that promised safer and more nourishing alternatives free of chemical contaminants and fortified with "natural" goodness. Their ranks were swelled by hordes of faddists who latched onto one or another nutrient as the panacea for a host of modern ills, from backache to boredom.

Millions of Americans, whose sufferings resisted medical treatment or who no longer trusted the doctors who applied them, took matters into their own hands and turned to nutrition. Others bombarded doctors with questions about nutrients and diet plans—questions for which medical school had provided no ready answers. Coming from behind, the medical profession periodically defended itself against what it regarded as nutritional quackery—always useless and sometimes harmful, and most certainly threatening to the status of medicine.

But while scorned by doctors, scientists, and officials of government and industry, the health-food movement made *nutrition* a household word. Many Americans now pause to read labels as they scurry
through the aisles of a supermarket, and stop to think before shoving
coins into a vending machine. More and more of us are taking stock
of how and what we eat and how it may affect our health.

National leaders were late getting into the act. After decades of
governmental dillydallying and buckling under industrial pressures,
action finally came, not from the United States Department of Agriculture or the Department of Health, Education, and Welfare, but from
Congress. As chairman of the Senate Select Committee on Nutrition
and Human Needs, George McGovern took on the big guns—first the
problem of obesity and the billion-dollar industry that caters to its cure,
and then the entire structure of the American diet and its devastating
effects on health and longevity. In 1977, the McGovern committee
culminated its investigation with the publication of a new set of nutritional guidelines for Americans intended to quell many of the nation's
major killers—heart disease, cancers of the colon and breast, stroke,
high blood pressure, obesity, diabetes, arteriosclerosis, and cirrhosis of
the liver, all of which have been linked to the current American diet.

The committee estimated that if its goals were reached by all
Americans, there'd be an 80-percent drop in the number of obese
Americans, a 25-percent decline in deaths from heart disease, a 50-
percent drop in deaths from diabetes, and a 1-percent annual increase
in longevity. To achieve only a part of this increase in life expectancy
would be an incredible feat. Since 1920, the life expectancy for 50-year-
old American men has increased by only nine months.

The Dietary Goals of the McGovern committee call for Americans
to eat less fat, especially less artery-clogging saturated fat, less cholesterol, less refined and processed sugars, less salt, less alcohol, fewer
calories, and more complex carbohydrates and roughage. The specific
recommendations of the Dietary Goals are depicted in Chart 1. This
chart shows the percentage of calories derived from various nutrients
in the current American diet and in the dietary scheme recommended
by the Senate Select Committee on Nutrition and Human Needs. Not
shown are two other important Dietary Goals advised by the committee: a reduction in salt intake to a maximum of 5 grams a day and a
reduction in cholesterol to 300 milligrams a day, about half the current
amount. The chart does not include alcohol, which adds another 210
calories per day to the average diet of drinking-age Americans. No
specific recommendation was made for increasing dietary fiber, but an

Chart 1 • RECOMMENDED DIET FOR AMERICANS

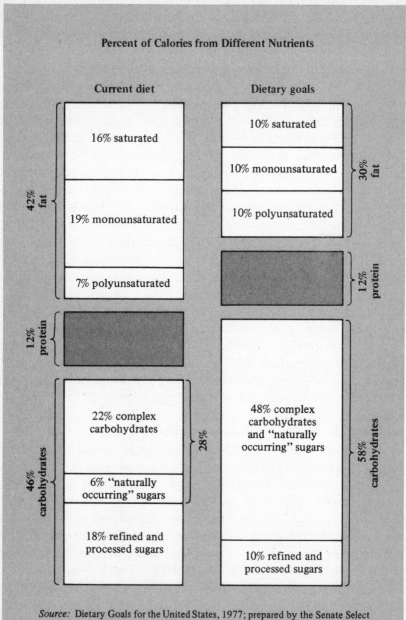

Percent of Calories from Different Nutrients

Current diet

Dietary goals

42% fat

16% saturated

19% monounsaturated

7% polyunsaturated

10% saturated

10% monounsaturated

10% polyunsaturated

30% fat

12% protein

12% protein

46% carbohydrates

22% complex carbohydrates

6% "naturally occurring" sugars

28%

18% refined and processed sugars

48% complex carbohydrates and "naturally occurring" sugars

58% carbohydrates

10% refined and processed sugars

Source: Dietary Goals for the United States, 1977; prepared by the Senate Select Committee on Nutrition and Human Needs.

increase in complex carbohydrates and natural sugars would lead automatically to more fiber in the diet.

To put these goals into effect, the McGovern committee recommended that people eat more fruits, vegetables, and whole grains; fewer foods rich in added sugars, refined flour, and fat; fewer egg yolks and other high-cholesterol foods, and less added salt and foods high in salt. The committee suggested choosing meats, poultry, fish, and dairy products that are lower in total fat, and specifically saturated fat, as well as lower in cholesterol. And it urged a cutback in calorically dense and nutritionally deficient "junk foods," especially sweet, fatty, and salty snacks and alcoholic beverages.

The concepts are hardly revolutionary. Many public-health experts have been saying as much for decades. But the meat, dairy, and egg industries took loud offense, and the American Medical Association (which has often opposed major public-health initiatives for the population as a whole, advising instead that you "see your doctor" for individualized advice) decried the goals as unproven, unnecessary, and premature.

Protest notwithstanding, the McGovern committee had started something. Within two years, the Departments of Agriculture and HEW had essentially adopted the Dietary Goals. The Department of Agriculture established a new Human Nutrition Center, with an internationally known biologist and former Harvard professor, Mark Hegsted, at the helm. Dr. Hegsted published in 1980 the first of a series of food guides to help people choose more healthfully from among the 12,000 products that may confront them in their neighborhood supermarket. And HEW released a Surgeon General's report on preventive medicine, "Healthy People," that advocates, among other things, a Dietary Goals diet. Even the recalcitrant National Institutes of Health, the leaders of the nation's medical research establishment, have come forward with dietary advice to help prevent heart disease and some cancers. Early in 1980, the USDA and HEW published "Nutrition and Your Health: Dietary Guidelines for Americans," a pamphlet based on the philosophy of the McGovern committee, and followed it with a menu plan developed by the Human Nutrition Center (see page 26). This new approach to nutrition is expected to be the foundation for future revisions in nutritional labels on food packages to enable Americans to choose more wisely when they shop for food.

So premature or not, the Dietary Goals are beginning to reshape the nutritional philosophy of America, if not yet the eating habits of most Americans. As Dr. Hegsted pointed out in a preface to the Dietary

Goals: "The diet of the American people has become increasingly rich —rich in meat, other sources of saturated fat and cholesterol, and in sugar. . . . The diet we eat today was not planned or developed for any particular purpose. It is a happenstance related to our affluence, the productivity of our farmers and the activities of our food industry. The risks associated with eating this diet are demonstrably large. The question to be asked, therefore, is not why should we change our diet but why not? . . . Heart disease, cancer, diabetes and hypertension are the diseases that kill us. They are epidemic in our population. We cannot afford to temporize."

The American Diet May Be Hazardous to Your Health

Three facts may surprise you.

1. Past infancy, people have no "natural instinct" to help them distinguish between wholesome and unnourishing foods. So even without chemically concocted products and advertising that starts the saliva flowing for "empty" calories, we'd have to apply thought and intelligence to choosing a nutritious diet.

2. Most of the peoples of the world, including those in a number of developed countries, do not eat the way we do. Their diet is relatively rich in starches and vegetable sources of protein and low in meats, fats, and sugars. They also don't suffer from any chronic health problems. But as affluence increases, meat—the international status symbol— becomes a more prominent part of the diet, and deaths from heart disease rise along with its increased consumption. This is happening now in Japan, where postwar industrialization and affluence have permitted increased meat consumption. The traditional low-meat Japanese diet had contained only a quarter to a third the amount of fat found in typical American diets, and nearly all of that fat was artery-sparing unsaturated fat.

Nations that share our dietary habits, particularly the Scandinavian countries, industrialized Europe, and Canada, also share our diseases and deaths. And when persons from "protected" nations migrate to the United States and adopt our diet, they inherit our diseases. Genetic heritage and cultural background have little influence. Diet is nearly all.

3. Americans didn't always eat like this. Though we live longer now

than at the turn of the century, the increase in life expectancy is almost entirely due to the conquest of infectious diseases through improved sanitation, antibiotics, and immunizations. Meanwhile, the death rates for chronic, diet-related diseases have increased dramatically.

Today we eat far more meat, fish, and poultry, drink much more alcohol and soft drinks, and use loads more sugar than we did in 1910, when the U.S. Department of Agriculture began keeping systematic track of the food supply. At the same time, consumption of milk, grain products, fresh fruit, and vegetables declined dramatically. Most of our protein—70 percent—comes from fat- and cholesterol-rich animal sources, whereas at the turn of the century half came from plants (grains, beans, and the like) that contained little fat and no cholesterol.

According to the Center for Science in the Public Interest, a Washington-based consumer group, the net result of these dietary changes has been a 34-percent increase in fat consumption, from 32 percent of calories in 1910 to 43 percent by 1981; a 100-percent increase in consumption of sugar and other caloric sweeteners, from 12 to 24 percent of calories; and a 40-percent decrease in consumption of complex carbohydrates (starches), from 37 percent to 22 percent of calories. Thus, today 3 of every 5 calories Americans eat are from fats or added sugars. Because our modern diet is relatively low in whole grains, fruits, and vegetables, it is also deficient in dietary fiber. And our generous intake of animal foods has overburdened our diet and blood vessels with cholesterol. Although consumption of eggs, our most common concentrated source of cholesterol, has dropped greatly since its peak in 1945, it is today only slightly below the per-capita consumption level of 1910. And processed foods—more than half of what we eat—are loaded with salt and other sodium-containing compounds.

Total calories *have* dropped slightly—by about 3 percent—since 1910, but Americans are now so sedentary that less is still far too much. Two in 5 Americans are overweight, even though the average adult American consumes fewer calories than is recommended for good nutritional health. In fact, since nutritionally empty fat and sugar calories comprise so large a share of our caloric total, some overweight Americans may actually be short on essential nutrients.

A few encouraging trends have recently emerged in American eating habits. For example, national food-consumption surveys conducted by the Department of Agriculture show that since 1965 average calorie intake has dropped among children and adults of all ages and both sexes. Per person, we are eating somewhat less fat now than in

Table 1.1 • TRENDS IN THE AMERICAN DIET:
CHANGES IN ANNUAL CONSUMPTION PER PERSON

Foods	Time period	% change	Time period	% change
Beef	1910–1976	+72	1976–1981	−19.4
Butter	1910–1976	−76	1976–1981	−3.7
Candy	1968–1976	−18	1976–1980	+7.4
Cheese	1910–1976	+388	1976–1981	+9.3
Chicken	1910–1976	+179	1976–1981	+21.1
Coffee	1946–1976	−44	1976–1981	−17.6
Eggs	1945–1976	−32	1976–1981	−2.0
Fish, fresh and frozen	1960–1976	+42	1976–1981	−4.9
Flour and cereal products	1910–1976	−54	1976–1981	+.7
Fruit, fresh	1910–1976	−33	1976–1981	+5.4
Fruit, processed	1910–1976	+500	1976–1981	−2.0
Ice-cream products	1910–1976	+1,426	1976–1981	−3.5
Margarine	1910–1976	+681	1976–1981	−5.9
Milk	1910–1976	−12	1976–1981	−6.9
Potatoes, fresh	1910–1976	−74	1976–1980	+2.5
Potatoes, frozen	1960–1976	+465	1976–1981	0
Soft drinks	1960–1976	+157	1976–1981	+25.3
Sugar and other sweeteners	1875–1976	+221	1976–1981	+.88
Vegetables, fresh	1945–1976	−16	1976–1981	+6.1

Source: Adapted from Letitia Brewster and Michael F. Jacobson, *The Changing American Diet,* Center for Science in the Public Interest, based on statistics from United States Department of Agriculture (Washington, D.C.: Center for Science in the Public Interest, 1978). Updated 1983.

1965, and more of it is polyunsaturated vegetable oil. But more than a third of the fat we eat is saturated. Compared with 1965, Americans today are eating more poultry, fish, and margarine—foods relatively low in saturated fats and cholesterol—and less butter, milk, cream, cheese, eggs, and ice cream, which are rich in these artery-clogging nutrients. Our passion for beef, which peaked in 1976, began dropping in 1977, because of prices, but has continued in a general downward decline, dropping nearly 20 pounds per person per year by 1985.

Consumption of canned and frozen vegetables is up, but fewer fresh vegetables are eaten. We are actually eating more potatoes, but all the increase is due to frozen potatoes processed for frying, the least nutritious way to eat this otherwise low-fat vegetable. As with vegetables, total fruit consumption is up, but the proportion of fruit that we eat fresh—without added sugar and with natural fiber intact—is down.

Although we've cut back some on refined sugar, there's been a dramatic increase in food processors' use of corn sweeteners, leading to an overall rise in per-capita total sugar consumption since the mid-1960s. Those who satisfy their sweet tooth with honey instead of refined sugar should note that honey is 99.9 percent sugar. The amount of vitamins and minerals in honey is of no practical nutritional significance. (See page 122.)

In the "junk foods" department, consumption of soft drinks—both artificially sweetened and sugar-sweetened carbonated sodas and fruit-flavored drinks—is up dramatically since 1965. Per-capita consumption of alcoholic beverages, especially wine and beer, has also risen, along with pastries, potato chips, and their ilk. More Americans today are deriving more of their calories from nutritionally deficient foods than ever before.

Whatever Happened to "Three Square"?

Of equal importance is the recent change in the *way* our foods are consumed. It is a rare modern family that shares more than one meal a day.

Breakfast is a hit-or-miss affair. If any breakfast is eaten at all, more often than not it consists of presweetened cereal and milk or a vitamin-enriched breakfast bar (really a cookie in disguise) for the youngsters and juice, toast, and coffee for the adults. Three-quarters of American families do not eat breakfast together. In up to half the families, one or more persons regularly skip breakfast. And in 40 percent of families, the parents have nothing to do with the children's breakfast.

For lunch, nearly everyone is on his or her own. Mother, perhaps dieting, may skip it entirely or eat only yogurt. Father is usually in a restaurant or on a cafeteria line (have you ever noticed that these usually start with the desserts?). And the children who eat at school may trade or discard the contents of lunch boxes or shun the unappetizing meals in the school cafeteria. For many youngsters, lunch is a candy bar or bag of potato chips and soda pop from the school vending machine.

Supper is the one meal families are likely to eat together, and it is generally the largest meal of the day. Unfortunately, large amounts of caloric energy are least needed when the day's activities are nearly over. But even supper has become highly diluted in terms of nutritional control and content. In half the nation's households both parents work, and supper often consists of a heat-and-serve meal or something from the local take-out. Very few dinners are prepared "from scratch" with a single intelligence in charge of nutrients. Few cooks know the nutritional value of the prepared foods they use.

Eating out has become the American way of life, no longer reserved for "special occasions." By the mid-1970s, 25 percent of American meals were eaten outside the home. In this decade, experts predict that this percentage will double. By 1985, restaurant meals accounted for 39 percent of every dollar Americans spent on food. And a quarter of those restaurant meals were eaten at fast-food establishments, where high-calorie, high-fat, and high-salt foods are offered. Even in "good" restaurants, diners have no way of knowing the nutrient content or ingredients used in the foods they order.

Snacking has become endemic. Children may get cookies and milk midmorning in school, with more of the same at home at three o'clock. Adults have morning and afternoon coffee breaks—liquid refreshment often accompanied by a sweet roll. After dinner in front of the TV, it's more snacks. Seventy-five percent of Americans have a snack before bed.

With so many people choosing such a large proportion of their daily calories on their own, sound nutritional knowledge has become vitally important. It is no longer enough that the "homemaker" know what's good to eat. Even in the "old days," such nutritional knowledge was limited. In a Maryland survey of homemakers and 4-H youths in 1971, most persons questioned did not know that vitamins and minerals have no calories; gelatin and meat do not have the same kind of protein; and hard mental work does not greatly increase caloric needs. In 1973, a Pillsbury Company survey revealed that only about half the housewives they interviewed could come close to describing a nutritionally balanced meal. Yet four out of five said they thought their families consumed adequate nutrients.

Even so, a significant number of Americans are changing their eating habits. Several recent surveys indicate that we have become more aware of what we're eating and have begun to change our consumption patterns. For example, in a Department of Agriculture survey of 1,400 representative households in 1976, in about half the homes, one or more persons said they were changing their diet due to health concerns.

Some of the dietary changes are reflected in current death statistics. Deaths from heart disease began to drop in the 1970s for the first time in our history. The age-adjusted death rate from all causes has also dropped, indicating that the decline in the proportion of heart deaths is not simply due to a relative increase in some other cause of death.

No one yet knows to what extent dietary changes have influenced the declining death rate, but there's every reason to believe they are an important factor.

The Basics of the New Nutrition

Three principles guide the new approach to eating.

Variety. Variety in the diet is essential if you want to obtain the proper balance of needed nutrients and to avoid possible excesses of toxic substances. Besides, a varied diet is more interesting than an unvaried one. Despite our affluence and ready access to foods of diverse ethnic derivations, the standard American diet concentrates on relatively few types of foods. There are many highly nutritious foods—various fruits, grains, beans, and other vegetables—that few Americans currently ingest. And there are dozens of tasty new ways to combine familiar ingredients that you may never have thought of before. Scores of cookbooks have been published in recent years to guide you in preparing unfamiliar foods, and magazines and newspapers these days are continually publishing recipes that cater to more healthful dining, even for the most discriminating gourmet. You can also adapt your own favorite dishes to incorporate the goals of the new nutrition without any significant sacrifice in taste or texture. You'll find tips to more healthful ways of preparing the old standbys throughout Part I, "What to Eat."

Moderation. The new nutrition is not an all-or-nothing phenomenon, but a matter of putting more emphasis on some foods and less on others. Unless you have a health problem that requires you to steer clear of certain foods, there's no reason why you need to give up any food you especially adore. A salami sandwich every day for lunch would be ill advised (too much fat and salt). A salami sandwich once a month won't hurt you. A dish of ice cream for dessert every night is not healthy (too much fat and sugar and too many calories). But there's nothing wrong with ice cream once a week. It's a question of tradeoffs —if you eat a high-fat food for breakfast, choose those low in fat for the rest of your meals that day.

Moderation also means portion control. If you eat ½ pound of steak at a sitting, you'll be taking in too much fat and cholesterol, and too many calories to meet the Dietary Goals. But if your serving is 2 or 3 ounces, you can stay within the new guidelines. Note the portion sizes recommended for adults following the Basic Four scheme, and commit them to memory (see Table 1.2). You need a lot less food for

Table 1.2 • THE BASIC FOUR FOOD GROUPS: WHAT'S "A SERVING"?

Food	Amount per serving*	Servings per day
Milk Group		
Milk	8 ounces (1 cup)	Children 0–9 years: 2 to 3
Yogurt, plain	1 cup	Children 9–12 years: 3
Hard cheese	1¼ ounces	Teens: 4
Cheese spread	2 ounces	Adults: 2
Ice cream	1½ cups	Pregnant women: 3
Cottage cheese	2 cups	Nursing mothers: 4
Meat Group		
Meat, lean	2 to 3 ounces cooked	2 (can be eaten as mixtures of animal
Poultry	2 to 3 ounces	and vegetable foods; if only vegetable
Fish	2 to 3 ounces	protein is consumed, it must be bal-
Hard cheese	2 to 3 ounces	anced—see Chapters 2 and 24 on pro-
Eggs	2 to 3	tein and vegetarian diets)
Cottage cheese	½ cup	
Dry beans and peas	1 to 1½ cups cooked	
Nuts and seeds	½ to ¾ cup	
Peanut butter	4 tablespoons	
Vegetable and Fruit Group		
Vegetables, cut up	½ cup	4, including one good vitamin C
Fruits, cut up	½ cup	source like oranges or orange juice
Grapefruit	½ medium	and one deep-yellow or dark-green
Melon	½ medium	vegetable
Orange	1	
Potato	1 medium	
Salad	1 bowl	
Lettuce	1 wedge	
Bread and Cereal Group		
Bread	1 slice	4, whole grain or enriched only, in-
Cooked cereal	½ to ¾ cup	cluding at least one serving of whole
Pasta	½ to ¾ cup	grain
Rice	½ to ¾ cup	
Dry cereal	1 ounce	

*These amounts were established by the U.S. Department of Agriculture to meet specific nutritional requirements. For the milk group, serving sizes are based on the calcium content of 1 cup of milk. For the meat group, serving size is determined by protein content. Thus, rather than eat 2 cups of cottage cheese (milk group) or 4 tablespoons of peanut butter (meat group), it would make more sense to eat half those amounts and count each as half a serving in their respective groups. If cottage cheese (½ cup) is consumed as a meat substitute, you may count it as a full meat serving and a quarter of a milk serving.

good health than you may think.

Evolutionary change. Whatever you do, don't read this book and go tearing through your kitchen and recipe file tossing out this and that because you now deem it to be "unhealthy." Eventually, you may want to completely overhaul your diet. But if you make the changes too abruptly, you're likely to resent them and you'll probably build up cravings for various beloved foods you've banished from your menu.

While some people can make large, abrupt changes in their lives, most find evolutionary—rather than revolutionary—change easier to adapt to and more likely to last. For example, rather than feeding all your whole milk to the cat, start mixing it half and half with skim, gradually increasing the proportion of nonfat milk as you get accustomed to the taste. The same with butter: mash a bar in a bowl with a bar of margarine. Then reshape them into two sticks that are half and half. Gradually increase the proportion of margarine until butter is left out completely. Likewise, with salt. If you suddenly stop cooking with salt and refrain from adding it at the table, you're likely to find your foods unpalatable. But if you gradually cut back on the amount of salt you use, you'll hardly notice the difference.

Start thinking about how to make sensible selections within the framework of the Basic Four. Of the various possibilities in each category, choose those foods that are lower in fat, especially in saturated fats, lower in cholesterol, lower in added sweeteners, and lower in salt. In making such choices, you will necessarily increase the amount of fiber and complex carbohydrates in your diet. You will probably also reduce the number of calories without even trying! If you are careful, you can choose ordinary, delicious foods for each of the four categories, and, sticking to the prescribed portion sizes, you can consume most of the essential nutrients in recommended amounts and wind up with a 1,200 to 1,600-calorie-a-day diet. Many people would lose a fair bit of weight on such a scheme. If you're not interested in losing weight, you can eat larger portions, eat more servings in each category (especially of grains, fruits, and vegetables), and/or flesh out your remaining calorie needs with "treats" in the fifth category—fats, sweets, and alcohol (pastries, jams, salad dressings, wine, and other empty-calorie extras).

The Center for Science in the Public Interest has devised a modification of the Basic Four scheme that places more emphasis on the foods that are lower in fat, cholesterol, salt, and added sugars and higher in fiber, natural vitamins and minerals, and starches. CSPI's program, as described in Table 1.3, shows how you can have your cake and eat it

Table 1.3 • NEW AMERICAN EATING GUIDE

Anytime	In moderation	Now and then
	Beans, Grains, and Nuts *(4 or more servings per day)*	
Bread and rolls (whole grain)	Cornbread[8]	Croissant[4,8]
Bulgur	Flour tortilla[8]	Doughnut[3 or 4,5,8]
Dried beans and peas	Granola cereals[1 or 2]	Presweetened cereals[5,8]
Lentils	Hominy grits[8]	Sticky buns[1 or 2,5,8]
Oatmeal	Macaroni and cheese[1,(6),8]	Stuffing (with butter)[4,(6),8]
Pasta, whole-wheat	Matzoh[8]	
Rice, brown	Nuts[3]	
Sprouts	Pasta, refined[8]	
Whole-grain hot and cold cereals	Peanut butter[3]	
Whole-wheat matzoh	Pizza[6,8]	
	Refined, unsweetened cereals[8]	
	Refried beans[1 or 2]	
	Seeds[3]	
	Soybeans[2]	
	Tofu[2]	
	Waffles or pancakes with syrup[5,(6),8]	
	White bread and rolls[8]	
	White rice[8]	

[1]Moderate fat, saturated.   [3]High fat, unsaturated.   [5]High in added sugar.   [(6)]May be high in salt or sodium.   [8]Refined grains.
[2]Moderate fat, unsaturated.   [4]High fat, saturated.   [6]High in salt or sodium.   [7]High in cholesterol.

Fruits and Vegetables
(4 or more servings per day)

All fruits and vegetables except
   those at right
Applesauce (unsweetened)
Unsweetened fruit juices
Unsalted vegetable juices
Potatoes, white or sweet

Avocado[3]
Cole slaw[3]
Cranberry sauce[5]
Dried fruit
French fries[1 or 2]
Fried eggplant[2]
Fruits canned in syrup[5]
Gazpacho[2,(6)]
Glazed carrots[5,(6)]
Guacamole[3]
Potatoes au gratin[1,(6)]
Salted vegetable juices[6]
Sweetened fruit juices[5]
Vegetables canned with salt[6]

Coconut[4]
Pickles[6]

Milk Products
(3 to 4 servings per day for children, 2 for adults)

Buttermilk (from skim milk)
Low-fat cottage cheese
Low-fat milk (1%)
Low-fat yogurt
Nonfat dry milk
Skim-milk cheeses
Skim milk
Skim-milk and banana shake

Cocoa with skim milk[5]
Cottage cheese, regular[1]
Frozen yogurt[5]
Ice milk[5]
Low-fat milk (2%)[1]
Low-fat yogurt, sweetened[5]
Mozzarella, part-skim[1,(6)]

Cheesecake[4,5]
Cheese fondue[4,(6)]
Cheese soufflé[4,(6),7]
Eggnog[1,5,7]
Hard cheeses: blue, brick,
   Camembert, cheddar, muenster,
   Swiss[4,(6)]
Ice cream[4,5]
Processed cheeses[4,6]
Whole milk[4]
Whole-milk yogurt[4]

Table continues on next page

[1]Moderate fat, saturated. [3]High fat, unsaturated. [5]High in added sugar. [6]May be high in salt or sodium. [8]Refined grains.
[2]Moderate fat, unsaturated. [4]High fat, saturated. [6]High in salt or sodium. [7]High in cholesterol.

Table 1.3 continued

Poultry, Fish, Meat, and Eggs
(2 servings per day; vegetarians should eat added servings from other groups)

Anytime	In moderation	Now and then
Cod	Fried fish[1 or 2]	Fried chicken, commercial[4]
Flounder	Herring[3,6]	Cheese omelet[4,7]
Gefilte fish[(6)]	Mackerel, canned[2,(6)]	Whole egg or yolk (limit to 3 a week)[3,7]
Haddock	Salmon, canned[2,(6)]	Bacon[4,(6)]
Halibut	Sardines[2,(6)]	Beef liver, fried[1,7]
Perch	Shrimp[7]	Bologna[4,6]
Pollock	Tuna, oil-packed[2,(6)]	Corned beef[4,6]
Rockfish	Chicken liver[7]	Ground beef[4]
Shellfish, except shrimp	Fried chicken in vegetable oil (homemade)[3]	Ham, trimmed[1,6]
Sole	Chicken or turkey, boiled, baked, or roasted (with skin)[2]	Hot dogs[4,6]
Tuna, water-packed[(6)]	Flank steak[1]	Liverwurst[4,6]
Egg whites	Leg or loin of lamb[1]	Pig's feet[4]
Chicken or turkey, boiled, baked, or roasted (no skin)	Pork shoulder or loin, lean[1]	Salami[4,6]
	Round steak or ground round[1]	Sausage[4,6]
	Rump roast[1]	Spareribs[4]
	Sirloin steak, lean[1]	Red meats, untrimmed[4]
	Veal[1]	

Source: Developed by the Center for Science in the Public Interest. A full-color poster of this guide can be obtained from CSPI, 1501 16th Street NW, Washington, D.C. 20036.

[1] Moderate fat, saturated.   [3] High fat, unsaturated.   [5] High in added sugar.   [6] May be high in salt or sodium.   [8] Refined grains.
[2] Moderate fat, unsaturated.   [4] High fat, saturated.   [6] High in salt or sodium.   [7] High in cholesterol.

too, as long as it's not too often! For each food category, the organization has listed examples of foods that can be consumed regularly without compromising the objectives of the Dietary Goals, those that should be consumed in moderation, and those that should be eaten only now and again.

Less than 30 percent of the calories in "anytime" foods come from fat, and these foods are usually low in salt and sugar. The "now and then" foods mostly contain at least 50 percent fat calories, including a large amount of saturated fat. A few foods in this category are very high in salt or sugar. Those under the "in moderation" heading either have medium amounts of fat with low to moderate amounts of saturated fats, or they have larger amounts of mostly unsaturated fat. The numbers next to many of the items (especially those in the "in moderation" and "now and then" columns) are your clue to the real or potential nutritional shortcomings of the food. Check the key at the bottom of the chart.

After reading this book you may want to construct your own Basic Four eating guide, based on your personal needs and tastes. But be sure to leave yourself plenty of room in the "anytime" column for new and exciting foods you're likely to discover as you gradually change the way you eat and expand your dietary horizons.

Menu Planning for a Healthier Diet

If you don't yet have confidence in your ability to plan your own menu within the new nutrition guidelines, you might adopt or adapt the menu plans on pages 24–25 that were designed with adequate nutrition, variety, and moderation in mind.

The Human Nutrition Center of the U.S. Department of Agriculture has also devised some meal plans to help people meet the general dietary guidelines established in 1980 with the Department of Health, Education, and Welfare (see pages 26–27). These are the center's recommendations.

- Eat a variety of foods.
- Maintain ideal weight.
- Avoid a lot of fat, saturated fat, and cholesterol.
- Avoid a lot of sodium and salt.
- Avoid a lot of sugar.
- Eat foods with starch and fiber.
- Drink only moderate amounts of alcohol.

MENUS FOR REACHING THE DIETARY GOALS

The following information was developed by the Bureau of Nutrition of the New York City Department of Health based on menus that were tested successfully on 1,100 men over a 12-year period. The daily menu provides approximately 2,000 calories: 16.5 percent from protein; 55.5 percent from carbohydrates (including 8 percent from refined sugars); 28.8 percent from fats (including 7 percent from saturated fatty acids and 9 percent from polyunsaturates); and 268 milligrams of cholesterol. If you need fewer than 2,000 calories to maintain your weight, you could skip the desserts (other than fresh fruit) at lunch or dinner, substitute skim milk for low-fat (1 percent) milk, and/or reduce portion sizes slightly. A better idea, though, would be to increase your physical activity so that you can stay trim on 2,000 calories a day.

Sample Menus

Menu Pattern	I	II	III
		Breakfast	
FRUIT	Orange	Orange/grapefruit juice	Grapefruit, ½
EGG OR SUBSTITUTE	—	Egg, 1	Peanut butter
		Toast, 1 slice	Toast, 2 slices
CEREALS, GRAINS	Hot oatmeal, 1½ cups	Cereal, 1 cup	Hot cereal, 1 cup
LOW-FAT MILK	Milk, 8 ounces	Milk, 8 ounces	Milk, 8 ounces
LOW-FAT BEVERAGE	Beverage	Beverage	Beverage

Lunch

FRUIT	Pineapple juice	—	—
PROTEIN FOOD	Lean ham, 2 ounces	Tuna salad, 2 ounces	Split-pea soup
BREAD	Rye bread, 2 slices	Whole-wheat bread, 2 slices	Roll
SALAD WITH DRESSING	Lettuce wedge with dressing	Fruit salad with dressing	Tossed salad with blue cheese dressing
LOW-FAT DESSERT	Sponge or angel food cake	Sherbet	Applesauce
LOW-FAT BEVERAGE	Beverage	Beverage	Beverage

Dinner

PROTEIN FOOD	Broiled fish, 2½ ounces	Chili con carne with beans, 1 cup	Roast chicken, 2½ ounces
POTATO OR SUBSTITUTE	Macaroni with tomato sauce, 1 cup	Rice, 1 cup	Large baked potato
VEGETABLES	Cooked greens	Broccoli	Baked squash
	Raw vegetable salad with dressing	Tomato salad	Cole slaw
BREAD	Bread, 1 slice	Bread, 1 slice	Bread, 1 slice
FRUIT	Fruit compote	Fresh fruit	Fruited gelatin
LOW-FAT MILK	Milk, 8 ounces	Milk, 8 ounces	Milk, 8 ounces

Snacks

FRUITS	Fruits, 2	Fruits, 2	Fruits, 2

INCLUDED DAILY	Vegetable oil for salad dressing and cooking, 2 tablespoons
	Margarine with liquid vegetable oil as the main ingredient, 1 pat
	Refined sugars, including jellies and syrups, not more than 1½ tablespoons

The menus are planned for adults but can be adapted for family use. The 1,600-calorie menu for adult females can meet the needs of school-aged children by adding one to two glasses of low-fat or skim milk a day. For teenaged girls, add two to three glasses of milk a day. For teenaged boys, add two to three glasses of milk to the 2,400-calorie menu designed for the adult male. Two days of menus, plus recipes for the starred items, are included here. You can obtain the complete seven-day guide with explanatory text and lists of acceptable menu choices. Copies of "Ideas for Better Eating" are for sale (Stock No. 001-000-04217-3) by the U.S. Government Printing Office, Superintendent of Documents, Washington, D.C. 20402.

MENU I

1,600 Calories	2,400 Calories

Breakfast

Cantaloupe, ¼ medium	Cantaloupe, ¼ medium
Egg (soft-cooked), 1 large	Corn muffins, 2 average
Corn muffin, 1 average	Margarine (soft), 2 teaspoons
Milk (1%), ½ cup	Jelly, 2 teaspoons
	Milk (whole), 1 cup

Lunch (eaten out)

Ham and cheese sandwich	Pork chop, loin (lean), 1 large
Ham, 1 ounce	Black-eyed peas, ½ cup
Swiss cheese, 1 ounce	Rice, ½ cup
Rye bread, 2 slices	Hard roll (enriched), 1 large
Mayonnaise-type salad dressing, 2	Margarine (soft), 1 teaspoon
teaspoons	Sliced peaches (in syrup), ½ cup
Lettuce	Apple cider, ¾ cup
Tossed salad (lettuce, tomato, carrots,	
green onion), 1¼ cups	
Italian dressing, 1 tablespoon	
Orange, 1 medium	
Water, tea, or coffee	

Dinner

Flounder Florentine*, 1 serving	Flounder Florentine*, 1 serving
Potato (baked), 1 medium	Potato (baked), 1 medium
Sour cream, 2 tablespoons	Sour cream, 2 tablespoons
Green peas (fresh or frozen), ½ cup	Green peas (fresh or frozen), ½ cup
Whole-wheat roll, 1 small	Whole-wheat roll, 1 small
Margarine (soft), 1 teaspoon	Margarine (soft), 1 teaspoon

1,600 Calories	*2,400 Calories*
Vanilla yogurt (low-fat), 4 ounces	Vanilla yogurt (low-fat), 8 ounces
Strawberries (unsweetened), ½ cup	Strawberries (unsweetened), ½ cup
Water, tea, or coffee	Water, tea, or coffee

Snacks

English muffin (enriched), 1 whole	English muffin (enriched), 1 whole
Marmalade, 1 tablespoon	Margarine (soft), 2 teaspoons
	Marmalade, 1 tablespoon

MENU II

1,600 calories	*2,400 calories*

Breakfast

Orange juice, ¾ cup	Orange juice, ¾ cup
Whole-wheat pancakes*, 2	Whole-wheat pancakes*, 3
Blueberry sauce*, ½ serving	Blueberry sauce*, 1 serving
Milk (1%), 1 cup	Margarine, 2 teaspoons
Water, tea, or coffee	Milk (1%), 1 cup
	Water, tea, or coffee

Lunch (eaten at home)

Beef taco*, 1	Beef tacos*, 2
Fresh fruit cup (oranges, apples, banana), ¾ cup	Fresh fruit cup (oranges, apples, banana), ¾ cup
Milk (1%), ½ cup	Milk (1%), 1 cup

Dinner

Roast pork loin (lean only), 4 ounces	Roast pork loin (lean only), 4 ounces
Tossed salad (lettuce, tomato, carrots, green onion), 1¼ cups	Tossed salad (lettuce, tomato, carrots, green onion), 1¼ cups
Italian dressing, 1 tablespoon	Italian dressing, 1 tablespoon
Sweet potato (baked), 1 small	Sweet potato (baked), 1 medium
Collard greens, ½ cup	Collard greens, ½ cup
Biscuit, 1	Biscuit, 2
Margarine (soft), 1 teaspoon	Honey, 1 tablespoon
Water, tea, or coffee	Margarine, 2 teaspoons
	Water, tea, or coffee

Snacks

Graham crackers, 4 squares	Graham crackers, 4 squares
Juice, 8 ounces	Juice, 12 ounces
	Apple, 1 medium

Flounder Florentine

1 pound frozen skinless
flounder fillets, thawed, or
fresh fillets
1½ cups boiling water
10 ounces frozen chopped spinach or 1 pound fresh spinach,
chopped
1 tablespoon finely chopped
onion

½ teaspoon marjoram
2 tablespoons flour
1 cup skim milk
½ teaspoon salt
Pepper, dash
2 tablespoons grated Parmesan
cheese

Place the fish fillets in 1 cup boiling water. Cook uncovered, 2 minutes. Drain. Place the spinach and onion into a saucepan with ½ cup
boiling water. Separate spinach with a fork. When water returns to a boil,
cover and cook 2 minutes. Drain well; mix with the marjoram. Put spinach
in an 8 × 8 × 2-inch glass baking dish. Arrange cooked fish on top of
spinach. Mix flour thoroughly with ¼ cup of milk. Pour remaining milk
into a saucepan and heat. Add flour mixture slowly to hot milk, stirring
constantly. Cook, stirring constantly, until thickened. Stir in salt and
pepper. Pour sauce over fish and sprinkle with Parmesan cheese. Bake at
400 degrees until the top is lightly browned and the mixture is bubbly,
about 25 minutes. Yield: 4 servings (about 140 calories per serving).

Whole-Wheat Pancakes

1⅓ cups whole-wheat flour
2 teaspoons baking powder
¼ teaspoon salt
1 egg, slightly beaten
1⅓ cups milk

1 tablespoon (packed) brown
sugar
1 tablespoon oil
Blueberry sauce (recipe below)

Grease the griddle if not well seasoned or nonstick. Heat the griddle
while mixing the batter (water sprinkled on it should bounce when it's
ready to use). Mix together the flour, baking powder, and salt. Beat egg,
milk, sugar, and oil together. Add the liquid mixture to the flour mixture,
stirring only to moisten the dry ingredients (batter should be slightly
lumpy). For each pancake, pour about ¼ cup batter onto the hot griddle.
Cook until the pancake is covered with bubbles and its edges are slightly
dry. Turn and brown other side. Serve with blueberry sauce. Yield:
4 servings (2 pancakes each, about 245 calories per serving without
sauce).

Blueberry Sauce

2 teaspoons cornstarch
½ cup water
¾ cup crushed unsweetened blue-

berries
2 tablespoons honey
2 teaspoons lemon juice

Mix the cornstarch with a small amount of water in a saucepan and stir until smooth. Add the remaining water, blueberries, and honey. Bring the mixture to a boil over medium heat, stirring constantly. Cook the mixture until it is thickened. Remove the saucepan from the heat; stir in the lemon juice. Serve the sauce warm over pancakes. Yield: 4 servings (¼ cup each, about 50 calories per serving).

Beef Tacos

12 taco shells, fully cooked
1 pound lean ground beef
¼ cup chopped onion
1 8-ounce can tomato sauce
  (or 1 cup homemade sauce)

2 teaspoons chili powder
1 cup chopped tomatoes
1 cup shredded lettuce
½ cup (2 ounces) shredded
  natural sharp cheddar cheese

Heat the taco shells as directed on the package. Brown the ground beef and onion in a frying pan. Drain off the excess fat. Stir in the tomato sauce and chili powder. Bring to a boil. Reduce heat. Cook 10 to 15 minutes uncovered, stirring occasionally, until the mixture is dry and crumbly. Fill heated taco shells with approximately 2 tablespoons of meat mixture. Mix tomato, lettuce, and cheese, and spoon about 2 tablespoons over beef in taco shells. Yield: 6 servings (2 tacos each, about 340 calories per serving).

How to Get Reliable Nutrition Advice

Anyone can call himself or herself a "nutritionist"—someone with at least four years of education and training in the field, someone with a medical degree and some formal nutrition education, someone with a degree (M.D., Ph.D., Sc.D., M.A., B.S., and a host of others) whose training is in an entirely unrelated field, and someone with no degree or formal training who has just decided to be a "nutritionist." Unfortunately, the voices of unschooled quacks are often heard over those with sound background and knowledge. Fortunately, for those wanting to avoid the eccentricities and misinformation of self-styled nutritionists, there are reliable alternatives.

One of the best is the registered dietitian (R.D.). Once relegated almost exclusively to the kitchens of hospitals, schools, and other institutions, increasing numbers of dietitians in recent years have begun working directly with the public, offering professional personal nutrition counseling. A registered dietitian has completed a prescribed course of study in dietetics or nutrition at an accredited college or university, plus an internship in a hospital or other professional setting, or three years of specialized work experience, or a master's degree in nutrition or a related field with six months' work experience. In addition, an R.D. must pass a registration examination and must maintain proficiency and up-to-date knowledge through continuing education. Most qualified dietitians belong to the American Dietetic Association (ADA), which established the above educational requirements. The ADA also has associate members, who are dietitians-in-training. Qualified nutritionists might also belong to one of the following organizations: the Society for Nutrition Education (SNE), the American Society of Clinical Nutrition, or the American Institute of Nutrition (AIN).

As so aptly noted in *Environmental Nutrition Newsletter,* a monthly newsletter edited by two R.D.s, "an ethical nutritionist does not promise cures or guarantee results. . . . Nor do qualified nutritionists believe in superfoods having special, health-giving properties. While there are, of course, foods with a high nutrient density, the emphasis should always be on the overall quality of the diet, not on a few special foods. . . . Ethical, well-trained nutritionists do not recommend an array of expensive vitamin, mineral, or protein supplements since the nutritional needs of nearly all people can be met through the diet." Nor does the reliable nutritionist rely on "spurious diagnoses" of conditions like "adrenal insufficiency" or "hypoglycemia," which can rarely be confirmed by appropriate medical tests performed by physicians without a vested interest in some dietary scheme.

The new breed of dietitian works as a private practitioner on a consulting basis, usually through referral by a physician. Some work independently and can be reached through listings in the Yellow Pages, the local medical society, or departments of nutrition at community colleges, universities, or university-based medical centers. You may also obtain a referral list of private-practice dietitians in your area by writing to the American Dietetic Association, 430 North Michigan Avenue, Chicago, Illinois 60611. A consulting dietitian can provide general nutrition advice or, with a doctor's referral, specific advice individualized to your particular situation—your health problems, family circumstances, life style, and abilities. The consulting nutritionist delves into your current eating habits, your routine, and your medical needs. A trial meal plan is developed and revised as needed. A wide selection of foods and simple menu planning, shopping schemes, and meal preparations are emphasized. The emphasis is on a realistic, enjoyable nutritional plan that you can follow easily for the rest of your life. A consulting dietitian can help you if your problem is obesity, diabetes, heart disease, high blood pressure, liver disease, ulcer, gout, etc., or if you're "just" an ordinary healthy person who's interested in staying that way.

For general nutrition information, there are many reliable sources that supply excellent material—including menu plans and recipes—at no cost or for just a minimal charge. Among them are local health departments (some, like New York City, have a Bureau of Nutrition); county cooperative extension services (where a staff nutritionist can provide telephone advice), located throughout the nation in affiliation with land-grant colleges and universities; departments of nutrition at community colleges, universities, and medical centers; local chapters of the American Heart Association, American Dietetic Association, and American Diabetes Association; and in some areas, local medical societies.

You might also consider subscribing to such newsletters as the following: *Tufts University Diet & Nutrition Letter,* prepared and published 12 times a year by Tufts University School of Nutrition; for a subscription, write to P.O. Box 10948, Des Moines, Iowa 50940; *Nutrition & Health News,* published quarterly by the Center for Human Nutrition at the University of Texas Health Science Center at Dallas, 5323 Harry Hines Blvd., Dallas, Texas 75235; *Nutrition and Health,* prepared and published six times a year by the Institute of Human Nutrition, Columbia University College of Physicians and Surgeons, 701 West 168 Street, New York, New York 10032; *Environmental Nutrition Newsletter,* prepared by two dietitians and published twelve times a year by Environmental Nutrition, Inc., 52 Riverside Drive, New York, New York 10024.

For those who are more politically oriented, the following independent "action" newsletters may prove stimulating: *Nutrition Action,* published twelve times a year by the Center for Science in the Public Interest, 1501 16th Street NW, Washington, D.C. 20036 (annual subscription fee includes membership in the organization, two nutrition posters, and a 10-percent discount on other of the center's health publications); *Nutrition Week,* published fifty times a year by the Community Nutrition Institute, 2001 S Street NW, Washington, D.C. 20009.

FOR FURTHER READING

Dietary Goals for the United States, prepared by the Senate Select Committee on Nutrition and Human Needs, sold under Stock No. 052–070–04376–8 by the Superintendent of Documents, U.S. Government Printing Office, Washington, D.C. 20402.

Food 2, a 48-page paperback in full color that reviews up-to-date facts about weight loss and provides sensible and safe ideas for effective weight control. It includes 42 taste-tested recipes that are low in calories. Published by the American Dietetic Association in cooperation with the United States Department of Agriculture.

Sold by the American Dietetic Association, 430 North Michigan Avenue, Chicago, Illinois 60611.

Nutrition and Your Health: Dietary Guidelines for Americans, a 23-page booklet published in 1985 by the United States Departments of Agriculture and Health and Human Services. Available free (Item No. 520P) from the Consumer Information Center, Pueblo, Colorado 81009.

John W. Farquhar, M.D., *The American Way of Life Need Not Be Hazardous to Your Health* (New York: Norton, 1978). The author is a Stanford University cardiologist and preventive-medicine specialist with a practical approach to healthful living.

Judith J. Wurtman, Ph.D., *Eating Your Way through Life* (New York: Raven Press, 1979). The author is a nutrition educator on the staff of the Massachusetts Institute of Technology.

Dr. Zak Sabry and Ruth Fremes, *Nutriscore* (New York: Methuen/Two Continents, 1976). Dr. Sabry is a biochemist and nutritionist now at the Food and Agriculture Organization in Rome, and Ruth Fremes is a Canadian home economist.

Eva May Hamilton and Eleanor Noss Whitney, *Nutrition: Concepts and Controversies* (St. Paul: West, 1979). The authors are nutritionists at the Florida State University. This is a college text for nonnutrition majors.

Jean Mayer, Ph.D., *A Diet for Living* (New York: David McKay, 1975; also in paperback from Pocket Books). The author, physiologist and former professor of nutrition at Harvard School of Public Health, is now president of Tufts University.

Ronald M. Deutsch, *Realities of Nutrition* (Palo Alto, Calif.: Bull, 1976). The author is a nutrition writer (one of the few reliable ones without professional credentials in nutrition).

Letitia Brewster and Michael F. Jacobson, Ph.D., *The Changing American Diet* (published in 1978 by the Center for Science in the Public Interest, 1501 16th Street NW, Washington, D.C. 20036).

Cheryl Corbin, *Nutrition* (New York: Holt, Rinehart & Winston, 1980). A health action plan developed by the nutritionist for the Preventive Medicine Institute in New York City.

The Prudent Diet, a 32-page booklet available free from the Bureau of Nutrition, New York City Department of Health, 93 Worth Street, Room 714, New York, New York 10013.

Michael F. Jacobson, Ph.D., *The Complete Eater's Digest and Nutrition Scoreboard* (New York: Anchor Press, 1985). An up-to-date consumer's factbook on healthful eating that rates the nutritional value of available foods and discusses safety of processed foods.

Jane E. Brody, *Jane Brody's Good Food Book* (New York: Norton, 1985, and Bantam, 1987). A complete guide to putting good nutrition into practice in your daily life, with 386 recipes and menu plans.

2 ✍ THE BIG PUSH
FOR PROTEIN

TEN surprising facts about protein:

1. Most of us eat at least twice as much protein as we really need for good nutrition.

2. You can get fat eating too much protein. Excess protein is of no use to the body except as an energy source—calories.

3. Most of the common sources of protein in the American diet are high in fat and calories. In fact, most contain a much greater percentage of calories from fat than from protein.

4. Excess protein puts a strain on your liver and kidneys, which have to process what the body doesn't need and get rid of it. Excess protein also promotes bone loss and resulting fractures.

5. On a per-pound basis, your requirements for protein *decline* with age. Pound for pound, infants need nearly three times as much protein as adults.

6. The protein you eat cannot be stored by your body; it needs a new supply daily.

7. After infancy, you can get all the protein your body needs even if you never eat meat, milk, fish, cheese, poultry, or eggs. But a healthy diet based solely on vegetables cannot rely on a single source of plant protein.

8. You must consume "complete" protein within the same meal for your body to get full value from the protein you eat. Most animal proteins are "complete" whereas most vegetable proteins are "incomplete." However, two or more incomplete proteins can be combined in a meal to form complete protein, or tiny amounts of complete protein can be used to supplement an incomplete one.

9. Nearly all vegetables—including green, yellow, and starchy ones—contain some protein, which, over the course of a day, contributes significantly to meeting your protein requirement.

10. The amount of protein listed on food packages as "Percentage

of U.S. Recommended Daily Allowance" can be very misleading. Most people actually need only one-half to two-thirds that amount each day.

Too Much Protein

Americans excrete the most expensive urine in the world. If it were economical to collect and dry it, tons of nitrogen could be harvested from the nation's toilet bowls each day.

Where does all this *nitrogen* come from? From the excess protein most Americans consume. Nitrogen is the element that distinguishes tissue-building protein from the other two main classes of nutrients: fats and carbohydrates. But if you eat more protein than the body needs, the excess nitrogen is excreted as urea in your urine and the rest of the protein molecule is used for energy or stored as fat.

The kidneys of most normal, healthy people can handle a nitrogen excess without difficulty. But if you have pre-existing (often hidden) kidney damage or if your kidneys are already under strain for other reasons, the job of excreting unneeded nitrogen can be overburdening. This is why people with kidney failure are placed on low-protein diets. And since kidney function declines with age, old people especially should limit their protein intake to the amount actually needed. Anyone who goes on a high-protein reducing diet (not the best of ideas anyway—see also Chapters 5 and 16) should be sure to drink large quantities of liquid (ten glasses a day) to help flush out the kidneys.

Excess protein can also be a hazard to premature infants, whose kidneys are usually not well developed. Dr. Gerald Gaull, professor of pediatrics at Mount Sinai Medical Center in New York City, points out that cow's milk, which contains two times the protein of human milk, can overtax the kidneys of some infants. Some studies suggest that infants can develop neurological problems from the build-up of ammonia that occurs when their kidneys fail to process all the urea.

Excess protein may also cause your body to lose needed calcium, the mineral that supports bones and teeth, and increase body fat.

What the Body Does with Protein

Of course, protein is an essential nutrient for us all, and what was said above should not be taken to suggest that it is not a critically important part of the diet. Indeed, the word itself, coined in 1838 by Gerardus Johannes Mulder, a Dutch chemist, is taken from the Greek meaning "in first place." He chose the name because he thought that life could not go on without it. Although we now know that we cannot live on protein alone, we have also discovered during the last century and a half many essential functions for dietary protein.

Every cell in your body contains some protein. Excluding water, 50 percent of the body's weight is protein—hundreds of different kinds of proteins, each with special properties and functions. Protein is part of muscle, bone, cartilage, skin, blood, and lymph. All enzymes and many hormones are proteins. The only body substances that normally lack protein are bile and urine.

The protein of muscle allows this tissue to contract and hold water. The protein in hair, skin, and nails is hard and insoluble, providing a protective coating for the body. The protein in blood vessels is elastic, allowing them to expand and contract to maintain normal blood pressure. Protein is also the rigid framework for the minerals of bones and teeth.

With protein, the body forms new tissues, replaces worn-out ones, regulates the balance of water and acids and bases, and transports nutrients in and out of cells. Protein is needed to make antibodies, which help us combat foreign invaders like disease-causing bacteria. Proteins transport oxygen and nutrients in the blood and are essential to the clotting of blood and the formation of scar tissue.

The protein you eat is not used as such to fulfill these roles. Rather, dietary protein must first be broken down into its component parts in the digestive tract and then absorbed into the bloodstream. These components travel in the blood to all parts of the body wherever cells might need them. In tissues throughout the body, new proteins are built up from these components to meet the body's needs.

The building blocks of proteins, called *amino acids,* are nitrogen-containing chemicals that get strung together in ever-larger units—usually 100 to 300 individual amino-acid molecules—until a complete protein is formed. The particular combination of amino acids and the order of the amino-acid necklace determine the properties of the resulting protein. Because there are so many possibilities for constructing proteins, it is our most versatile nutrient.

Living tissue contains 22 different kinds of amino acids. The human body can take apart amino acids derived from the diet and reconstruct new ones from their basic elements, carbohydrates and nitrogen. However, 9 of the amino acids we need we cannot manufacture. These are called *essential amino acids;* they must be supplied in their final form as part of the protein we eat.

The essential amino acids are methionine, threonine, tryptophan, isoleucine, leucine, lysine, histidine, valine, and phenylalanine. This rather forbidding list is presented merely to help you understand what follows and to appreciate proposals for supplementing certain foods with particular amino acids.

How to Get "Good" Protein

Most animal proteins, including meats, fish, poultry, dairy products, and eggs, contain reasonable amounts of all the essential amino acids plus a healthy supply of the nonessential ones. They are therefore called *complete proteins.* By themselves, they provide balanced protein which the body can use to meet its own protein needs. An exception among animal-derived proteins is gelatin. Gelatin is missing two essential amino acids, tryptophan and lysine. Thus, if you eat a gelatin dessert by itself as a snack, your body derives no useful protein.

In addition, certain animal proteins contain less than an ideal amount of one or another essential amino acid, and, by themselves, they cannot support continued growth. These are called *partially complete proteins:* among them, the protein in some fish, which has relatively little methionine, and the milk protein casein, which is short on arginine that is essential during infancy.

Proteins from vegetable sources are even more *incomplete.* They contain small amounts of one or another essential amino acid, most commonly lysine, methionine, or tryptophan. If a particular vegetable protein is eaten by itself, your body cannot take full advantage of it as a protein source. Only part of the vegetable's total protein can be used as protein. However, by eating two or more vegetable proteins that make up for each other's deficiencies, you can, in effect, create a complete protein for your body to use. Such combinations are called *complementary proteins.*

For example, if you eat a food made from corn, which is low in the essential amino acids tryptophan and lysine, together with beans, which are low in methionine but have plenty of lysine and enough tryptophan, you end up with as complete a protein as is found in a piece of steak. Or, if you smear peanut butter, which is low in methionine, on a piece of wheat bread, which has plenty of methionine but little

Chart 2 • COMPLEMENTARY VEGETABLE PROTEINS: POSSIBLE COMBINATIONS

If you combine vegetable proteins in the same meal in any of the ways suggested below, you will obtain complete protein equivalent to the protein in meat and other animal foods.

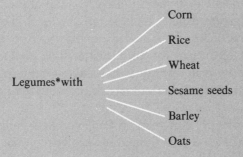

Legumes*with

- Corn
- Rice
- Wheat
- Sesame seeds
- Barley
- Oats

*Appropriate legumes include soybeans, peanuts, black-eyed peas, kidney beans, chickpeas, navy beans, pinto beans, lentils, split peas, and lima beans.

lysine and isoleucine, you again have a complete protein. A sandwich made with two tablespoons of peanut butter supplies more than a third of the recommended daily protein intake for a 60-pound child. (See the Chart 2 for suggestions on how to turn vegetables into complete proteins.)

Another way to take full advantage of vegetable proteins is to eat them with a small amount of an animal protein. Complete or partially complete animal proteins can be eaten merely as condiments to round out the protein in the vegetables that are the main part of your meal. This is, in fact, how most of the world gets its protein. In China and Japan, rice, an important source of protein—albeit an incomplete one —is usually served with a protein-containing food derived from soybeans, such as bean curd (tofu), to form complete protein. In India, lentils are the complement. In addition, very small amounts of meat, fish, poultry, or eggs are usually included in the meal. This is why a Chinese meal for four or six can be made from only half a pound of meat and provide adequate protein for all. Oriental-style cooking is a fine budget stretcher and a healthy way to eat since it contains very little saturated fat and cholesterol, both of which promote the development of heart disease.

Western examples of completed protein are a little milk on gelatin dessert, some grated cheese on a mound of spaghetti, or spaghetti with sauce that contains clams or ground beef. Other combinations that complete the protein from vegetable sources include cereal and milk, macaroni and cheese, the rice and milk in rice pudding, a noodle casserole with tuna. You can greatly increase the protein value of baked goods by adding skim milk. Two tablespoons of dried milk powder for each cup of wheat or rye flour increases the protein value of the bread by about 45 percent.

MAKING THE MOST OF A LITTLE MEAT

The following family favorites use ½ pound of lean, well-trimmed meat to feed the four of us. Vegetables in the stir-fried pork can be varied according to taste to create many different dishes. Also, chicken, beef, or a firm fish can be used in place of the pork. The recipe, incidentally, may seem more complicated than it really is. Once you get used to stir-frying, you should find it as easy as making an omelet. All ingredients can be prepared in advance and refrigerated, with only 15 minutes or less of last-minute preparation.

Stir-fried Pork with Vegetables

2 tablespoons cornstarch
1 tablespoon imported soy sauce
2 tablespoons dry sherry
½ pound well-trimmed pork butt or loin, cut across grain into thin strips about ¼ inch by 2 inches
¼–½ cup broth (use the larger quantity for firmer vegetables)
1 tablespoon imported soy sauce
1 tablespoon sherry
½ teaspoon sugar
4 cups cut-up vegetables, either single ingredient or combination (see note)
2 tablespoons oil
2 chopped scallions, including some green part
1 large clove garlic, minced
2–3 quarter-size slices ginger root, minced (omit if not available; do not substitute powdered ginger)
¼ teaspoon salt

Combine the cornstarch, first tablespoon soy sauce, and 2 tablespoons sherry in a bowl. Add the pork, and marinate for 1 hour. Make the sauce by combining broth, second tablespoon soy sauce, 1 tablespoon sherry, and sugar; set aside. While the pork is marinating, prepare the vegetables (slice carrots diagonally, cut broccoli florets into bite-sized pieces and slice stems thinly, cut green beans into 2-inch lengths, etc.). Heat the wok or skillet until it is very hot. Add 1 tablespoon oil, heat 30 seconds longer. Add scallions, garlic, and ginger, stir a few seconds, and add pork and salt. Stir-fry until pork has lost its pink color (about 3 to 4 minutes), then remove from pan and set aside. Add remaining tablespoon oil to pan, heat, and add vegetables (slow-cooking ones like carrots first, faster-cooking ones like bean sprouts later). Stir to coat with oil, then add the sauce and stir-fry until the vegetables are tender-crisp. Return the pork to the pan and stir-fry briefly to mix well. Serve with rice, bulgur, or pasta. Yield: 4 servings.

Note: Vegetable possibilities include carrots, onions, scallions, broccoli, red or green sweet peppers, celery, water chestnuts, bamboo shoots, bean sprouts, snow peas, green beans, Chinese cabbage, bok choy, etc. All should be sliced thinly or cut into bite-sized pieces, as appropriate.

Pasta with Vegetable-Meat Sauce

½ pound lean ground beef
1–2 tablespoons vegetable oil
2 cloves garlic, minced
1 medium onion, chopped
½ green pepper, chopped
½ pound mushrooms, sliced
1 pound zucchini, sliced ¼ inch thick
½ cup grated carrots (optional)
2 tomatoes, chopped (or small can tomato sauce)
1 teaspoon dried basil
½ teaspoon orégano
Salt and freshly ground black pepper, to taste
½–¾ pound spaghetti, linguine, or macaroni, cooked and drained
Grated Parmesan cheese (optional)

Brown the beef in a skillet. Remove the meat and discard any fat. Heat the oil in the skillet and add the garlic and onion. Sauté for 2 minutes, then add the green pepper, mushrooms, zucchini, and carrots and cook 5 minutes longer. Add tomatoes and seasonings and cook another 5 minutes. Add the browned meat to the vegetables, stir to combine, and serve over the pasta. Serve with Parmesan cheese, if desired. Yield: 4 servings.

The following recipes, compliments of Giant Food, Inc. and the National Heart, Lung, and Blood Institute, turn gelatin into a protein-rich dessert or snack.

Fluffy Yogurt Gelatin

1 small package fruit-flavored gel-   1 cup plain low-fat yogurt
  atin

Prepare the gelatin according to the package directions. When the gelatin has started to set, whip with a beater until light and fluffy. Stir in the yogurt until thoroughly combined with the gelatin, and place the mixture in the refrigerator until set. Yield: 4 to 6 servings.

Strawberry-Pineapple Frozen Yogurt

¼ cup cold water   1 cup mashed or puréed fresh
1 envelope (1 tablespoon) unfla-   strawberries
  vored gelatin   1 cup crushed pineapple (packed
½ cup sugar   in juice), drained
2 cups plain low-fat yogurt

Add the cold water to a small saucepan. Sprinkle the gelatin over the water and wait 5 minutes. Heat gelatin over low heat until it is dissolved. Add the sugar, and stir until well mixed. Let the mixture cool. Stir in the yogurt. Refrigerate in shallow dish until somewhat thickened (about 45 minutes). Add the strawberries and pineapple, and whip until light and airy (about 2 minutes with an electric mixer). Gently pour the mixture into a freezer tray without dividers or into cupcake papers and freeze until firm, about 2 hours. Let stand at room temperature about 10 minutes before serving. Yield: 8 servings.

Note: You can use this recipe with other fresh fruits as well as fruits canned in fruit juices.

The body has no storage organ for protein. Protein needs to be supplied daily, although a few days without protein does not cause serious harm in an otherwise well-nourished person. But even after just one day without protein in your diet your body will begin to break down the protein in nonessential tissues like muscles and use it to reconstruct the proteins needed by organs vital for survival.

The body can use protein most efficiently if protein is consumed frequently during the day. Six small meals containing some protein allow the body to make better use of the nutrient than if you eat it in two or three large meals. And again, because protein is not stored, even for several hours, *complete protein—a balanced combination of all the essential amino acids plus nonessential ones—must be consumed in the same meal.*

Animal Protein Is Overplayed

The human species would have died out early in its evolution if it had depended on a continual and plentiful supply of animal protein, such as Americans eat today. As did our prehistoric ancestors, you can live very well mostly on vegetable protein with only an occasional "feast of meat." And, as you will see in Chapter 24 on vegetarian diets, you can live entirely on vegetable protein and never eat meat or any other animal food.

There's been little change in the total amount of protein eaten by the average American since the early part of the century when the U.S. Department of Agriculture began keeping such statistics. However, the *sources* of American protein have changed in potentially dangerous ways. Whereas flour and cereal products used to supply most of our protein, today animal flesh far and away leads the list. From 1909 through 1913, meat, fish, and poultry supplied only 30 percent of the protein consumed by the typical American. By the mid-1970s, animal flesh was giving us 42 percent of our protein and flour and cereal products only 17 percent (see Chart 3). The contribution of dairy products to our protein intake has also increased, from 16 to 22 percent. Animal flesh and dairy products together now comprise a staggering 70 percent of our total protein whereas nutritionists recommend that a properly balanced diet should derive a third of its protein from animal sources and two-thirds from plant sources (see Table 2.1).

The richest sources of vegetable protein are *legumes—dried peas and beans,* including lentils, black-eyed peas, soybeans, chickpeas, kidney beans, pinto beans, black beans, and their many ethnic relatives. (Fresh green peas and beans are not high-protein foods.) Cooked in water or stock, these provide almost as complete protein as animal foods do. Among them, soybeans and foods made from soybeans (such as bean curd) contain protein that most closely resembles animal protein.

Chart 3 • WHERE OUR CALORIES COME FROM

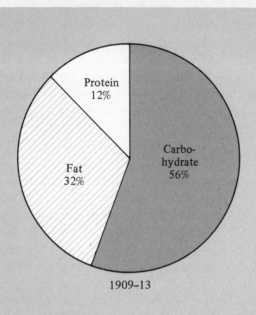

1909–13

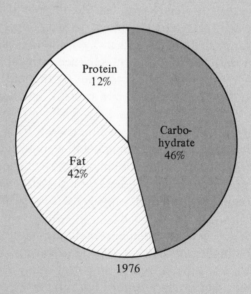

1976

Source: 1978 Handbook of Agriculture Charts,
USDA, Agriculture Handbook No. 551, p. 56.

Table 2.1 • WHERE WE GET OUR PROTEIN:
AMOUNT CONSUMED PER PERSON IN 1978

Product	Pounds per year	Grams protein per day
Red meat	150	24
Flour	112	17
Milk and milk products	310	14
Poultry	57	9
Eggs	35	6
Cheese	17	5
Potatoes	125	5
Fish	13	4
Vegetables	164	3
Peanuts	7	2
Other	—	3
	Total	92

Source: Economics, Statistics, and Cooperatives Service,
United States Department of Agriculture.

All dried peas and beans can be a healthy substitute for animal protein in anyone's diet. The amino-acid balance of the peas and beans can be improved by consuming them with rice, corn, or any grain or cereal food. This is what the Mexicans do when they eat tortillas (cornbread) with beans. In the southeastern United States, the combination of rice and black-eyed peas is a good example of complementary vegetables as proteins.

Nuts, seeds (sesame, sunflower, etc.), *and peanuts* (which are legumes) also are rich sources of vegetable protein. But unlike peas and beans, nuts, seeds, and peanuts contain too much fat—albeit unsaturated fat—to be used as a frequent major source of protein. However, they are excellent as complements to other vegetable proteins. When nuts or peanuts are combined with grains or rice, or when seeds are eaten with legumes, a completely balanced protein results. Thus, the Middle Eastern dish hummus, made from mashed chickpeas and ground sesame seeds, is a complete protein. So is soybean curd (tofu) with sesame seeds, rice pilaf with nuts, or even a bread stuffing with nuts.

Here's one dish that needs only a salad and a green or yellow vegetable to round out the meal.

Red Beans and Rice

1 tablespoon margarine
½ cup chopped onion
½ cup chopped celery
1 clove garlic, minced
1½ cups cooked kidney beans
(or 1 16-ounce can)

2 cups cooked rice
1 tablespoon chopped parsley
Salt and freshly ground pepper, to taste

Melt the margarine in a skillet. Sauté the onion, celery, and garlic until they are softened. Add the remaining ingredients, stir to combine, and simmer for about 5 minutes to blend the flavors. Yield: 3 servings as a main dish; 6 servings as a side dish.

The following version, reprinted with permission from *Environmental Nutrition,* is suitable for a company meal.

Company Beans with Rice

1 medium onion, coarsely chopped
1–2 cloves of garlic, crushed
2 tablespoons oil
2 medium tomatoes, finely chopped
1 medium zucchini or other summer squash, coarsely chopped
½ teaspoon orégano

1 1-pound can of any kind of beans (kidney, pink, garbanzo, etc.), drained
Salt to taste (optional)
3–4 cups cooked rice (white or brown)
1 cup shredded cheese (like cheddar)

Sauté onion and garlic together in oil until onion softens. Add tomatoes, zucchini, and orégano. Cover and let simmer until vegetables soften. Add beans. Simmer together until vegetables are just done and mixture is thoroughly heated. Add salt if desired. Pour over cooked rice and cover with shredded cheese. Serves 4 as a main dish.

Other kinds of vegetables also provide some protein, although we tend to forget them in figuring out how much protein we eat in a day. For example, ½ cup of green peas, a large potato, or ⅔ cup of broccoli, spinach, or corn kernels has as much protein as a tablespoon of peanut butter, or half a glass of milk, or two-thirds of a medium egg. And sweet potatoes, which are also often overlooked as a protein source, have about 2 grams of protein in each potato. (See Table 2.5.)

What Comes Along with Protein

Nobody eats protein all by itself. It would taste dreadful. Rather, the foods we commonly think of as protein sources contain other nutrients as well, particularly fats and carbohydrates. Protein may not even be the principal ingredient. In fact, it usually is not. These foods merely contain more protein than other foods not commonly considered good sources of protein.

When choosing protein foods, you should have some idea of the "baggage" that comes along with it. *Many animal proteins contain more fat than protein,* and ordinarily half or more of this fat is saturated fat. If you look at foods in terms of the percentage of calories supplied by the different nutrients, you'll discover the following:

In a T-bone steak, about 20 percent of the calories are protein; the remaining 80 percent are fat. At the very best, an extremely well-trimmed T-bone steak will still contain 50 percent of its calories as fat.

In cheddar and other hard cheeses, only a quarter of the calories are protein; three-fourths of the calories are fat.

In whole milk, protein is 21 percent of the calories; fat provides 48 percent.

In tuna packed in oil, protein is 34 percent of calories and fat is 64 percent. If all the oil is drained off, however, protein then becomes 58 percent and fat 37 percent of calories.

In fillet of sole, which is much leaner than tuna, 90 percent of the calories is protein and only 10 percent is fat.

Chicken is also a lean source of protein. The quality of the protein is as good as steak, but without skin 64 percent of the calories in chicken are protein and 31 percent are fat. Thus, ounce for ounce, chicken provides more protein than steak, but steak has two and a half times as many calories and twice the amount of fat.

In other protein foods, particularly vegetable proteins, carbohydrates rather than fats supply the bulk of the calories:

Skim milk (all the butterfat removed) is 40 percent protein and 60 percent carbohydrates.

In kidney beans, 25 percent of the calories are protein, 70 percent carbohydrates.

Whole-wheat bread is 16 percent protein, 80 percent carbohydrates.

Oatmeal is 15 percent protein and 70 percent carbohydrates.

But peanut butter, which contains a lot of vegetable oil, is 17 percent protein, 13 percent carbohydrates, and 66 percent fat.

Since in the ideal diet, protein should comprise only 10 to 15 percent of your daily calories, fats no more than 30 percent, and carbohydrates 55 to 60 percent, it makes good nutritional sense to put more emphasis on the low-fat vegetable sources of protein and less on the fattier animal proteins.

There is also a *caloric advantage* to leaner sources of proteins, if —like so many Americans—you need to watch your weight. A gram of fat provides the body with 9 calories of fuel, but a gram of carbohydrates (or a gram of protein) yields only 4 calories. Thus, a half cup of creamed cottage cheese (4 percent butterfat) provides approximately the same amount of protein as a 2½-ounce hamburger. But the hamburger has nearly three times the fat, and 50 percent more calories. You do even better if you use low-fat (1 percent) cottage cheese, which has even fewer calories, but still has the same amount of protein as the hamburger.

The foods in Table 2.2 all provide approximately the same amount of protein—18 grams, about a third of the protein a 150-pound adult should eat in a day. But because of the difference in their fat content, they vary widely in the amount of calories they contain.

As the last two items in Table 2.2 indicate, there's a clear advantage to trimming the fat off your meat and leaving it behind for Jack

Table 2.2 • FATTY PROTEINS ARE LOADED
WITH CALORIES

Food	Amount	Calories
Chicken, roasted, no skin	2.2 ounces	114
Cod, broiled	2.2 ounces	107
Pork loin, lean only	2.1 ounces	162
Boiled ham	3.3 ounces	220
Frankfurter	3 franks	456
Egg, boiled or poached	3 eggs	240
American cheese	2.7 ounces	288
Milk, whole	17.5 ounces	338
Milk, skimmed	17.5 ounces	180
Peanut butter	4.5 tablespoons	422
Tuna in oil, drained	2.2 ounces	122
Sirloin, regular, broiled	2.7 ounces	300
Sirloin, lean only, broiled	2.0 ounces	115

Sprat's wife, the dog, or the garbage. Similarly, ounce for ounce, low-fat dairy products contain the same amount of protein but far fewer calories than the regular unskimmed products.

How Much Protein Do You Really Need?

There's another valuable lesson to be learned from Table 2.2. Look at the amounts listed in the middle column. You'll see that *for most meats, chicken, and fish, it takes only slightly more than a 2-ounce portion to fulfill a third of the day's protein needs for a 150-pound adult.* Yet how many of us eat only 2 ounces of steak? More likely, your portion is 5 ounces (more than 500 calories) or more. This provides half the protein needed by a 180-pound adult in a day, and that's not counting the amount of protein in the rest of the meal. If you're eating three meals a day, there's no need to pack in this much protein—and this many calories—all at once.

However, if your meal is a casserole or an Oriental-style meat-and-vegetable dish with rice, an adult portion will contain only about 2 ounces of meat, fish, or chicken, which is more than adequate to meet protein needs and to provide a satisfying amount of food.

The amount of protein each person requires is basically determined by size and age. The Food and Nutrition Board of the National Academy of Sciences has established *Recommended Dietary Allowances (RDAs) for protein* for people of different ages and weights. Although there is some scientific disagreement about the adequacy of the protein RDAs, they represent the best estimates from available data. The allowances are based on studies of the amount of nitrogen people consume and the amount they lose in their urine. These "nitrogen balance" studies reveal the minimum daily protein requirement. In calculating the RDA for protein, the academy added another *45 percent* to the minimum requirement, which means that the RDA provides a substantial margin of safety for most people. There's no need for an ordinary healthy person to eat more protein than the RDA suggests, and four people out of five can get along well with a third less.

Here's how to figure out how much protein you should be eating each day. The academy lists the RDA in terms of the number of grams of protein you should eat for every kilogram of your ideal body weight. (A gram equals 0.035 of an ounce; there are 28 grams in 1 ounce.) Ideal body weight—what you really *should* weigh—is used in the calculation because your need for protein is determined by the amount of lean tissue in your body, not by how much fat your body contains. Since most people don't know their weight (real or ideal) in kilograms, I have converted the academy's kilogram listings into pounds of body weight (see Table 2.3). To determine how many grams of protein you should be eating each day, multiply the appropriate number in the table by the number of pounds you weigh (or *should* weigh, if you are too fat).

But there is a problem. Unless the food is packaged and the label lists the number of grams of protein in a typical serving, most people have no idea how much protein is in the various foods they eat. For those interested in a detailed analysis of the nutritive content of Ameri-

Table 2.3 • DAILY RECOMMENDED DIETARY
ALLOWANCE (RDA) FOR PROTEIN

Ages (in years)	Grams protein (per pound ideal body weight)
Infants	
0–0.5	1.00
0.5–1	0.90
Children	
1–3	0.81
4–6	0.68
7–10	0.55
11–14	0.45
15–18	0.39
Adults	
19 and over	0.36
Pregnant women	0.62
Nursing women	0.53

Note: Here are some sample calculations to determine a day's protein needs:

For a 5-year-old child who weighs 50 pounds: $0.68 \times 50 = 34$ grams.

For a 160-pound man: $0.36 \times 160 = 57.6$ grams.

For a 110-pound 12 year old: $0.45 \times 110 = 49.5$ grams.

For a 125-pound pregnant woman: $0.62 \times 125 = 77.5$ grams.

According to the Food and Nutrition Board of the National Academy of Sciences–National Research Council, the amounts of protein determined in this fashion should be adequate to meet the needs of virtually all healthy persons.

can foods, the United States Department of Agriculture publishes a handbook that lists 2,483 food items, giving the kind and amount of nutrients in typical-sized servings. The handbook, called "Nutritive Value of American Foods" (Agriculture Handbook No. 456, Stock No. 001–000–03184–8), can be purchased from the Superintendent of Documents, U.S. Government Printing Office, Washington, D.C. 20402. An abbreviated but still highly useful list is contained in the Agriculture Department's Home and Garden Bulletin No. 72, "Nutritive Value of Foods," also sold by the Superintendent of Documents.

Tables 2.4 and 2.5 have been extracted from Handbook No. 456 to give you an idea of how much protein you're likely to get, first,

Table 2.4 • PROTEIN IN "PROTEIN" FOODS

Food	Serving size	Grams protein
Bacon	2 medium slices	3.8
Beef, chuck roast	3 ounces cooked	24.0
Beef, lean ground	¼ pound raw	23.4
Bologna	3 slices (3 ounces)	10.2
Cheese, American	1 ounce slice	6.6
Cheese, cheddar	1 ounce	7.1
Cheese, cottage	½ cup	15.0
Chicken, fryer	1 drumstick	12.2
Eggs	2 medium	11.4
Fish sticks	3 sticks (3 ounces)	14.1
Flounder	3 ounces	25.5
Frankfurter	1 (2 ounces)	7.1
Ham, boiled	3 slices (3 ounces)	16.2
Kidney, beef	½ cup cooked	23.1
Lamb, rib chop	3 ounces	17.9
Liver, chicken	1 liver	6.6
Mackerel	3 ounces	18.6
Milk, skim	1 cup	8.8
Peanut butter	2 tablespoons	8.0
Pizza, cheese	¼ 14-inch pie	15.6
Pork, loin	3 ounces	20.8
Pork sausage	2 links (2 ounces)	5.4
Scallops	3 ounces fried	16.0
Shrimp	3 ounces fried	11.6
Tuna, canned	3 ounces drained	24.4
Turkey	3 ounces	26.8
Veal, stew meat	3 ounces	23.7
Yogurt	1 cup	8.3

Table 2.5 • PROTEIN IN OTHER FOODS

Food	Serving size	Grams protein
Banana	1 medium	1.3
Barley	¼ cup raw	4.1
Bean curd (tofu)	1 piece	9.4
Beans, kidney	½ cup cooked	7.2
Beans, lima	½ cup cooked	6.5
Beans, navy	½ cup cooked	7.4
Bean sprouts (mung)	½ cup	2.0
Bran flakes (40%)	1 cup	3.6
Bread, rye	1 slice	2.3
Bread, white	1 slice	2.4
Bread, whole wheat	1 slice	2.6
Broccoli	½ cup	2.4
Bulgur	1 cup cooked	8.4
Corn	½ cup kernels	2.7
Farina	1 cup cooked in water	3.2
Lentils	½ cup cooked	7.8
Macaroni	1 cup cooked	6.5
Muffin, corn	1 medium	2.8
Noodles, egg	1 cup cooked	6.6
Oatmeal	1 cup cooked in water	4.8
Pancakes	3 4-inch cakes	5.7
Peas, green	½ cup cooked	4.3
Potato	7 ounces baked	4.0
Rice, brown	1 cup cooked	4.9
Rice, white	1 cup cooked	4.1
Sesame seeds	1 tablespoon	1.5
Soup, bean with pork	1 cup with water	8.0
Soup, chicken noodle	1 cup with water	3.4
Soup, cream of mushroom	1 cup with milk	6.9
Soup, tomato	1 cup with milk	6.5
Soup, vegetable	1 cup with water	2.2
Soybeans	½ cup cooked	9.9
Spaghetti	1 cup cooked al dente	6.5
Squash, acorn	1 cup baked	3.9
Sweet potato	5 ounces baked	2.4
Walnuts	10 large	7.3
Wheat flakes	1 cup	3.1
Wheat, shredded	2 biscuits	5.0

from the foods that Americans eat as sources of protein and second, from foods we usually regard as vegetables, "carbohydrates," or side dishes.

Based on the RDA, an 8-year-old child who weighs 60 pounds would need 32 grams of protein a day. This amount could be obtained by eating any of the following combinations:

Chicken (2 ounces)		18 grams
Cottage cheese (½ cup)		15 grams
	Total	33 grams protein

or

Hamburger (2½ ounces cooked)		18
Peanut butter (2 tablespoons)		8
Bread (2 slices)		5
Banana (1 medium)		1
	Total	32 grams protein

or

Milk (2 cups)		18
Cheese (1-ounce slice)		6
Bread (2 slices)		5
Potato (1 baked)		4
	Total	33 grams protein

Similarly, a 120-pound woman could meet her RDA of 43 grams of protein by eating one of the following combinations: 3½ ounces of broiled fish and 2 ounces of chicken; or 2½ ounces of tuna, one egg, ¾ cup of kidney beans, ½ cup of broccoli, and one medium potato.

And for a 170-pound man, the RDA of 61 grams of protein could be satisfied by a 3-ounce pork chop, ½ cup of cottage cheese, and 3 ounces of tuna; or 3 ounces of chicken, 1 cup of oatmeal, ½ cup of peas, 1 cup of macaroni with 1 ounce of cheese, 1 cup of buttermilk, and ¾ cup of rice.

The above possibilities are not intended to be recommended menus. Rather, they are listed to give you an idea of the variety of ways in which you can fulfill your protein requirement, and to demonstrate how little of the concentrated sources of protein you must eat to meet your body's needs. Remember, if you get all the protein you need for the day from foods like meat, fish, chicken, cheese, or eggs, you're not even counting the protein in the milk you drink, the nuts you snack on, and the breads, cereals, and vegetables that accompany your meals.

Some Problems with Proteins

Proteins from different sources differ in how well they can be digested and absorbed by the human digestive tract. In some foods, the amino acids are structured in a way that resists the digestive action of enzymes in the gastrointestinal tract. The protein in cereals, legumes, and nuts is less digestible than that in meat and eggs, and the amino acids from vegetable proteins are less well absorbed than those from animal proteins.

Since the RDA takes into account variations in the digestibility of different proteins for people eating a diet containing both animal and vegetable proteins, the lower usability of vegetable proteins is not likely to result in a shortage of protein for most people. However, vegetarians who eat little or no animal protein must be careful to consume their full RDA for protein each day to assure that they are getting adequate amounts of usable protein.

Some circumstances disturb the body's need for and ability to use dietary protein. Even when the amount of protein in your diet is adequate, inactivity, illness, injury, and emotional stress cause your body to lose more protein than it synthesizes. A healthy person who spends his days in bed loses nitrogen (protein) rather rapidly—12 to 18 grams a day. This is the result of muscle tissue wasting away. Have you ever noticed how thin your arms and legs look after you have spent a week in bed with flu? That's not just lost water or fat—it's also lost protein. Fever, severe pain, diarrhea, surgery, wounds, and burns also result in an excessive loss of body protein.

The protein RDA contains an allowance to cover differences in individual needs for protein due to ordinary life stresses like minor infections or injuries, loss of sleep, or psychological strain. However, for persons who are seriously injured or very ill, some doctors now recommend feeding extra protein to compensate for their excessive protein loss and to enhance their ability to recover. Extra protein fed by tube into the stomach or directly into a vein can speed the healing of wounds and burns and enhance natural defenses against infectious organisms and cancer cells.

The usefulness of various proteins can also be affected by the way they are processed or cooked. Refining grains to make white flour lowers the usable protein because much of the lysine, already in short supply in grains, is lost when the germ is removed from the grain. Thus, products made from whole wheat provide more protein than those prepared from refined white flour.

Heat can also adversely affect protein availability. Puffing of wheat at high temperatures destroys some of the lysine. Overheated pork is digested more slowly and less completely than meat that is properly cooked (to an internal temperature of 140 to 160 degrees). With soybeans, moderate heating increases the amount of amino acids the body can absorb, but overheating diminishes it. However, the digestibility of the protein in dried milk is improved by heat used to evaporate the water. The browning reaction used in preparing certain breakfast cereals (for example, Wheat Chex and Corn Flakes) renders about a third of the protein unusable.

Certain protein-rich foods, such as peanuts, should not be eaten raw because they contain toxic substances or enzymes that must first be destroyed by heat before the food can be used by the body. However, raw (unroasted) peanuts can be used if, in preparing the food, they will be cooked for at least a few minutes at a high temperature.

Getting Your Money's Worth in Protein

Even if we are not on a tight budget, most of us complain about the steadily rising cost of food, especially of meat and fish, which are among the main sources of the nation's protein. By substituting vegetable proteins for some of the more costly animal foods, you can stretch your food dollar much further.

Ounce for ounce, the protein in bologna costs four times as much as the protein in peanut butter. The protein in pork chops is five times as expensive as the same amount of protein from kidney beans. And the protein in bacon is more expensive than fish fillets or a beef rump roast. Table 2.6 shows the relative cost of 20 grams of protein—about one-third the daily amount for an adult male—from different foods. The figures, based on December 1985 prices, were derived by the U.S. Departments of Agriculture and Labor. While they may be slightly different from the current food prices, they should give you a relative idea of how you might best spend your protein dollar.

Table 2.6 • WHAT DO YOU PAY FOR PROTEIN?

Food	Amount (20 grams protein)	Cost (December 1985)
Dried beans, cooked	1¼ cups	$.16
Eggs	4 large	.25
Peanut butter	5 tablespoons	.26
Beef liver	4 ounces	.26
White bread	8 slices	.28
Chicken, whole	¼ small broiler	.33
Turkey, whole	2½ ounces meat	.34
Pork, picnic	5 ounces	.34
Milk	20 ounces	.34
Ground beef, lean	4 ounces	.35
Tuna, canned	2¾ ounces	.36
Ham, whole	3 ounces meat	.45
Chicken breasts, with bone	4½ ounces	.47
Salmon, pink, canned	2¾ ounces	.47
Chuck beef roast	3 ounces meat	.47
American cheese	3 ounces	.51
Cheddar cheese, natural	3 ounces	.55
Pork loin roast	3 ounces meat	.58
Rump roast, boneless	4 ounces	.59
Ocean perch, frozen fillets	4½ ounces	.62
Round beefsteak	3½ ounces	.62
Ham, canned	4 ounces	.65
Frankfurters	3 medium	.71
Sardines, canned	3¾ ounces	.75
Pork chops, bone in	5 ounces	.76
Haddock, frozen fillets	4½ ounces	.81
Pork sausage, bulk	8 ounces	.84
Bacon, sliced	8 ounces	1.00
Beef rib roast, with bone	5¼ ounces	1.00
Yogurt, fruit flavored	16 ounces	1.17
Porterhouse steak, with bone	5½ ounces	1.17

3 ✺ FATS: ESSENTIAL NUTRIENTS OR HEALTH HAZARDS?

WITH ALL the importance Americans place on protein, it may surprise you to learn that, as a percentage of daily calories, we eat three to four times more fat than protein. Most of this fat is unnecessary for good nutrition and good dining, and is detrimental to our health. Studies of cuisines and health statistics throughout the world strongly suggest that the high-fat American diet is a bad habit that we all can and should try to break.

In considering what fat does for—and against—us, it's important to distinguish between body fat and dietary fat. *You don't need to eat any fat to acquire body fat. Your daily need is for a mere tablespoon of dietary fat to maintain good nutrition.* Yet the average American adult consumes 6 to 8 tablespoons of fat a day! Even those who bypass the butter and margarine and go easy on salad dressings probably eat far more fat than they realize because so much fat is hidden in foods we don't usually think of as fatty.

Your body can make fat from the other two major nutrients, proteins and carbohydrates, if your diet contains more calories than you need for energy on a daily basis. This is how you "get fat." *Body fat* is a storage depot for calories; your body uses the stored calories when it needs more energy than your diet supplies. That's why, conversely, you lose body fat on a low-calorie diet.

Fat does have its uses. Deposits of body fat help to support and cushion vital organs, protecting them from injury. Since fat is a poor conductor of heat, the layer of fat under your skin provides insulation against extremes of heat and cold. In the cold, the fat layer helps your body maintain its normal temperature. Fat deposits in muscles are a source of energy for the muscles, including the heart muscle. (You're probably familiar with these muscle fat deposits as the marbling in

meat, which is the animal's muscle tissue.) The oils in your skin and
hair follicles prevent dryness and give your complexion a healthy glow.
Fats also provide the construction material for hormonelike regulatory
substances called prostaglandins. Prostaglandins are essential constituents of cell membranes throughout the body and help to regulate the
body's use of cholesterol. And without some body fat, a woman's
sex-hormone balance and menstrual cycle may be disrupted.

Dietary fats also have important functions. First and foremost,
polyunsaturated fats (mostly from vegetable oils) are a source of the
essential fatty acid, linoleic acid, without which the body cannot make
fats properly. Two other polyunsaturated fatty acids, arachidonic and
linolenic, are sometimes considered essential. But in a pinch, if they are
not supplied in the diet, the body can manufacture its own supply of
both of them from linoleic acid. If polyunsaturated fatty acids are
missing from an infant's diet, the baby's liver develops abnormalities
and the skin becomes red and irritated. For an adult it can take a long
time, perhaps a year, before a lack of polyunsaturated fats shows up as
deficiency symptoms. About 1 to 2 percent of your day's calories should
be linoleic acid, which is found in corn oil, safflower oil, and soybean
oil, among other vegetable oils (but not olive or coconut oil). Even strict
low-fat diets should contain at least 1 tablespoon of such a polyunsaturated oil each day. *Saturated fatty acids, however, are not needed
in the diet at all.*

Dietary fats are also needed to transport certain fat-soluble vita-
mins into your body and through the walls of the digestive tract.
Without some fat in your diet, you would not absorb vitamins A, D,
E, and K because they don't mix with water.

The fats you eat are a concentrated source of energy for your body,
supplying 9 calories per gram—more than twice the energy provided
by proteins and carbohydrates. For those concerned about keeping
down their weight, this fact is a mixed blessing: while from the body's
perspective fats are an efficient way to store energy, they are also an easy
way to accumulate excess calories in your diet. A pound of pure fat
contains more than 4,000 calories, compared to just over 1,800 in a
pound of pure protein or carbohydrate. So it's easy to eat too many fat
calories long before your stomach feels full.

The concentrated energy in fat also means that to lose pounds of
body fat (which is all a dieter should lose), the caloric deficit in your
diet has to be greater than if you were trying to get rid of stores of
protein or carbohydrate. A pound of body fat (some water and protein

is mixed with the fat) contains about 3,500 calories. To shed 1 pound of excess fat, your diet must build up an energy deficit of 3,500 calories. That's why it takes so long to achieve a real and lasting weight loss of fat (as opposed to losing water that may be held temporarily in your tissues). If, for example, each day you eat 500 fewer calories than your body uses, after a week you will have lost 1 pound of fat. A young woman weighing about 115 pounds would have to fast totally (except for water) for two days to burn up a pound of body fat. (See Part IV, "What to Do about Your Weight.")

Fats are popular constituents of the diet because they make foods taste better, providing flavor, aroma, and texture. Pure protein is dry and dreadful-tasting; a little fat greatly improves its appeal. But, as you've seen in the previous chapter, most of the foods Americans regard as good sources of protein, such as meat and cheese, actually contain far more calories of fat than of protein. Even so-called lean meat contains substantial amounts of fat.

Fat in the diet also helps to satisfy the appetite and, because fat is emptied from the stomach and digested more slowly than other nutrients, delays the return of hunger. This is why many Americans complain that they get hungry again only an hour or two after eating a Chinese meal. Most Oriental dishes, which emphasize more rapidly digested carbohydrates (vegetables and rice), contain little fat.

However, dietary fats also "dilute" the nutrient value of a given food by increasing the number of calories that food provides without giving a commensurate increase in vital nutrients. Using this concept of "nutrient density," Drs. R. Gaurth Hansen and Bonita W. Wyse of Utah State University in Logan, Utah, can show that you get far greater food value from a plain baked potato than you would from French fries or potato chips, both of which contain a lot of calories from the fat used in cooking (see Chart 4). In other words, for the same number of calories you get many more nutrients from the baked potato than from either the fries or the chips.

The Fatty American Diet Is Changing

Americans have made significant changes in the past quarter century in how much fat and cholesterol they eat. Whether for reasons of economics, health, or weight control, the average American today eats less saturated animal fat, less cholesterol, and more polyunsaturated

Chart 4 • HOW HIDDEN FAT DILUTES NUTRIENT VALUE

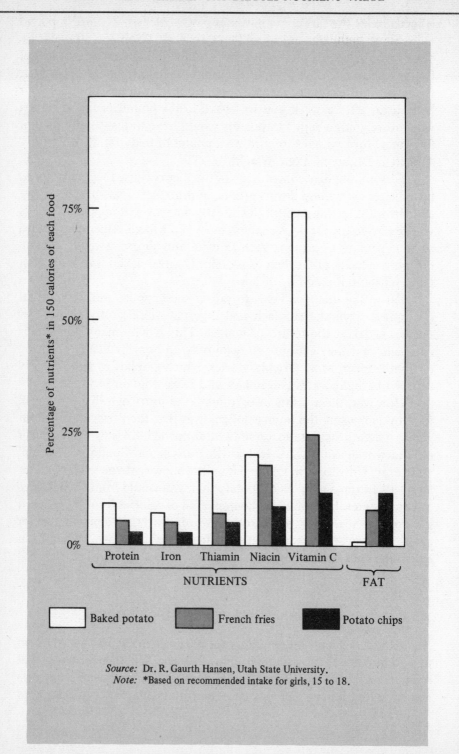

Source: Dr. R. Gaurth Hansen, Utah State University.
Note: *Based on recommended intake for girls, 15 to 18.

vegetable fat than he or she consumed a generation ago (see Chart 5).

Some highlights of the changes in recent years:

Consumption of eggs, a concentrated source of cholesterol, has dropped 35 percent, from a peak of 403 per person in 1945 to 261 in 1984.

Per-capita consumption of milk-fat solids, a source of saturated butterfat, is down nearly 40 percent, from 33 pounds in 1940 to 21 pounds in 1984.

For lard (pork fat), the decline has been even more dramatic— from 14 pounds per person in 1940 to about 2 pounds in 1984, an 85-percent drop in this source of saturated animal fat.

And while the use of animal-derived fats has dropped, consumption of less saturated and cholesterol-free fats and oils from vegetable sources has risen dramatically. Per-capita consumption of vegetable oils and cooking fats and margarines has leaped 183 percent, from 18 pounds in 1940 to 51 pounds in 1982.

Correspondingly, since the early 1960s, there has been a 10-percent drop in the average blood cholesterol level in American adults. Each 1-percent drop in cholesterol is associated with a 2-percent decline in heart attack risk, and since 1968, deaths from cardiovascular disease have been on a continuous decline. In 1975, for the first time since 1967, the total number of deaths from cardiovascular disease dropped below 1 million (even though the average age of the population was older in 1975, which means more, rather than fewer, heart-related deaths were expected). How much of the decline, if any, can be attributed to the dietary change is unknown, but experts believe diet is an important contributing factor. (Other factors, such as less cigarette smoking, improved control of high blood pressure, and increased physical activity, are probably also playing important roles in reducing coronary deaths.)

Clearly, Americans are doing something right, but we are hardly home free. Fats and cholesterol are still far too prominent in the American diet, and cardiovascular disease still claims many lives before the Biblical three score and ten.

Cholesterol, a Crucial Chemical

Cholesterol and saturated fat are the subjects of the most intense and persistent controversy in human nutrition today. Vast amounts of scientific data indicate that a diet rich in animal fats and cholesterol is

Chart 5 • WE EAT TOO MUCH FAT

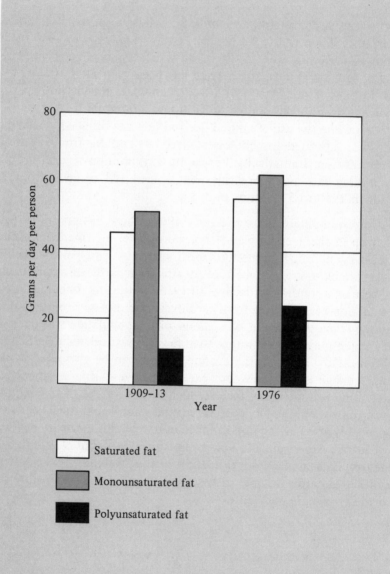

strongly related to a high risk of dying young of heart and other diseases. Although the evidence is very strong, there is still no direct, incontrovertible proof that the risk of premature death can be lowered by dietary change. Lacking such proof, some argue that reducing our intake of fat and cholesterol is unwarranted.

But if you're waiting to change your diet until there's an airtight case against fats and cholesterol, you may die waiting. The studies that could theoretically establish such proof have not been begun, and because of the expense and time involved, they will probably never be done. Sooner or later, you will have to make your decision based on less than the best possible evidence. And most health experts say the evidence already in hand is sufficiently convincing.

Faced with an epidemic of heart and blood-vessel disease, more than a quarter of a century ago public-health-minded physicians began an intensive search for the cause. What they found placed the responsibility not on some uncontrolled microorganism or insidious environmental poison, but on the "good life" enjoyed by mid-twentieth-century Americans. They pinpointed such characteristics of the American life style as the reduced need for physical exertion at work, at home, and in between; the cornucopia of rich and fattening goodies on the American table; the increasing reliance on a legal drug—nicotine—for relaxation; and the stresses peculiar to a fast-paced, ever-changing pattern of life. All of these, separately and together, fostered this epidemic of premature illness and death.

At the heart of the epidemic—accounting for fully half the deaths in this nation—is a disease called atherosclerosis, the accumulation of "crud" in arteries until the arteries become so clogged that blood cannot flow through them properly. It's similar to what happens inside an old water main: eventually the opening gets blocked up with accumulated minerals.

The deposits inside arteries consist mainly of cellular debris and a fatty substance called cholesterol, which is produced as a part of fat by all animals, including ourselves. Cholesterol is a vitally important substance. It is made primarily in the liver (and, to a lesser extent, in the small intestine) and sent through the bloodstream to cells throughout the body. Our cells, some of which also produce their own cholesterol, use it to make strong cell membranes, to mold the sheaths that protect nerve fibers, and to produce vitamin D and certain hormones, including the sex hormones. The liver also uses cholesterol to make bile acids needed for digesting fats. In a single day, the liver typically churns out 1,000 milligrams of cholesterol to meet the body's needs.

But although cholesterol is an essential body chemical, after six months of age you don't need it as a nutrient. Even if your diet contained not 1 milligram of cholesterol, your body would make enough of it out of fats and carbohydrates to satisfy all its needs. The typical American diet, however, supplies about 600 milligrams of cholesterol a day over and above that made by the liver. While this is a lot less than the liver makes on its own, it seems to be critical in exceeding the body's ability to keep down the amount of cholesterol circulating in the blood. The body's own cholesterol production decreases when cholesterol is eaten, but not enough to compensate for the amount consumed. Blood cholesterol levels therefore rise. In general, when groups of people are studied, the more cholesterol there is in their usual diet, the higher the levels of cholesterol in their blood.

But more than by the cholesterol you eat, the amount of cholesterol circulating in your blood is influenced by the amount and kinds of fats you consume. Specifically, diets rich in so-called saturated fats tend to raise the level of blood cholesterol, whereas polyunsaturated fats and monounsaturated fats help to lower it.

Ninety-five percent of dietary fat consists of complex molecules called *triglycerides,* which in turn are made up of three smaller substances called *fatty acids.* Fatty acids come in three types: saturated, monounsaturated, and polyunsaturated. If you think of a fatty-acid molecule as a baseball diamond, the degree of saturation reflects how loaded the bases are. It refers to how many places exist on the fatty-acid molecule for additional atoms of hydrogen. A *saturated* fatty acid has no more room for added hydrogen; a *monounsaturated* fatty acid can accept two more hydrogen atoms, and one that is *polyunsaturated* can take four or more additional hydrogen atoms (see Table 3.1).

Animal fats generally contain a high proportion of saturated fatty acids, whereas most *vegetable fats* contain mainly unsaturated (mono- or polyunsaturated) fatty acids. (There are some important exceptions: coconut and palm "oils," both vegetable fats, are highly saturated. More about these later.) In addition, all animal fats contain cholesterol, but *no cholesterol is naturally present in any vegetable foods.* Vegetable fats do contain sterols, but unlike cholesterol, vegetable sterols are not absorbed by the human digestive tract.

The more saturated a fat is, the harder—or firmer—it is at room temperature. Thus, butterfat, with 59 percent saturated fatty acids, and beef fat, 54 percent saturated, are solids at room temperature. But vegetable oils are liquids. Safflower oil, for example, has only 11 percent saturated fats and 89 percent unsaturates (mostly polyunsaturates), and

Table 3.1 • TYPES OF FATS

Kind of fatty acid	Examples
Saturated	Butter
	Cheese
H–C–C–C–C–H (with H atoms bonded above and below each carbon)	Chocolate
	Coconut and coconut oil
	Egg yolk
	Lard
	Meat
	Milk
	Palm oil
	Poultry
	Vegetable shortening
Monounsaturated	Avocado
	Cashews
H–C–C–C=C–C–C–H (with H atoms bonded to carbons)	Olives and olive oil
	Peanuts and peanut oil
	Peanut butter
Polyunsaturated	Almonds
	Corn oil
H–C–C=C–C–C=C–C–H (with H atoms bonded to carbons)	Cottonseed oil
	Filberts
	Fish
	Margarine (most)
	Mayonnaise
	Pecans
	Safflower oil
	Salad dressing
	Soybean oil
	Sunflower oil
	Walnuts

Note: Saturated fats tend to raise the level of cholesterol in the blood, polyunsaturated fats and monounsaturated fats tend to lower it.
C, a carbon atom.
H, a hydrogen atom.
−, a single bond.
=, a double bond.

olive oil has 16 percent saturates and 84 percent unsaturates (mostly monounsaturates).

The various types of fats and where they're found will be discussed in greater detail later in this chapter. For now, the important thing to remember is that saturated fatty acids (except for stearic acid in cocoa butter) increase the amount of cholesterol in your blood, and polyunsaturates and monounsaturates reduce it. Recent studies have also shown that the kind of fats in fish, called omega-3 fatty acids, can also lower blood cholesterol, even though fish fat is partly saturated and contains some cholesterol. Even low-fat fish and shellfish have a protective effect. In the next chapter, you'll see how to adjust your diet to tip the balance of fats in your heart's favor.

The "Good" Cholesterol and the "Bad"

But, alas, the picture is not so simple. Not all cholesterol found in the blood is the same. You've heard of people who eat all the "wrong" things and don't seem to develop a high blood cholesterol or who show no signs of heart disease despite an advanced age. You may also have heard of others who are stricken with heart attacks very early in life —in their thirties or forties—despite a diet one could hardly call fatty.

In recent years, medical scientists have uncovered some remarkable facts about cholesterol that largely account for these and other apparent contradictions. These facts also explain how the various factors known to be associated with heart disease may do their dirty work. The new understanding, which is still evolving, centers on an elaborate transportation network that carries cholesterol from the liver, through the blood, into the cells, and back again. Basically, it works like this:

Cholesterol, being a fatty substance, is not soluble in water and does not travel through the blood by itself. Rather, it's carried in an envelope of *lipoprotein* (literally, fatty protein) that is also formed in the liver. Three main types of lipoproteins are important to cholesterol transport. *High-density lipoproteins (HDLs)* are sometimes casually referred to as the "good kind" of cholesterol. As a rule, HDLs don't cause atherosclerosis and, in fact, seem to protect against it, apparently by removing cholesterol from artery walls and returning it to the liver and by helping the liver excrete unneeded cholesterol as bile through the intestinal tract.

Two other types of cholesterol carriers, the *low-density lipoproteins (LDLs)* and the *very-low-density lipoproteins (VLDLs)*, have the opposite effect. They keep cholesterol in circulation and depend on scavenger cells to clear out excess cholesterol from the blood. Some of these scavenger cells are found in the muscle layers of the artery walls, and this is believed to be how the arteries become clogged with cholesterol-laden deposits.

The main role of LDLs (VLDLs become LDLs after they deliver triglyceride to the body's fat depots) is to supply cells with needed cholesterol. When cells need cholesterol, they produce molecular "latches," called receptors, on their surfaces that hook up with LDLs. When the cholesterol from the LDL in the blood passes into the cell, the cell's own production of cholesterol shuts down. And when the cell has all the cholesterol it needs, it stops producing LDL receptors.

Sometimes, however, this finely tuned feedback mechanism goes awry. Some people's body cells, because of an inherited abnormality, can produce only half or none of the normal number of LDL receptors. As a result, the cells don't receive the proper signal to shut down their own cholesterol machinery and instead continue to manufacture cholesterol despite a large amount available in the blood. Such people develop severe atherosclerosis and are prone to heart attacks very early in life.

On the other side of the coin, physicians have recently identified a genetic "abnormality" that appears to make some people highly immune to heart disease. Such people may have cholesterol levels as high or higher than other heart-attack-prone Americans, but an unusually large proportion of their blood cholesterol is carried by HDLs, the protective lipoproteins. These people, described as having the "longevity syndrome," tend to live free of heart disease into their eighties or nineties or beyond.

For most of us, however, the following facts about lipoproteins are crucial.

• About 70 percent of the cholesterol in our blood is LDL cholesterol, the "bad" kind.

• When the diet contains large amounts of saturated fats, the liver produces lots of VLDLs and LDLs.

• Polyunsaturated fats, on the other hand, favor cholesterol transport by HDLs and decrease the proportion carried by LDLs and VLDLs.

• Obese persons may have relatively low levels of HDLs, but the percentage of these protective lipoproteins increases when these persons lose weight.

• Strenuous exercise, such as jogging or marathon running, increases HDL cholesterol, and may be part of the reason such exercise protects against heart disease.

• Before menopause, women have higher HDL levels than men of the same age, which may explain women's low rate of heart disease below age 50.

Except for primates, most mammals are relatively immune to developing atherosclerosis. As it turns out, the majority of their cholesterol is carried by HDLs. That's why carnivores like dogs can eat so much fat and cholesterol without keeling over from heart attacks. In fact, some heart specialists routinely toss their dogs such "table scraps" as egg yolks and trimmed fat instead of eating these cholesterol-laden foods themselves.

Cholesterol and Your Heart

In general, then, since the vast majority of us have mainly LDL cholesterol, the more cholesterol there is in our blood, the greater the likelihood that some will build up on the inner walls of our arteries as "plaques" of atherosclerosis. As the plaques get larger and larger, the opening through which the blood must flow gets narrower and narrower until eventually, all it takes is a small clot to completely shut down circulation through an artery.

If the artery happens to be one that nourishes the heart, this life-sustaining muscle is suddenly deprived of essential oxygen and cannot work. This is a heart attack, and it is frequently fatal. A similar blockage in an artery feeding the brain can result in a stroke. Clogged arteries in the legs can result in painful muscle spasms from even slight exercise because the muscles can't get enough oxygen. A chronic shortage of oxygen in the heart muscle causes the excruciatingly painful spasms of angina pectoris.

In a famous study of 12,000 middle-aged men in seven developed countries, Dr. Ancel Keys and his co-workers from the University of Minnesota found that the people of east Finland had the highest death rate from diseases of the coronary arteries—220 per 10,000 men in a five-year period—the highest percentage of saturated animal fats in their diet (22 percent of total calories were saturated fats, mostly from cheese, butter, and milk), and the highest blood cholesterol levels. The United States was not far behind in coronary deaths (185 per 10,000) and blood cholesterol levels.

But in Mediterranean countries like Greece and Italy, where the fat is mostly of vegetable origin and therefore unsaturated and lacking cholesterol, early death from coronary heart disease was far less common. And in Japan where only 10 percent of the diet is fat and most of that is polyunsaturated fat from vegetable sources (only 3 percent of total calories is saturated fat), the cholesterol levels were very low and the death rate from coronary artery disease was only 20 per 10,000.

Among those raised on a typical American diet, clogging of the arteries with cholesterol-laden plaques can begin in the first years of life and progress slowly throughout childhood and adulthood until the arteries are so narrow that symptoms of heart disease or sudden cardiac death occur. Among American soldiers killed during the Korean War at an average age of 22, 35 percent already had significant narrowing of their coronary arteries due to atherosclerotic plaques.

When people migrate from a country where saturated-fat consumption is low to one where it is high, their risk of developing heart disease early in life increases as they adopt the high-fat diet of their new country. Thus, Japanese migrants to Hawaii develop higher cholesterol levels and suffer more heart attacks than do the Japanese in Japan. And among Japanese migrants to California, the coronary death rates and cholesterol levels are higher still. About twenty experiments with humans have shown that an increase in cholesterol consumption usually raises blood levels of cholesterol as well.

Although in previous studies of Americans who were not placed on special diets it has been difficult to show a direct relationship between dietary cholesterol and heart disease, a long-term study of 1,900 American men published in January, 1981, showed that the amount and kind of fats and the amount of cholesterol consumed does, in fact, directly influence a person's risk of dying prematurely of coronary heart disease. The study, directed by Dr. Richard B. Shekelle of Rush–Presbyterian–St. Luke's Medical Center in Chicago, analyzed deaths among the men 20 years after their diets and other factors were first recorded. Those whose intake of cholesterol and saturated fat was lowest had a coronary death rate that was one-third lower than that of the men whose diets were richest in cholesterol and saturated fat.

There is some evidence that a reversal of atherosclerosis can occur in people who reduce their intake of saturated fats and cholesterol. A twelve-year study in two mental hospitals in Finland provides strong support for the health benefits of such a dietary change. In the first hospital, a cholesterol-lowering diet was instituted for six years, with soybean oil replacing the butterfat in milk and highly unsaturated margarines substituting for butter. At the end of the six years, this experimental diet was begun in the second hospital for a second six-year period, and the first hospital went back to its regular diet. In each hospital, during the time the experimental diet was in effect, the death rate from coronary heart disease dropped significantly. When the first hospital returned to its original diet high in saturated fats, the death rate from heart disease more than doubled.

A related study is now under way in North Karelia, Finland, where 186,000 Finns are cooperating to see if by lowering blood cholesterol levels through diet, among other heart-saving measures, the area can lose its dubious distinction of having the world's highest heart-attack rate. The study has already revealed a significant decline in strokes resulting from the changes in the Finnish high-fat life style.

In addition to lowering the risk of atherosclerosis, diets low in saturated fat and relatively high in polyunsaturated fat have been shown to reduce the clotting tendencies of blood platelets. This may be another way in which polyunsaturated fatty acids help to protect against heart attacks and strokes.

The studies described above are merely a sampling of the evidence gathered thus far in the heart's case against cholesterol. On the basis of such evidence, the Senate's Select Committee on Nutrition and Human Needs recommended in 1977 that Americans reduce their total fat intake by nearly a third—from a current 42 percent of daily calories to 30 percent. The committee also urged that we reduce saturated fats from 16 percent of calories to 10 percent, and that the remainder of fats be divided equally between monounsaturates and polyunsaturates (10 percent each). The committee also recommended a halving of cholesterol consumption from 600 milligrams per day to 300.

Some, like the late Nathan Pritikin (who was neither a physician nor a nutritionist, but an engineer), founder of the Longevity Center in Santa Monica, California, advocate a far more stringent restriction in fats and cholesterol than is recommended by the McGovern committee and other experts cited in this book. Pritikin, who died at age 69 with almost plaque-free coronary arteries, urged a daily fat intake of no more than 10 percent of calories and cholesterol intake of 100 milligrams a day at most. While there is no known harm in such a diet, neither is there clear-cut evidence that so severe a restriction is needed to protect the blood vessels of the average healthy American. Given the current structure of the typical diet and the realities of supermarket choices and restaurant menus, not to mention conditioned taste buds, most people would find it difficult to adhere to the levels Pritikin recommended. However, preliminary findings by Pritikin researchers indicate that the strict diet and exercise program he recommended can reverse many of the symptoms of such chronic diet-related diseases as atherosclerosis, diabetes, and high blood pressure.

Are Eggs Bad for You?

As the most concentrated source of cholesterol in the typical American diet, the yolk of a single large egg contains between 250 and 275 milligrams of cholesterol. If one follows the guidelines of the various public-health policy organizations that have recommended a maximum intake of 300 milligrams of cholesterol per day, eating but one egg a day doesn't leave room for much else in the way of cholesterol-containing foods.

Since eggs have long been a central part of the American diet and since, except for their burden of cholesterol, eggs are a rich and well-balanced source of essential nutrients, many people have resisted the antiegg propaganda. And, in fact, a number of experiments suggest that eating eggs has no effect on overall cholesterol levels. Eggs in various quantities were fed to volunteers for weeks or months, but most of the volunteers showed no significant increase in their blood cholesterol levels. These observations have prompted a number of scientists—and the egg industry—to claim that there is no good case against eggs.

In one such study, supervised by Dr. Fred A. Kummerow of the University of Illinois, eggs were added to the diets of patients who had been hospitalized for heart surgery. Two eggs a day added to the patients' diets for 20 to 54 days produced no change in the average cholesterol level. In another study, conducted by Drs. Grant Slater and Roslyn Alfin-Slater at the University of California at Los Angeles, young men were asked to eat two extra eggs a day and older men either one extra egg each day or two extra eggs every other day. The authors concluded that the added eggs did not affect blood cholesterol levels (the older men did show a rise after three weeks of one extra egg a day but a drop in cholesterol after two eggs every other day).

However, critics of these studies point out that the diets of the subjects were not controlled, no account was taken of what the eggs might have substituted for, the subjects' diets were high in cholesterol to begin with (so that the impact of the additional egg or two might be expected to be minimal), and changes in weight of the subjects, which can affect cholesterol levels, were not considered.

On the other side of the controversy, a carefully controlled eighteen-month study from the Harvard School of Public Health showed that as egg yolk was added to the diets of men in a Boston mental hospital, blood cholesterol levels rose. Contrary to the beliefs of some egg enthusiasts, this rise was not prevented by the lecithin contained in the egg yolk, nor by any kind of dietary fat. When fed along with different oils, the highest blood cholesterol levels resulted from coconut oil, which is highly saturated; the next highest levels accompanied olive oil, a monounsaturated oil; and the least increases in blood cholesterol occurred with the polyunsaturated safflower oil. But in all cases, adding eggs to the diet added cholesterol to the blood.

A more recent study by scientists at the National Heart, Lung and Blood Institute in Bethesda, Maryland, revealed some illuminating details about the potentially damaging effect of egg yolks on blood cholesterol levels. The study, which also involved feeding a lot of eggs each day to volunteers, showed that even if the total level of cholesterol in the blood did not rise in response to the egg diet, the balance between the cholesterol-carrying lipoproteins was adversely affected. The researchers found that eating eggs led to a dramatic increase in a type of HDL cholesterol that behaves in the body like harmful LDL cholesterol. Although most HDL cholesterol appears to protect against heart disease, this other type, which the researchers call HDL-c, is even more damaging to blood vessels than LDL cholesterol.

Thus, even though some people can eat a lot of eggs without their blood cholesterol levels rising, the really important effect may not be the total amount of cholesterol in the blood, but the way cholesterol is carried around. This study, incidentally, was partly sponsored by the American Egg Board, an industry-supported group that promotes eggs.

Fats and Cholesterol: Not Guilty?

Some researchers and physicians disagree with the emphasis others have placed on fats and cholesterol as contributors to diseases of the heart and blood vessels. They cite various studies of Americans that failed to show a link between diet and blood levels of cholesterol. And, not surprisingly, the industries that purvey foods high in saturated fats and cholesterol work hard to publicize this minority view.

Among the arguments is the fact that we cannot point to a particular individual and predict what effect diet will have on that person's chances of developing atherosclerosis. An individual's genetic predisposition certainly influences the extent of the damage the environment can cause. Some people are so susceptible that they get into trouble even if they adhere to the proscriptions that would protect most of us. And others are blessed with constitutions that enable them to eat or do all the wrong things without suffering any of the horrible consequences to which the rest of us are prone.

Unfortunately, while analysis of the relative amounts of HDL and LDL cholesterol in a person's blood can give some important clues, it's currently impossible to say with certainty who is and who is not "immune" to heart disease. (Probably, as indicated by the death statistics, most of us are *not* immune.) Given this uncertainty, the advocates of dietary change say, the most sensible approach is for everyone to cut back on the potentially harmful foodstuffs. In every aspect of life, the pleasures of a few must be sacrificed for the safety of the many. Why not, they ask, when it comes to overconsumption of fats and cholesterol?

As Dr. Henry Blackburn, heart researcher and head of the Laboratory of Physiological Hygiene at the University of Minnesota, points out, changing the diet to lower the average blood level of cholesterol is without harmful effects and is likely to reduce the nation's death rate from atherosclerosis. While a diet low in saturated fats and cholesterol is no guarantee of protection for an individual, it can weight the odds in your favor.

Of course, fats and cholesterol are not the only dietary constituents that could influence a person's risk of developing atherosclerotic diseases. Many researchers have studied such factors as the hardness of water, the amount of sugar in the diet, dietary fiber, various vitamins, caffeine, and what have you, sometimes finding possible links to heart disease. Those with a vested interest in products containing animal fats and cholesterol tend to emphasize these other findings and thereby distract attention from the animal fats and cholesterol in the foods they purvey. But despite extensive studies of, say, the role of sugar in heart disease, no dietary factor has yet been shown to be more strongly linked to premature death and disease than saturated fats and cholesterol.

Fats and Cancer

The same high-fat diet associated with heart disease also may increase the risk of developing certain cancers, according to the findings of recent studies. Included are two cancers that frequently strike Americans: cancer of the colon, the nation's leading life-threatening cancer, and cancer of the breast, the leading cancer killer of American women. Cancer of the endometrium, the lining of the uterus, also seems related to a high-fat diet.

These cancers are uncommon among peoples like the Japanese, who eat little fat of any kind. But when the Japanese migrate to the

United States, their risk of developing these diseases rises as they adopt
the Western way of eating. A study of Seventh-Day Adventists showed
that those who at one time in their lives had eaten meat (high in fat)
were two to three times more likely to develop colon cancer than those
who had stuck to a vegetarian diet all their lives.

As for breast cancer, throughout the world there is a fivefold to
tenfold difference in the death rate between countries with high-fat diets
such as ours and those with low-fat diets such as Japan.

Researchers here and in England have shown that when the diet
contains lots of fats and cholesterol, bacteria that live in the gut break
down these foodstuffs into substances that can cause cancer directly or
that promote the action of other cancer-causing chemicals. Since such
diets usually contain relatively little bulky, fibrous foods, the stool tends
to be concentrated and to stay longer than usual in the colon, exposing
colonic tissues to these carcinogens. A recent study in London showed
that when cholesterol was added to the diet of laboratory rats, it promoted the growth of colon cancer caused by another chemical.

In addition, some of the substances produced from cholesterol by
intestinal bacteria can mimic the action of female sex hormones and
may thus promote the growth of cancer in hormone-sensitive tissues
like the breast and the endometrium. Furthermore, people who eat lots
of fats are more likely to be obese than those whose diets are leaner.
Obesity is one of the factors associated with a high risk of developing
cancers of the breast and endometrium. Chemical reactions in body fat
result in the formation of substances that act like the female sex
hormones and may stimulate the growth of breast and endometrial
cancers.

Are Polyunsaturated Fatty Acids Harmful?

As with heart disease, there are dissenting views on the purported
link between diets high in animal fats and cancer. For example, research conducted at the University of Maryland, and covering the last
sixty years in this country, analyzed the relationship between fat intake
and cancer. The researchers found no relationship between animal fats
and cancer, but they did uncover a possible link between processed
vegetable fats and cancer. Since 1909, they said, the consumption of
animal fat has dropped somewhat, whereas the amount of vegetable fat
Americans consume has increased significantly. The Maryland researchers pointed a suspicious finger at the process of "hydrogenating"
natural vegetable oils to make them into solid shortenings and im-

proved cooking oils. *Hydrogenation* makes an unsaturated oil more saturated. Other studies have indicated that the chemical change induced in fatty acids by hydrogenation can affect the function of cell membranes, possibly making it easier for cancer-causing chemicals to get into cells.

A study by an international team of researchers of people with colon cancer revealed that, counter to expectations, the cancer patients had lower blood cholesterol levels than persons free of cancer. The findings suggest that large amounts of polyunsaturated fatty acids in the diet may indeed clear cholesterol from the blood but also increase the formation of bile acids that can be converted by intestinal bacteria into cancer-causing chemicals.

In one large study in Los Angeles of veterans placed on a diet high in PUFA (*poly*unsaturated *f*atty *a*cids), deaths from heart disease dropped, but those from cancer rose (perhaps because many of the men were elderly and had to die of something). However, most of the cancers occurred in the men who stuck least closely to the PUFA diet. And three other such experiments involving large numbers of people showed no increased cancer risk associated with polyunsaturated fats. In addition, among the Africans, Eskimos, and Japanese, whose dietary fats are primarily polyunsaturated fish and vegetable oils, there is no increased cancer risk. However, animal studies suggest that diets high in total fat can promote tumor growth and that large amounts of PUFA have a greater tumor-promoting effect than saturated fats.

Other possible hazards of excessive amounts of PUFA include an increased risk of gallstone formation (as indicated in studies of monkeys), a greater need for vitamin E, and exposure to potentially hazardous oxidized forms of PUFA. Oxidation of polyunsaturated fatty acids results in the formation of highly reactive substances called free radicals that can damage cells and body proteins. However, the usual sources of PUFA in the American diet are themselves sources of vitamin E, which is an antioxidant that prevents the formation of free radicals.

Heating PUFA to very high temperatures in the laboratory can result in the formation of toxic and cancer-promoting substances. When such heated oils are fed to laboratory animals, they develop a host of problems, including loss of appetite, diarrhea, kidney and liver enlargement, and even death in some cases. However, oils that were heated to the lower temperatures used in commercial and home cooking contained few of these toxic substances and produced no significant ill effects in animals that ate them.

Another possible hazard of polyunsaturated fats results from the chemical change that occurs when polyunsaturates are partially converted to saturated fats to make margarines and vegetable shortenings. Some of the fatty acids end up with a chemical structure called "trans" that has been shown to raise blood levels of cholesterol in experimental animals even more than naturally saturated fats like butter and beef tallow. Baby pigs fed polyunsaturated fats containing trans fatty acids developed extensive clogging of their arteries. However, a subsequent study of laboratory animals showed no such effect on blood cholesterol even when very high levels of trans fatty acids were included in the diet.

On the positive side of the "poly" coin, in addition to suppressing cholesterol accumulation, polyunsaturated fatty acids may keep the lid on blood pressure. The U.S. Department of Agriculture studied rats that had inherited a tendency toward high blood pressure. Some of the animals were fed linoleic acid, the major polyunsaturated fatty acid in corn oil and some other vegetable oils. The blood pressure of the rats given a fat-free diet rose much higher than that of the animals fed linoleic acid.

Further research is needed to fully define the precise benefits and risks of the various unsaturated fats. At this point, most evidence suggests that *as long as the total amount of fat in the diet is low, the unsaturated fats do more good than harm,* if they indeed do any harm to people. Meanwhile, those wishing to take the fewest chances with their health might consider the following approach:

Reduce total fat intake by 25 percent or more. You can go down to as little as 10 percent of your day's calories as fat without introducing any risk to your health. (Currently, you'll recall, 43 percent of calories in the typical American diet are fat calories, so there's lots of room for improvement.)

Wherever possible, use vegetable oils in place of hard shortenings and animal fats.

But don't go overboard with polyunsaturates, sprinkling them here and there on the theory that if a little is good, more must be better. After reducing the total amount of fat you eat, vegetable oils should be used in place of saturated cooking and table fats, not in addition to them.

In general, the less fat you eat of any type, the better. For details, see the next chapter on low-fat cooking tips.

4 ☙ HOW TO EAT WELL THE LOW-FAT WAY

CONTRARY TO the opinions of some, a diet lower in fats generally, and saturated fats and cholesterol in particular, need not be boring and tasteless. Certain foods you've come to love may disappear from your day-in-and-day-out diet, but nothing need be banished forever. Unless your physician has placed you on a strict diet, you can—with some modifications—"have your cake and eat it too."

The following guidelines are designed to help you live within the Dietary Goals spelled out by the McGovern committee, one of twenty organizations that have recommended a reduction in fat and cholesterol. The aim is to reduce total fat intake to 30 percent or less of daily calories, more or less equally divided between saturated, monounsaturated, and polyunsaturated fats. In addition, cholesterol intake should not exceed 300 milligrams a day when averaged out over the course of a week or two.

Meat, Fish, and Poultry

• Forget the symbol of American affluence—meat at every meal —and instead eat red meat at most only once a day. Vegetable sources of protein (see Chapters 2 and 24), which contain little fat and no cholesterol, can substitute for animal protein in some meals. Chicken, turkey, and fish, which contain less total fat *and* less saturated fat than beef and pork, are preferred sources of animal protein. In any case, keep portions small—a 3-ounce serving is more than enough for most adults.

• Choose lean cuts. Check meat for marbling—the white visible fat that runs through the red meat—and avoid well-marbled cuts.
For *beef,* the leanest cuts are eye of round, shoulder (arm), rump, chuck with round bone, and sirloin tip roasts; flank, round, tenderloin, and sirloin tip steaks; dried and chipped beef; extra-lean ground beef (regular ground beef has three times as much fat); lean stew meat, and

Table 4.1 • THE PERCENT OF FAT CALORIES IN YOUR FOOD

75% or More

Avocado

Bacon

Beef—choice grade of chuck rib, sirloin, and loin untrimmed, hamburger (regular)

Coconut

Cold cuts—bologna, Braunschweiger, salami

Coleslaw

Cream—heavy, light, half-and-half, sour

Cream cheese

Frankfurters

Headcheese

Nuts—walnuts, peanuts, cashews, almonds, etc.

Olives

Peanut butter

Pork—sausage, spareribs, butt, loin, and ham untrimmed

Salt pork

Seeds—pumpkin, sesame, sunflower

50% to 75%

Beef—rump, corned

Cake—pound

Canadian bacon

Cheese—blue, cheddar, American, Swiss, etc.

Chicken, roasted with skin

Chocolate candy

Cream soups

Eggs

Ice cream (rich)

Lake trout

Lamb chops, rib

Oysters, fried

Perch, fried

Pork—ham, loin, and shoulder (trimmed lean cuts)

Tuna with oil

Tuna salad

Veal

40% to 50%

Beef—T-bone (lean only), hamburger (lean)

Cake—devil's food with chocolate icing

Chicken, fried

Ice cream (regular)

Mackerel

Milk, whole

Pumpkin pie

Rabbit, stewed

Salmon, canned

Sardines (drained)

Turkey pot pie

Yogurt (whole milk)

30% to 40%

Beef—flank steak, chuck pot roast (lean)

Cake—yellow, white (without icing)

Chicken, roasted without skin

Cottage cheese, creamed

Fish—flounder, haddock (fried), halibut (broiled)

Granola

Ice milk

Milk, 2%

Pizza

Seafood—scallops and shrimp (breaded and fried)

Soups—bean with pork

Tuna in oil (drained)

Turkey, roasted dark meat

Yogurt (low fat)

Table 4.1 continued

20% to 30%

Beef—sirloin (lean only)	Pancakes
Corn muffin	Shake, thick
Fish—cod (broiled)	Soups—chicken noodle, tomato,
Liver	vegetable
Oysters, raw	Wheat germ

Less than 20%

Beans, peas, and lentils	Fruits
Bread	Grains
Buttermilk	Milk, skim
Cabbage, boiled	Seafood—scallops and shrimp (steamed
Cakes—angel food, sponge	or boiled)
Cereals, breakfast (except granola)	Soups—split pea, bouillon, consommé
Cottage cheese, uncreamed	Tuna in water
Fish—ocean perch (broiled)	Turkey, roasted white meat
Frozen yogurt	Vegetables

corned beef and pastrami made from round. Once in a while, it's okay to eat fattier cuts: porterhouse, T-bone, sirloin, and rib (small end) steaks, or chuck blade and sirloin roasts. To improve the flavor of lean ground beef, add a little vegetable oil or grated raw potato to the meat before cooking.

There are no very lean cuts of *pork*. The leanest are the center-cut ham—fresh, smoked, or boiled sliced ham, loin chops, and pork tenderloin. Roast sirloin of pork and Canadian bacon can be eaten now and then.

All ordinary cuts of *veal,* except the breast, are very lean, though higher in cholesterol than beef and pork.

For *lamb,* the leanest cuts are leg of lamb, leg chop (also called lamb steak), and sirloin chop. Somewhat fattier are the loin, shoulder (arm) and rib chops, and lamb shank.

Small chickens (broilers and fryers), turkey, and Cornish game hens are the leanest *poultry.* Small, young birds are leaner than large, older ones. Chicken broilers have less than 10 percent fat, roasters have 12 to 18 percent, and large hens 20 to 30 percent. Therefore, for a large crowd, it's better to use two small birds instead of one big one. In all poultry, the white meat has less fat and less cholesterol than the dark meat. If you remove and discard the skin after you cook poultry, you cut the fat calories in half.

Most *fish* are low in total fat and especially low in saturated fat. High-fat fish include salmon, albacore tuna, mackerel, bluefish, herring, anchovies, sardines, shad, and trout. Medium-fat fish include bluefin tuna, rockfish, halibut, mullet, red snapper, and swordfish. Low-fat fish include cod, flounder, haddock, croaker, monkfish, sea bass, pike, and whiting. If you can afford the calories, it is okay to eat fish that is naturally fatty since certain oils in fish—the so-called omega-3 fatty acids—have been shown to reduce cholesterol in the blood and to inhibit the formation of blood clots, both of which should reduce the risk of heart attack. Omega-3 fatty acids may also inhibit cancer growth. Shellfish too can be a regular part of a healthy diet. They are no higher in cholesterol than meat and very low in fat, but most of the fat they do contain is omega-3 fatty acids. However, in canned fish, choose water-packed varieties since the oil added is not fish oil.

Game, including pheasant, wild duck, quail, rabbit, and venison, is also lean.

• Avoid meats with a high fat content. These include regular bacon, ham hocks, pigs' feet and ears, pork butt, picnic and shoulder ham, and spareribs; lamb riblets and ground lamb (unless lean); compressed veal patties; regular hamburger, brisket, club and rib (large end) steaks, rib roast, short ribs, and tongue; duck, goose, capon, and stewing hens; frankfurters, luncheon meats, canned meat, and sausages (four-fifths of the calories in these processed meats are fat calories).

High-cholesterol meats to avoid include all the organ meats— brains, sweetbreads, liver, kidneys, and heart. Liver, an important source of iron and many vitamins, can be eaten occasionally, as often as once a week by children and by women who menstruate. (See pages 196–198.) Sardines, anchovies, caviar, and fish roe are also high in cholesterol and should be avoided.

• Trim off all visible fat before cooking your meat. This includes fat pads under the skin of poultry and the "blanket" of fat butchers often wrap around roasts to keep them from drying out. Instead, you might try smearing the top of the roast with vegetable oil and basting often with stock or pan juices. Or sear the roast to seal in the juices by putting it in at a high temperature (450 degrees) for the first 15 or 20 minutes. However, low-temperature roasting gets rid of more of the unwanted fat. Roasts should be placed on a rack to allow the fat to drip away.

• Broil or roast meats, fish, and poultry rather than fry or stew them. This allows the fat to drip off, and you can then discard it. Fish can also be poached in skim milk, tomato juice, or water flavored with a little lemon juice, vinegar, or dry wine, and herbs and spices. Or poach fish in a traditional court bouillon.

Court Bouillon for Fish

4 cups water
1 carrot, diced
1 onion, sliced and stuck with a clove
Bouquet garni (2 to 3 sprigs of parsley, pinch of thyme, and bay leaf)

6 peppercorns
1 teaspoon salt
1 cup dry white wine or vermouth, or 6 tablespoons vinegar, or ¼ cup fresh lemon juice, or any combination of the three

Combine all the ingredients in a stainless steel or enamel pot, cover, and bring to a boil. Lower the flame, cover partly with the lid, and simmer for about 30 to 45 minutes. Strain. Yield: 4 cups.

• If you are making a stew or soup with fatty meat or poultry, prepare it several hours or a day ahead and chill it; then before you reheat and serve it, skim off the fat that hardens on top. The same can be done with pan juices used to make gravy. To make a last-minute gravy from pan juices, skim an ice cube through the juice to harden the fat; then remove the hardened fat before you thicken or serve the gravy. Or, for immediate skimming of broths or pan juices, you can use a specially designed measuring cup with a spout that starts at the *bottom* of the cup. Since the fat rises to the top almost immediately, you pour off the fat-free liquid first.

Dairy Products

• Limit your servings of dairy foods containing fat to two a day if you're an adult, and three to four for children. Eight ounces of milk, a cup of yogurt, or 1 ounce of hard cheese would be one serving.

• Switch to *low-fat* and *skim milk* and milk products. In the process, you'll take in less cholesterol as well as less fat. Regular whole milk is 3.5 percent butterfat; so a milk product that's advertised as 96.5 percent fat-free (100 minus 3.5) is no advantage. If you're used to whole milk, make the change gradually, cutting first to 2-percent milk for a few weeks, then 1-percent milk, and finally skim milk. If 2-percent milk is not available, make your own by combining whole milk with skim.

Evaporated skim milk can be substituted for cream.

You can use skim milk in place of whole in recipes that call for milk, including creamed soups and white sauce. In baking you can leave out the milk entirely and substitute fruit juice.

Or use *buttermilk* (contrary to its name, it's made from low-fat milk) for baking and in making pancakes. Some find buttermilk a delicious drink by itself. Buttermilk also can be blended with fresh fruit and a little sugar and vanilla and crushed ice to make a refreshingly delicious and nutritious low-calorie, low-cholesterol milk shake.

Yogurt should contain about 1 percent butterfat (99 percent fat-free). Check the label, since some brands are made with whole milk.

Ice milk and ice milk "soft serve" contain less than half the fat of ice cream (3 to 4 percent as opposed to 10 percent or more in ice cream); *sherbet* contains even less fat (about 2 percent); and "ices" have none. The "shakes" served in many fast-food establishments, though only about 3 percent fat, are often made with coconut oil, a highly saturated fat, or butterfat.

• Use milk or milk powder in your coffee. Half-and-half is 12 percent butterfat; light cream is 20 percent butterfat, and heavy whipping cream 38 percent butterfat! *Avoid processed cream substitutes* unless made from polyunsaturated fat. Most are made with coconut oil, which is far more saturated than butterfat. The same is true for whipped-cream substitutes (whipped toppings), artificial sour cream, and "imitation" cream cheese. The label may just say "vegetable oil," but it is no health bargain unless it is neither coconut nor palm oil.

• Restrict your intake of hard and processed *cheeses*. They are high in fat and cholesterol. In cheddar, for example, 75 percent of the calories are fat calories, and only 25 percent is protein. Most other hard cheeses and processed cheeses are also high in fat. As a percentage of weight, they are 30 to 40 percent butterfat, and as a percentage of calories they may be 80 percent fat. Swiss Chris and Swiss Lorraine are low-cholesterol but not low-fat cheeses. Even *part-skim-milk cheeses* are not necessarily low in fat. Fat is usually added back in the cheese-making process, bringing them up to the fat content of ordinary cheese, perhaps 20 percent butterfat. However, Parmesan and part-skim mozzarella, with 20 to 24 percent fat, may be used in small amounts.

There are now on the market several brands of *low-fat cheese* slices and "imitation" processed cheese spreads (called imitation by law because the butterfat has been replaced by unsaturated vegetable oil) that can be eaten as the main protein in your meal. But read the label to be sure coconut or palm oil wasn't used. Eat ordinary hard cheeses only infrequently, substituting 1 ounce of cheese for 2 ounces of red meat in your regular diet.

Cottage cheese (particularly the low-fat or uncreamed kinds), *farmer cheese* (made with skim milk), *pot cheese,* and part-skim *ricotta* are also okay as a meat replacement. Regular creamed cottage cheese has at least 4 percent butterfat; the low-fat or uncreamed kinds have half that or less.

However, *cream cheese is not okay.* Its fat content is more than 37 percent by weight. Whipped cream cheese has about a third less fat by volume (there's no difference by weight), but still too much fat. As a substitute, you might try yogurt cheese, tart in flavor but low in fat. You can easily make your own.

Yogurt Cheese

2 cups plain low-fat yogurt   1 laige piece of cheesecloth (or a tea towel)

   Put the yogurt in the center of the cloth and gather the edges, tying off the yogurt with a rubber band. Hang the cloth from the faucet (or over a bowl) overnight. By morning, the water (whey) will have dripped out of the yogurt and you'll be left with a cheesy spread. (If you catch the whey, you can use it as a nutritious addition to soups and bread dough.) Yogurt cheese can be "dressed up" with chopped chives, onions, green pepper, or herbs or spices, as desired. Yield: 1 cup.

• In recipes calling for sour cream, which is at least 18 percent fat, use yogurt instead. Yogurt is especially good for salad dressings and party dips. But since yogurt is easily liquefied, it should be added carefully and not stirred, beaten, or heated too much. Or you can prevent the yogurt from separating if you first mix 1 tablespoon of cornstarch with 1 tablespoon of yogurt and then stir the mixture into 1 cup of yogurt.

Here's another low-fat substitute for sour cream:

Sour Minus Cream

1 cup creamed cottage   1 tablespoon vinegar or lemon
   cheese   juice
2 tablespoons skim milk   ¼ teaspoon salt

   Put all ingredients in a blender container and blend at medium-high speed. May be served cold or added to hot dishes at the last moment. Yield: 1 cup.

Eggs

• Because the yolk of a single large egg contains nearly your entire day's quota of cholesterol, you should limit your consumption of egg yolks to three or four a week, including those in prepared and processed foods. (Unfortunately, it is usually impossible to know how much egg yolk is in processed foods that contain eggs.) However, you can have as many egg whites as you wish—they're an excellent, low-calorie source of protein. In salads made with hard-boiled eggs, it's easy to leave out the yolk.

• In preparing eggs for a meal, discard every other yolk. In other words, make your omelet with two whites and one yolk. You can do the same with pancakes and French toast.

• In recipes that call for one or two eggs, you can substitute two egg whites for one whole egg or three egg whites for two whole eggs in the recipe. However, you cannot make such a substitution in recipes that require lots of eggs, such as a sponge cake or soufflé.

• Egg noodles are okay, but if you eat a lot of pasta, it's better to substitute noodles made without egg yolks.

• If you have a dog, the yolks you don't eat will give your pet a glossy coat and assuage your guilt about throwing away "good food."

• A more costly (and to my mind, less tasty) approach is to use cholesterol-free egg substitutes—either liquid eggs in which the yolk has been replaced by vegetable oils and other ingredients—or powdered artificial eggs, particularly for baking and cooking. Check the frozen-food section of your market for the liquid egg substitute.

Fats and Oils

• When you cook, bake, or season your food, don't use saturated animal fats such as butter, lard, suet, salt pork, and chicken fat. Also avoid solid vegetable shortenings. Substitute *polyunsaturated vegetable oils* and *margarine*. The total fat and calorie content are the same, but the saturated fat content is much lower and there is no cholesterol in pure vegetable fats.

• There are all kinds of margarines, so it pays to know how to choose the best. Some are highly unsaturated, others are nearly as

Table 4.2 • CHOLESTEROL CONTENT OF COMMON FOODS

Food	Amount	Cholesterol(mg)
Meat Group		
RED MEATS		
Bacon	2 slices	15
Beef (lean)	3 ounces	77
Frankfurter	2 (4 ounces)	112
Ham, boiled	2 ounces	51
Kidney, beef	3 ounces	315
Lamb (lean)	3 ounces	85
Liver, beef	3 ounces	372
Pork (lean)	3 ounces	70
Veal (lean)	3 ounces	84
FOWL		
Chicken, dark (no skin)	3 ounces	77
Chicken, white (no skin)	3 ounces	65
Eggs (whole or yolk only)	1 large	252
Turkey, dark (no skin)	3 ounces	86
Turkey, white (no skin)	3 ounces	65
FISH		
Clams, raw (meat only)	3 ounces	36
Crab, canned	3 ounces	50
Flounder	3 ounces	69
Haddock	3 ounces	42
Halibut	3 ounces	50
Lobster	3 ounces	71
Mackerel	3 ounces	84
Mussels	3 ounces	60
Oysters	3 ounces	42
Salmon, canned	3 ounces	30
Sardines	3 ounces	119
Scallops	3 ounces	45
Shrimp	3 ounces	128
Tuna, canned	3 ounces	55
Milk Group		
Butter	1 tablespoon	35
Buttermilk	1 cup	5
Cheese, cottage (4% fat)	½ cup	24
Cheese, cottage (1% fat)	½ cup	12
Cheese, cream	1 ounce	31

Table continues on next page

Table 4.2 continued

Food	Amount	Cholesterol(mg)
Cheese, hard	1 ounce	24–28
Cheese, spread	1 ounce	18
Chocolate milk (low-fat)	1 cup	20
Cream, heavy	1 tablespoon	21
Ice cream	½ cup	27
Ice milk	½ cup	13
Milk, skim	1 cup	5
Milk, 1% fat	1 cup	14
Milk, 2% fat	1 cup	22
Milk, whole	1 cup	34
Yogurt (low-fat)	1 cup	17
Bread Group		
Angel food cake	1 slice	0
Chocolate cupcake	2½-inch diameter	17
Cornbread	1 ounce	58
Lemon meringue pie	⅛ of 9-inch pie	98
Muffin, plain	3-inch diameter	21
Noodles, egg	1 cup	50
Pancakes	7 tablespoons batter	54
Sponge cake	$\frac{1}{12}$ of 10-inch cake	162

Note: Foods made only from plant sources, such as peanut butter, beans, vegetable margarines, grains, fruits, and vegetables, contain no cholesterol.
Source: Based on analyses by the U.S. Department of Agriculture.

saturated as butter. As a general rule, the softer the margarine, the less saturated it is. Thus, soft stick margarines are better than hard sticks, tub margarines are generally better than sticks, and liquid margarines (sold in a squeeze container) are even less saturated than the soft tubs.

The best margarines are labeled to show you their fat content. Ideally, the margarine should contain twice as much polyunsaturated (P) as saturated (S) fatty acids. If the label shows a P/S ratio, it should be 2 to 1 or higher. You can calculate this ratio yourself by dividing the amount of polyunsaturates by the amount of saturates in a serving (see Table 4.3).

Another clue to selecting a good margarine is the ingredients list. The first ingredient should be *liquid* vegetable oil, such as corn, safflower, or soybean. If the first ingredient is "partially hydrogenated" or "hardened" oil, don't buy it.

Table 4.3 • WHAT'S IN FATS AND OILS?

Type of fat (1 tablespoon)	Cholesterol (mg)	Fatty Acids (g)			
		Saturated	Monoun-saturated	Polyun-saturated	P/S ratio
Butter	31	7.1	3.3	0.4	0.08
Lard	13	5.1	5.3	1.3	0.2
Tub margarine					
Liquid safflower oil	0	1.6	2.6	6.7	4.5
Liquid corn oil	0	2.0	4.5	4.4	2.2
Stick margarine					
Liquid corn oil	0	2.5	4.4	3.9	1.6
Stick or tub margarine					
Partially hydrogenated					
or hardened oil	0	2.2	4.9	3.7	1.7
Imitation (diet) margarine	0	1.1	2.2	2.0	1.8
Mayonnaise	8	2.0	2.4	5.6	2.8
Vegetable shortening,					
hydrogenated	0	3.2	5.7	3.1	1.0
Corn oil	0	1.7	3.3	7.8	4.6
Cottonseed oil	0	3.7	2.6	7.1	1.9
Safflower oil	0	1.3	1.6	10.0	7.7
Sesame oil	0	2.1	5.5	5.7	2.7
Soybean oil	0	2.1	3.2	8.1	3.9
Soybean oil (lightly					
hydrogenated)	0	2.0	5.8	4.7	2.4
Sunflower oil	0	1.5	2.9	8.9	5.9
Olive oil	0	1.9	9.7	1.1	0.6
Peanut oil	0	2.3	6.2	4.2	1.8
Coconut oil	0	12.1	0.8	0.3	0.02
Palm oil	0	7.2	5.0	1.4	0.2

Source: American Heart Association.

For example, under "Nutrition Information per Serving" on the box of Mazola margarine, the entry for fat reads as follows:

Fat	11 grams
Percent of calories from fat	99%
Polyunsaturated	4 grams
Saturated	2 grams

And under "Ingredients," the label reads: "Mazola liquid corn oil, partially hydrogenated soybean oil, water . . ." Thus, Mazola, which has a P/S ratio of 2 to 1 and liquid vegetable oil as its main ingredient, would qualify as an acceptable margarine.

• Choose from among the most unsaturated vegetable oils (see Table 4.3). In order of preference, these are safflower, walnut, sunflower, corn (unhydrogenated), soybean, wheat germ, and cottonseed oils. Olive oil, a monounsaturated fat, can also be used since it too lowers blood cholesterol. However, be moderate in using peanut oil; although also monounsaturated, in monkey studies it has promoted the development of atherosclerosis.

• Develop a taste for the different vegetable oils. Sesame oil, with its nutty flavor, is wonderful for salads and sautéeing vegetables; safflower oil is mild and good for making mayonnaise; corn oil is richly flavored and good for baking. Soy and peanut oils are strong, but good for blending with lighter oils. Unless they will be used up within a month or two, it's best to refrigerate oils after opening to prevent rancidity. Never store them near the stove or in warm places.

• Get in the habit of checking the ingredients list of all processed foods (see Table 4.4). If the label lists as a prominent ingredient "vegetable oil" without specifying which kind, or if it states that the product may contain coconut or palm oil, avoid the product.

Table 4.4 • CHECK THE LABEL FOR FATS AND OILS

Ingredients That Are Okay

Carob	Hydrolyzed ingredients	Sesame oil
Cocoa	Monoglycerides	Skim milk
Corn oil	Nonfat dry milk	Soybean oil
Cottonseed oil	Nonfat milk solids	Sunflower oil
Diglycerides	Safflower oil	Walnuts

Ingredients to Avoid

Animal fat	Cream and cream sauce	Milk chocolate
Bacon fat	Egg and egg-yolk solids	Palm oil
Beef fat	Ham fat	Pork fat
Butter	Hardened fat or oil	Shortening
Chicken fat	Hydrogenated fat or oil	Turkey fat
Coconut	Lamb fat	Vegetable fat or oil*
Coconut oil	Lard	Vegetable shortening
Cod-liver oil	Meat fat	Whole-milk solids

Ingredients to Use Occasionally

Cocoa butter	Mustard seed oil	Peanut oil
Castor oil	Olive oil	

*Could be coconut or palm oil.

• Commercial baked goods—cakes, doughnuts, muffins, and butter rolls—are usually made with saturated fats. Avoid those that say just "vegetable oil" or specify coconut or palm oil or animal fat. It's better to make your own, using a polyunsaturated oil or margarine. Better yet, have fruit for desserts and snacks.

• In baking, use a polyunsaturated margarine for the fat. Or you can replace each cup of solid shortening or butter called for in the recipe with ⅔ of a cup of vegetable oil. The texture will be different, but you can even make a pie crust with oil: use ⅓ cup oil and 1⅓ cups flour for a single crust; ½ cup oil and 2 cups flour for a double crust.

• Instead of using commercial salad dressings, make your own, either from scratch or from a packaged mix, using polyunsaturated vegetable oil, mayonnaise (although mayonnaise contains a small amount of egg yolk, it is high in polyunsaturates), mayonnaise-type salad dressing, yogurt, or buttermilk. You might even experiment with an herb dressing using vinegar or lemon juice without any oil.

• When sautéeing or frying foods that don't need a lot of oil (for example, an egg, French toast, pancakes, or liver), brush the pan with oil just to coat it, use a nonstick spray made from vegetable oil, or use a nonstick pan that requires no greasing.

• Don't reuse frying oils that have darkened in color, or that flow more slowly than they did originally, or that foam to the top of the pot when you put the food in. In fact, unless you do a great deal of frying (not advisable if you're trying to cut down on fat) for a large family on a limited budget, it's best not to reuse frying oils at all. If you do, make sure they are not brought to the smoking point and strain them through cheesecloth after each use.

• It makes little difference whether you use cold-pressed or heat-pressed oils, except in price. Because less of the oil is extracted in cold-pressing, these oils cost more. Although refined oils may contain less vitamin E than unrefined ones, they also have had removed such unwanted substances as pesticide residues and malodorous chemicals.

Miscellaneous Tips

• Calories and cavities aside, *chocolate* candies and icings are on the watch-out list. Those made with hardened baking chocolate contain neutral fatty acids and are okay once in a while. Chocolate powder, which contains almost no fat, can be used freely. However, liquid baking chocolate contains saturated vegetable oils and should be avoided. Unless you know that a chocolate candy has not been made with saturated vegetable oils, it's best not to eat it. Also avoid candies containing cream or coconut centers.

• *Nuts* and *seeds* (e.g., sunflower and sesame) are all okay; they contain a high proportion of polyunsaturated fats and no cholesterol. However, they are high in total fat and calories, so should not be consumed to excess if you're cutting down on fat. As far as the type of fat is concerned, the best nuts are walnuts, followed by pecans, almonds, and peanuts.

• *Peanut butter* is also high in total fat and in calories. Eat it in place of meat, but not too frequently. A serving would be 2 tablespoons (equivalent to half a "meat" serving). Old-fashioned, "real," or home-made peanut butter is preferable to the processed variety, in which the oil has been partly hydrogenated to keep it from separating. Many of the processed brands are also high in sugar and salt, which you can omit if you make your own.

• *Avocados* also have a lot of fat, albeit unsaturated fat. An eighth of an avocado contains as much fat as a single slice of bacon or a pat of butter. Thus, they should all be thought of as fat, not as a vegetable (in the case of avocado) or protein (in the case of bacon).

• All fats, whether saturated or not, contain the same amount of calories by weight—4,000 per pound, or 250 an ounce. One tablespoon of an ordinary fat or oil has 100 calories. Low-calorie margarines or salad dressings are made by whipping air and/or water into the product, thus reducing the fat content and number of calories in a volume measure. A reduced-calorie margarine may contain 50 or 70 calories a tablespoon instead of 100. If you are watching your weight, you might look into these low-calorie fats, but be sure that in choosing a margarine labeled "diet" or "imitation" (called so by law because of its lower fat content) the first ingredient is liquid vegetable oil.

Dining Out

I agree with Dr. Myron Winick, director of the Institute of Human Nutrition at Columbia University and editor of the newsletter *Nutrition and Health,* who says you don't have to abandon fine dining nor join the brown-baggers to eat prudently. What you do have to do is learn how to make sensible choices and watch out for the booby traps on menus.

For example, Dr. Winick suggests that you avoid items described in any of the following terms: buttery, buttered or butter sauce; sautéed, fried, pan-fried, or crispy; creamed, cream sauce, or in its own gravy; au gratin, Parmesan, in cheese sauce, or escalloped; au lait, à la mode, or au fromage; marinated, stewed, basted, or casserole; prime, hash, pot pie, and hollandaise.

On the other hand, feel free to indulge in dishes described as follows: pickled, tomato sauce, steamed, in broth; in its own juice, poached or garden fresh; roasted, stir-fried, or cocktail sauce.

DINING OUT THE LOW-FAT WAY

The following recommended menu selections were prepared by the Institute of Human Nutrition, Columbia University College of Physicians and Surgeons, and published in the institute's newsletter, *Nutrition and Health.*

Appetizers

Fresh fruits and vegetables as "crudités" or juices; seafood cocktail.
Avoid sour or sweet cream and seasoned butter or oils.

Soups

Clear consommé or broth with noodles or vegetables.
Avoid cheese, cream soups, egg soups, and onion soup.

Salads

Green and tossed salads. As chef salad, may include chicken, turkey, seafood, tuna, lean roast beef, lean ham. Clear gelatin molds. Cole slaw, potato salad, and Waldorf salad should be prepared with a minimum of mayonnaise.
Avoid cheese and creamy dressings.

Fish

Any variety prepared without fat.
Avoid tartar sauce.

Poultry

Chicken, turkey, Cornish hen, prepared without fat, with skin removed.
Avoid goose, duck, and fried or batter-dipped coatings.

Red Meat

Always lean, hind-quarter cuts of beef, lamb, and pork; all cuts of veal.
Avoid prime cuts, gravy, breaded coatings, any ground beef.

Fruits

As much as you like.
Avoid cream or whipped toppings.

Vegetables

If plain, as much as you like. Beans and peas without oil or sauce. Walnuts and sunflower seeds.

Bread

All sandwich bread, breadsticks, hard rolls, French and Italian breads, Syrian pita bread, wafers, and toasts.
Avoid biscuits, croissants, corn muffins, bran muffins, blueberry muffins, and butter rolls.

Desserts

Angel food cake, gelatin desserts, frozen fruit ices, and low-fat dairy products.
Avoid cream and nondairy milk substitutes.

Beverages

Low-fat milk products, carbonated and alcoholic beverages, fruit juices, coffee, and tea.
Avoid cream and nondairy milk substitutes.

Extras

Pickles, relishes, mustard, Worcestershire and steak sauce, catsup, lemon juice, vinegar, spices, and herbs.

Most restaurants use animal fats or saturated vegetable fats to prepare their foods. But if you're dining in an Oriental restaurant, you can lift the restriction on fried foods (as long as you don't go overboard), since unsaturated oils (particularly soybean) are usually used.

In general, the more simply a dish is prepared, the less fat it contains. Concentrate your choices on poultry, fish, and seafood. Don't hesitate to ask for what you want. Order your fish broiled without butter. Ask for your salad dressing on the side so you can add a reasonable amount yourself. Or order oil and vinegar for your dressing, which you put on by yourself. Ask for skim milk and margarine in place of milk, cream, and butter. Order your meat and potatoes served without gravy or sauce.

Where to Find Low-Fat Recipes

Scores of cookbooks and recipe booklets have been published in recent years to cater to the new interest in low-fat cookery. Many have been put together by health organizations and companies that market polyunsaturated products. Free recipe booklets can be obtained from the following organizations:

"Recipes" for fat-controlled, low-cholesterol meals, American Heart Association, 7320 Greenville Avenue, Dallas, Texas 75231 (check your directory for local chapters).

"Cook with Love, Cook with Corn Oil," Consumer Service Department, Best Foods, a Division of CPC International, Inc., International Plaza, Englewood Cliffs, New Jersey 07632.

"Dietary Control of Cholesterol" and "Cooking with Egg Beaters," Fleischmann's Margarines, 625 Madison Avenue, New York, New York 10022.

"The Prudent Diet" (a booklet) plus pamphlets "Prudent International Recipes" and "Prudent Entertaining," Bureau of Nutrition, New York City Department of Health, 93 Worth Street, Room 714, New York, New York 10013.

For a cookbook filled with hundreds of easy-to-follow, tasty recipes, you might try *The American Heart Association Cookbook* published by David McKay Company, Inc., New York, in hard cover and by Ballantine with a paper cover. A revised and updated fourth edition was published in 1986 by Ballantine. Some of my family's perennial favorites come from this book. I'm especially grateful for the quick, nutritious, and delicious breakfast idea of "Cinnamon Toasties."

Cinnamon Toasties

4 slices of white or whole-wheat bread
1 cup low-fat cottage cheese

Cinnamon-sugar
Sliced fruit (optional)

Toast the bread and spread the slices with the cottage cheese. Sprinkle cinnamon-sugar on top of the cheese, and place the slices under the broiler for a few minutes until hot. Can be topped with fruit—for example, sliced bananas, strawberries, or peaches—before broiling. Yield: 4 servings.

Since breakfast seems to be a problem for so many people trying to reduce the amount of fat and cholesterol they eat, I'll share with you some of my other discoveries.

Hearty Oatmeal

4 cups skim milk (or 2 cups
  milk, 2 cups water)
2 cups oats (not instant)
¾ teaspoon salt
½ cup raisins

1 or 2 apples, peeled and slivered
  Cinnamon to taste or 1 teaspoon brown sugar (optional)

Mix the first five ingredients together in a saucepan. Bring to a boil, turn heat down, and cover and simmer, stirring often, for about 10 minutes or until the oatmeal reaches the desired consistency. Sprinkle with cinnamon or, if you can take the added calories, top with brown sugar, and serve. Yield: 4 servings.

Low-Cholesterol French Toast

2 whole eggs and 2 egg whites
¼ cup skim milk
2 teaspoons sugar
½ teaspoon cinnamon
¼ teaspoon salt

8 slices white or whole-wheat bread, cut in half
Sliced fruit
Syrup or sugar (optional)

Mix the eggs, egg whites, milk, sugar, cinnamon, and salt in a shallow bowl or pie plate. Dip half slices of bread into the mixture. Fry the bread on a hot griddle that has been lightly greased with vegetable oil or margarine until the bread is browned on both sides. Serve with sliced fruit (banana is my favorite, or strawberries in season) and, if you can afford the calories, a dribble of syrup or a sprinkle of sugar. Yield: 4 servings.

Wholesome Pancakes

⅔ cup whole-wheat flour
⅓ cup white flour
¼ cup wheat germ (optional)
½ teaspoon baking soda
1 teaspoon baking powder
2 teaspoons sugar
¼ teaspoon salt

1 cup buttermilk
½ cup skim milk
1 whole egg plus 1 egg white
1 tablespoon oil
Sliced fruit
Cinnamon-sugar, to taste

In a bowl mix together the first seven ingredients. In separate bowl, mix together the next four ingredients and add to the first seven ingredients, stirring to break up the lumps. Fry on a lightly greased griddle. Serve with sliced fruit and sprinkle with cinnamon-sugar. Serves 4 (makes about 16 4-inch pancakes).

Variation: Before the pancake sets on the first side, spread some peeled slivered apple or sliced banana on top and dribble a little batter over the fruit to prevent sticking. Sprinkle with cinnamon before flipping. This is sweet enough to eat without syrup.

On especially busy mornings, I serve unsweetened cold cereal (oat cereals generally give the best protein value) with skim milk, topped with half a sliced banana and some raisins.

My personal breakfast favorite is concocted from the night before's leftovers: rice, noodles, kasha (buckwheat groats), or bulgur (cracked wheat) stir-fried with vegetables and bits of meat, chicken, or fish (see page 111), or—if there are no such bits left over—a scrambled egg white or slivers of the boiled ham or turkey breast that we keep on hand for sandwiches. I also have found that the remains of a hearty, homemade soup can be a filling, nutritious, and quick low-fat breakfast.

With all these choices, weeks often go by before I realize I haven't had eggs for breakfast for a long time. And I used to breakfast on whole eggs at least four times a week!

Remember, though, that the prudent diet is not a rigid corset from which you can never escape. It doesn't hurt now and again to put pleasure ahead of prudence and splurge on special occasions, as long as the exceptions don't become the rule. If you are aware of the major fat-and-cholesterol offenders, you can cut down where it's easy to cut down, and adopt a philosophy of moderation in your eating habits. In all likelihood, you'll discover many new "lean" dining pleasures to replace the old fatty ones, which may gradually lose their appeal. But you don't have to give up everything you now love to preserve your health. You can have those blinis with caviar, sour cream, and chopped egg on New Year's Eve or that piled-high ice cream sundae dripping with whipped cream on your birthday, so long as such indulgences are infrequent and you are reasonably careful the rest of the time. In other words, if you really are prudent, you *can* have your cake and eat it too.

FOR FURTHER READING

Janet James and Lois Goulder, *The Dell Color-coded Low Fat Living Guide* (New York: Dell, 1980).

Joyce Daly Margie, Robert I. Levy, M.D., and James C. Hunt, M.D., *Living Better— Recipes for a Healthy Heart* (Radnor, Pa.: HLS Press, Chilton Book Company, 1981).

5 ❧ CARBOHYDRATES HAVE GOTTEN A BAD PRESS

IN A SOCIETY raised on the slogan of "a chicken in every pot" or—of late—a steak on every plate, it's no wonder that people have little regard for such basics as rice and potatoes. These, along with bread, pasta, and related starchy foods, are commonly considered long on calories and short on nutrition.

Well, if you haven't already guessed it, a revision of these attitudes and a reintroduction to the world of healthful carbohydrates are long overdue. Contrary to what most Americans think, carbohydrates are not "fattening." Ounce for ounce, they have the same number of calories as pure protein and less than half the calories in fat. And carbohydrate foods can be a rich source of vital nutrients. It may surprise you to know, for example, that the lowly potato is a nutritional bargain when measured against its caloric content. A medium potato (about 5 ounces) has about 110 calories, 4 to 5 percent of the daily caloric total needed by the average adult. At the same time, the potato supplies nearly 5 percent of the protein, 5 percent of the iron, 8 percent of the phosphorous, 10 percent of the thiamin, 11 percent of the niacin, and 50 percent of the vitamin C, as well as large percentages of vitamin B_6, copper, magnesium, iodine, and folacin needed daily by the average adult.

When you compare the calories in starchy foods to those in our venerated sources of protein, you're in for a further surprise: the comparable 5 ounces of steak has about 500 calories, four and a half times as much as the potato that the dieter skips as "too fattening." Five ounces of cooked white rice has 154 calories; kidney beans, 167; spaghetti, 210; and bulgur (cracked wheat), 238. Even 5 ounces of bread, at 390 calories, has fewer calories than 5 ounces of marbled steak. Why? Because steak is fatty and these other carbohydrate foods are not. You're better off going easy on the steak and eating the potato or the bread.

Carbohydrates—at least, the natural, unrefined kind in whole grains, beans, fruits, and vegetables—are the only food category *not* linked to any leading killer diseases.

What Are Carbohydrates?

Carbohydrates are made up of the elements carbon, hydrogen, and oxygen. There are two basic kinds of carbohydrates—the *starches*, called complex carbohydrates, and the *sugars*, or simple carbohydrates. Further, there are "natural" carbohydrates—both simple and complex —found in foods just as they come from the earth, and "refined" or "processed" carbohydrates, which are extracted from their natural sources and added to foods (often in concentrated amounts) that don't naturally contain them. (Alcohol, a refined substance that the body processes as a carbohydrate, will be discussed in Chapter 14.)

In nature, the vast majority of carbohydrates—both the complex starches and the simple sugars—come "packaged" in foods like corn, wheat, milk, apples, and oranges that contain a wide variety of essential nutrients, with a good ratio of nutrients to calories. However, many of the foods to which significant amounts of refined or processed carbohydrates are added, such as cookies, candy, cakes, and pies, are relatively low in nutrients for the large number of calories they contain. This is why the carbohydrates—that is, the refined sugars and starches—in these foods are commonly referred to as *empty calories*.

In addition to supplying vital nutrients like protein, vitamins, and minerals, natural carbohydrate foods are the only sources of an important nonnutrient—*dietary fiber*. Fiber is a carbohydrate from plants that cannot be digested by human beings. It goes through the human digestive tract—from the mouth to the large intestine—relatively intact. Some fibrous substances are digested by bacteria in the gut and then absorbed by the body, but all in all dietary fiber supplies relatively few or no calories. What it does supply is "roughage"—bulk that helps to satisfy the appetite and keep the digestive system running smoothly and eliminating wastes regularly. The truth—and considerable poetry —about fiber will be discussed at length in Chapter 7. For now, suffice it to say that many carbohydrate foods, particularly whole grains, beans, fruits, and vegetables, are excellent sources of healthful fiber.

Except for milk and milk products, which contain the sugar lactose, nearly all the carbohydrates we eat originally come from plants. All starches are plant materials, for starch is the plant's way of storing energy. The starchy beans and grains we eat are really the seeds for the next generation. They contain the food supply for the plant embryo after it germinates but before it's big enough to manufacture its own food through photosynthesis. As the sole source of nourishment for the new seedling, the grain is a storehouse of energy and essential nutrients.

All carbohydrates are made up of one or more molecules of sugar. The *sugars,* or simple carbohydrates, may be single molecules—*mono*saccharides, such as glucose, fructose, and galactose—or double molecules—*di*saccharides. The disaccharides are sucrose, a combination of glucose and fructose; maltose, a combination of two glucose molecules; and lactose, a combination of glucose and galactose. The various sugars will be discussed in greater detail in the next chapter.

Starches, branched chains of dozens of molecules of glucose, are called *poly*saccharides. All carbohydrates are readily broken down by digestive enzymes into their component sugars and absorbed into the bloodstream. The liver converts the monosaccharides fructose and galactose into glucose, which is commonly called "blood sugar."

Low-Carbohydrate Diets Are Dangerous

Glucose is the body's main energy source. It is the fuel the brain normally uses, and it is the main fuel for muscles. Without carbohydrates, your body is forced to run on fat and protein, a potentially dangerous situation. Fats burn inefficiently in the absence of carbohydrates, with the result that your blood becomes "polluted" with a fat waste product called ketone bodies. These are toxic compounds that can damage the brain and cause nausea, fatigue, and apathy. The kidneys are faced with the burdensome job of clearing them from the blood as fast as possible.

When your body must rely on proteins for energy, this vital nutrient is then not available for building and replacing body tissues. In addition, the nitrogen part of the protein molecule is left over and the kidneys must excrete it, a job that can overtax the kidneys of many people. This is why the faddish low-carbohydrate diets are potentially dangerous (see Chapter 16, "Why Diets Don't Work"). It's also why you're told to drink lots of water while on such diets. The water is essential to help the kidneys flush the accumulated poisons out of your system.

On a more balanced reducing diet, however, your body uses some of your stored fat (which is really all you want to lose) for energy, but the fat is burned more completely because it's burned in the presence of carbohydrates. Poisonous ketone bodies don't accumulate, and your body is not robbed of essential protein.

We Need to Eat More Carbohydrates

In the course of this century, an imbalance has crept into the American diet. Since the early 1900s, the percentage of our diet derived from carbohydrates has dropped, and the proportion of fat has risen dramatically. This fat is, as we have seen, an important factor in the nation's epidemic of heart disease and probably also in some common cancers, not to mention its contribution to obesity. The emphasis on fat stems primarily from our worship of animal sources of protein—meat, cheese, and other dairy products—and our denigration of the starchy foods like beans and grains.

Another unhealthful change relates to the *kinds* of carbohydrates in the American diet (see Chart 6). At the turn of the century, most of our carbohydrates were the *complex starches* in nutrient-rich grains and beans and the *natural simple sugars* in fruits and vegetables. Today a major portion of carbohydrates in the American diet comes from *refined and processed sugars* often found in relatively nutrient-deficient and high-calorie foods. As we shall see in the next chapter, this emphasis on "sweets" has been linked to a number of health problems, especially tooth decay and obesity.

Part of the problem is that there's no powerful, profit-making industry selling Americans on natural forms of complex carbohydrates at every commercial break on radio and TV. The growers of fruits, vegetables, grains, and potatoes are hard put to compete with the meat, dairy, and processed-foods industries for the consumer's attention.

The fall-off in consumption has been particularly dramatic for flour and cereal products. Today Americans typically consume half the amount of these foods their counterparts ate in 1910 (see Chart 7). At that time, flour (used in bread and pasta) and cereals were America's *chief* sources of protein, supplying 36 percent of the day's protein. Today they account for only 17 percent of protein consumed, having been replaced by fattier sources of protein, primarily meats.

And although we each eat more fruit now than early in the century, we actually eat a third less *fresh* fruit than we used to. Consumption of processed fruits, however, including those used in making fruit juices (which contain little or no natural fiber) and those canned in heavily sweetened syrup, has more than tripled.

We're doing somewhat better with vegetables. We each eat twice what we did in 1910, although the major increase took place in canned and frozen vegetables, rather than fresh ones. However, consumption

Chart 6 • SOURCES OF CARBOHYDRATES *(per capita per day)*

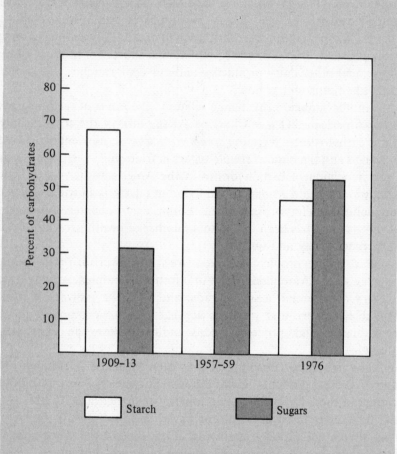

Source: Economic Research Service, U.S. Department of Agriculture

of fresh lettuce has increased fourfold, and consumption of fresh carrots and corn has tripled in the last half century. In general, canned fruits and vegetables have less nutrients than fresh or frozen ones (see Chapter 8).

Since the end of World War II, however, consumption patterns have gone from bad to worse. Except for citrus fruits, the amounts of natural carbohydrate foods we eat have dropped, some rather precipitously. Flour and cereal-grain products are down 31 pounds per person, potatoes down 21 pounds, fruits other than citrus down 30 pounds. Vegetables (excluding dark-green and deep-yellow ones) have dropped 12 pounds, and the dark-green and deep-yellow vegetables are down a third of a pound.

The sugar-consumption story is even sadder. Americans today are eating sugar at record levels—about 128 pounds per person a year, up from 40 pounds a century ago. Sweeteners now account for 24 percent of our daily calories, an increase from 11 percent since 1910. More than 70 percent of this sugar is sucrose—white, refined table sugar—and much of it is "hidden" in thousands of processed food items ranging from soup to nuts (see Chapter 6). But a lot of sugars are quite conspicuously consumed—in sweet baked goods, candy, ice cream, and other desserts and snacks that are very low on the nutrition totem pole.

What, then, should we be eating in the way of carbohydrates? Probably the most sensible recommendation is contained within the Dietary Goals of the Senate Select Committee on Nutrition and Human Needs. Instead of the 45 percent of total calories that carbohydrates currently account for, the Committee recommended that carbohydrates add up to 55 to 60 percent of our caloric intake. At the same time, however, the portion of calories derived from refined and processed sugars should drop—from 24 to 10 percent. The bulk—45 to 50 percent of calories or more—should be the complex carbohydrates (starchy foods) and naturally occurring sugars found in fresh fruits and vegetables. These would also displace a significant number of calories currently derived from artery-clogging fats.

Eating more complex carbohydrates and less fat-ridden animal protein can mean a substantial savings in your food budget. Consumers who say they buy foods like hot dogs and bologna for their families because it's all they can afford are wrong. They've fallen into the societal trap that lures people with the notion that meat is the best source of protein and should be consumed at every meal. In fact, the consumer who buys cheap meats is paying a very high price for protein because these meats are mostly fat (see Chapter 2).

Chart 7 • VEGETABLE, FRUIT, FLOUR, AND CEREAL CONSUMPTION

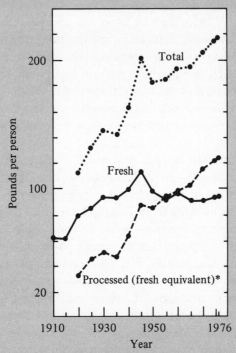

Vegetable Consumption

*The figures describing processed vegetable consumption on the graph are "fresh equivalent" weights. They exaggerate actual intake. Under fresh equivalency, for example, the weight of discarded corn cobs are included when figuring the "fresh equivalent" weight of canned corn. But by using "fresh equivalents," we can compare the consumption of vegetables in their fresh and their processed form.

**All figures used for processed fruits are "fresh equivalent" weights. These exaggerate apparent consumption. For example, under "fresh equivalency" 8 ounces of frozen orange juice concentrate is converted to the weight of fresh oranges needed to make up the concentrate—approximately 3 pounds. But, by using "fresh equivalents," we are able to compare the consumption of fresh and processed fruit.

Source: *The Changing American Diet*, Center for Science in the Public Interest, based on data from U.S. Department of Agriculture.

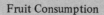

Fruit Consumption

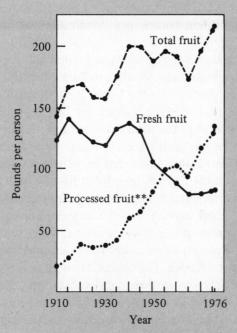

Flour and Cereal Product Consumption

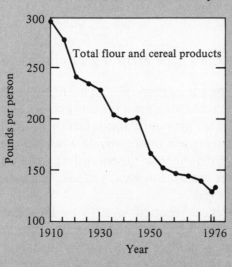

Developing a repertoire of meatless meals in which inexpensive protein is provided by properly balanced vegetable sources (see Chapter 24) can conserve your health as well as your money. Unlike animal sources of protein, most of which contain more fat calories than protein, most vegetable protein comes in a "container" of complex carbohydrates.

A greater emphasis on starchy foods and fruits and vegetables, the McGovern committee maintains, would produce a healthier America. Studies of populations throughout the world have shown that those in which atherosclerotic heart disease is relatively rare typically consume between 65 and 80 percent of the total calories in the form of carbohydrates derived from whole grains (cereals) and tubers (potatoes and their relatives). Southern Italians, who eat very little saturated fats but lots of carbohydrates in the form of bread and pasta, typically have far lower levels of triglycerides and cholesterol in their blood than northern Europeans, who eat fewer carbohydrates but more animal fats.

Increasing our consumption of whole grains, fruits, and vegetables will also mean a better supply of vitamins, minerals, and trace nutrients that are essential to good health. Foods that are high in fats and refined sugars are generally deficient in these vital substances. Our intake of dietary fiber would also be increased, a plus for our intestinal tracts, which tend to suffer from a variety of disorders on the highly refined diet typically consumed by affluent Americans. A final benefit involves weight control, for natural carbohydrates can help you cut back on calorie-dense fats and sweets.

Carbohydrates Can Help You Lose Weight

Considering all the admonitions you've heard about how *fattening* carbohydrates are, the above statement probably comes as a shock. You may be ready to accept the previously stated fact that carbohydrates are no more fattening than protein (both provide 4 calories per gram) and are considerably less fattening than the equivalent weight of fat (which provides 9 calories per gram). But how, you ask, can eating carbohydrates help make you thin?

Here is the evidence, reported in 1975 by Dr. Olaf Mickelsen, professor of nutrition at Michigan State University: "Contrary to what most people think, bread in large amounts is an ideal food in a weight reducing regimen. Recent work in our laboratory indicates that slightly overweight young men lost weight in a painless and practically effortless manner when they included *twelve slices of bread per day* [italics added] in their program. That bread was eaten with their meals. As a result, they became satisfied before they consumed their usual quota of calories. The subjects were admonished to restrict those foods that were concentrated sources of energy [that is, very high in calories]; otherwise, they were free to eat as much as they desired." In eight weeks, the average weight loss for the eight men who were given a high-fiber bread was 19.4 pounds; the eight who consumed a look-alike low-fiber bread lost an average of 13.7 pounds.

Now for the rationale. Carbohydrate foods—at least the starches, fruits, and vegetables—fulfill both your physical and your psychological need for food. They make you feel as though you've eaten something. They fill your stomach, stick to your ribs, give you something to chew on. In the case of fruits, they can satisfy a sweet craving without overloading you with calories, and they give you a nutrient bonus in the bargain. A plateful of spaghetti with meat sauce may not sound like a typical dieter's meal, but it can contain fewer calories and be more satisfying than a steak dinner or tuna salad. If the carbohydrates in your diet come from whole grains, fruits, and vegetables, you have the added advantage of the satisfying bulk and bowel regularity provided by the noncaloric fiber. In an experiment with adult laboratory rats who were fed diets virtually identical in calorie and fat content, those animals whose meals were rich in protein (as compared to carbohydrates) gained much more weight and put on more body fat than did the animals fed meals low in protein and high in carbohydrates. The University of Virginia scientists who conducted the experiment suggested that the typical American diet, which overemphasizes protein at the expense of carbohydrates, may be an important part of the reason why so many millions are overweight. Among possible explanations, the researchers suggested that on a low-protein, high-carbohydrate diet, more calories may be "burned up" as body heat and fewer stored as an energy reserve in the body's fat tissue.

And They're Good for Diabetics, Too

Diabetics have problems disposing of sugar in the blood, and many people believe that all carbohydrates are a problem for diabetics. In fact, Dr. William E. Connor and Sonja J. Connor of the Oregon Health Sciences University and Dr. Edward Bierman at the University of Washington have shown that a diet high in *complex* carbohydrates is useful in the treatment of diabetes. For one thing, it cuts down on the amount of fats diabetics might otherwise eat. Since diabetics are unusually prone to developing atherosclerosis, a low-fat, low-cholesterol diet can help prevent premature death and crippling heart and blood-vessel diseases. A second advantage is that in some diabetics a high-carbohydrate diet helps to improve their ability to process blood sugar, and in others it stabilizes their requirement for insulin. A diet low in fat and sugar but rich in complex carbohydrates and fiber is now commonly prescribed for diabetics, and for hypoglycemics.

A Field Guide to (Good) Carbohydrates

Not all starchy foods are equally nutritious. Some have less than others of the things that are good for you. Some have had much or all of nature's goodness refined out of them, leaving behind for you to eat little or nothing more than calories. The following is intended to help you select and prepare your foods so that you can get the most nutritional benefits from the calories you consume.

POTATOES

As you've already seen, potatoes as they come from nature are a nutritional bargain in terms of the calories they provide. In addition to vitamins, minerals, and trace nutrients, potatoes contain a small but significant amount of high-quality protein—3.2 grams per medium potato. An adult could derive nearly all needed nutrients from a diet of only potatoes. The Irish were so dependent on the potato as a source of nutrients and calories that when a potato blight struck in the nineteenth century and famine followed, 1 million Irish died, and more than 1 million others were forced to emigrate.

A medium-sized potato has about 110 calories, and a large one, 190—that is, if you hold back on the butter. Each pat (teaspoon) of butter or margarine you use adds 35 calories. Since a good baked potato has a scrumptious flavor of its own, you might try it with little or no added fat and just a sprinkling of salt or freshly ground pepper. Boiled potatoes are another treat, especially the little "new" potatoes. Try them with some chopped fresh parsley, dill, or chives and skip the butter. Since many of the potato's nutrients are in and just beneath the skin, you'll preserve them better if you boil the potatoes in their skin and, if you don't care to eat the skin, peel them after cooking. Studies by Consumers Union showed that a baked potato with its skin rivals the bean in nutritional value and is a better nutritional buy than rice, noodles, or white bread. Minus the skin, it's nutritionally comparable to these other starchy foods.

Frying potatoes, however, considerably changes the nutrient-to-calorie ratio—to your disadvantage. The high temperature of deep-frying destroys some of the vitamins, and the fat adds astronomically to the calories without enhancing the nutrient content. Seventy percent of the calories in French fries are fat calories. Whereas a ½-pound baked potato has about 170 calories, ½ pound of fries has 620! Potato chips are also mostly fat (and high in salt)—about nine chips add up

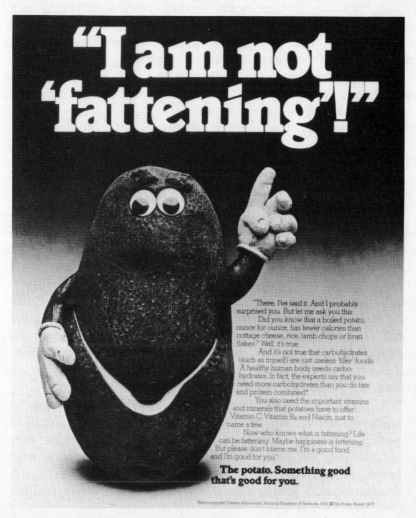

to 100 calories, an ounce has over 150, and ½ pound has more than 1,200 calories. Potato sticks are just as bad.

Sweet potatoes (without added sweetener or fat) have about a third more calories and slightly less protein than white potatoes. But they are very rich sources of vitamin A and contain more calcium, iron, potassium, and niacin than white potatoes.

FLOURS

Like potatoes, wheat and other grains as nature made them are a nutritional plus. But people, in their various attempts to "improve" on nature, frequently destroy much of what is best for them. A great nutritional travesty was wrought when people decided that *refined* white flour was more desirable than flour flecked with hard brownish specks. The goal was primarily one of gentility, not nutrition.

To appreciate what's lost in refining flour, it helps to know something about a kernel of grain as nature makes it. There are three main constituents in the whole-wheat kernel, and the nutrients are distributed throughout. Outermost is the *bran*—six layers of protective skin that consist primarily of noncaloric cellulose fiber, or roughage. The bran also contains many B vitamins—most of the niacin, B_6, pantothenic acid, riboflavin, and a third of the thiamin—and 19 percent of the protein. The bran is lost when grains are refined.

In a small area at the base of the kernel lies the *germ*—the embryo or sprouting section of the kernel—which contains vegetable oil (polyunsaturated fats) and vitamin E, most of the thiamin, smaller amounts of riboflavin, B_6, pantothenic acid, niacin, and 8 percent of the protein. The germ is often removed from milled wheat because its fat content limits the shelf life of the flour.

Most of the kernel is the central *endosperm,* which is primarily starch, the food supply for the sprouting seed. The endosperm contains three-fourths of the protein in the wheat kernel and large portions of two B vitamins, panthothenic acid and riboflavin, as well as smaller amounts of niacin, B_6, and thiamin.

All of the above constituents would be found in whole-wheat flour that is stone-ground. This most efficient milling process loses only 5 to 10 percent of the original grain, mostly the nutrient-deficient part of the bran called the "bee's wing." Other methods of grinding whole-wheat flour lose somewhat more of the nutrients. Graham flour, the basis for graham crackers, is simply a more coarsely ground whole-kernel flour than ordinary whole wheat.

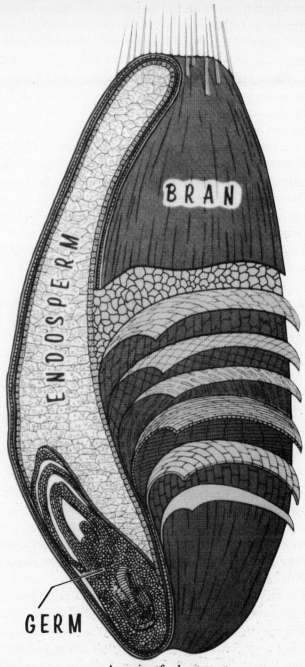

A grain of wheat.

Source: Kansas Wheat Commission.

Refined white flour, however, is pure endosperm; both the bran and the germ have been removed and only about 75 percent of the original kernel remains. Except for starch and protein, up to 80 percent of the essential nutrients in whole wheat are missing from white flour. White flour retains only a quarter of the vitamin E and 7 percent of the fiber of the original grain. *Bleaching* destroys even more of the vitamin E. Most white flour sold in the United States has been *"enriched"*— that is, some, but not all, of the vitamins and minerals removed during processing are added back. These are niacin, thiamin, riboflavin, and iron. But none of the natural fiber is replaced. White flour has one important advantage over whole wheat and other whole grains. The latter two contain a substance called phytic acid, which can combine with calcium, iron, and zinc and prevent the body from absorbing them. The significance to human health of the phytic acid in whole grains has not been clearly established, but most experts believe it presents no nutritional problem if high-fiber foods are consumed in moderation.

Contrary to what you might guess, ordinary pale-brown rye flour is ground just from the endosperm. The nutritious bran and germ are lost. However, the darker, more coarsely ground rye that's used to make pumpernickel is ground from the entire rye kernel. As a rule, though, you have no way of knowing just how much rye may be in a commercial bread, since rye has to be mixed with wheat flour to make a good bread dough.

BREAD

Despite the revival of interest in whole grains in the 1970s, three out of every four loaves of bread Americans buy are white breads. You get the most nutrients for your money if you buy whole-grain bread made from stone-ground flour. The next best thing is 100-percent whole-wheat or other whole-grain bread. Be sure to check the ingredients list on the label. Some commercial breads are made with eggs and milk, which bolsters their nutritional value.

If you're buying white bread, make sure it's enriched. That goes for Italian and French and bakery breads, as well as the factory-packaged loaves from the supermarket. If "brown breads" are your thing, remember they may contain little or no whole grain, just molasses for coloring. Check the label and buy for ingredients, not color.

The recently introduced high-fiber breads are usually lower in calories because a large percentage of their bulk is undigestible fiber, usually the bran from the wheat kernel. However, one brand, Fresh Horizons, uses wood fiber as its source of added roughage. There's no known harm in that, as long as you know that what you're paying for isn't nutritious wheat bran.

The best way to be sure you and your family are eating "good" breads is to make them yourself. Bread baking can be a very satisfying hobby that everyone in the family over the age of four can participate in. Most electric food processors will knead bread dough for you, although most bread makers I know—including my husband—find kneading by hand an enjoyable and "therapeutic" exercise.

Richard's Best Bread

2 cups skim milk, scalded
⅓ cup vegetable oil
⅓ cup sweetener (any combination of honey, sugar, brown sugar, molasses, or corn syrup)
2 teaspoons salt
2 envelopes dry yeast
½ cup tepid water
½ teaspoon sugar
2 well-beaten eggs
1 cup rolled oats
½ cup bran

6 cups flour, approximately (3 cups unbleached white plus 3 cups any combination of rye, whole-wheat, or buckwheat flours)
Flavorings, to taste (e.g., orégano, basil, thyme, sesame seeds, caraway seeds, anise, poppy seeds, fennel)
1 tablespoon melted margarine or oil
Cinnamon or nutmeg (optional)

Combine the milk, oil, sweetener, and salt in a large mixing bowl. Dissolve the yeast in the water, and add the sugar. When the yeast is bubbling and the milk mixture has cooled to tepid, combine and add the eggs. Add the oats and bran, and mix thoroughly. Start adding flour until the dough reaches the proper consistency—easy to handle and slightly moist but not sticky. Knead the dough for several minutes, adding more flour if necessary, and return the dough to mixing bowl. Cover with a damp towel, and set the bowl in a warm place (e.g., on top of the refrigerator or on a sunny window ledge). When the dough has doubled in size, punch it down and divide it into three parts. Add the desired flavorings, and form into loaves. Put the loaves into three 9×5×3-inch pans, and let them rise again about 1½ to 2 hours—longer if a lighter bread is desired. Brush the tops of the loaves with melted margarine or oil and, if desired, sprinkle with cinnamon or nutmeg. Preheat the oven to 350 degrees. Put in the loaves and reduce the heat to 325 degrees. Bake 35 to 40 minutes, or until the loaves have a hollow sound when tapped. Remove the loaves from the pans and place the loaves on a rack to cool. Yield: 3 loaves.

CEREALS

By now, it should come as no surprise to hear that whole-grain cereals are very nutritious. In general, whole-grain hot cereals are the best nutritional buy of any cereal. Farina, made from refined wheat, is missing much of the natural nutrients; if you buy it, be sure it's enriched. Oatmeal made from steel-cut or rolled oats (the old-fashioned kind, not the instant variety—the label may reveal the milling process used) leads the pack in food value, since oats contain the most protein of any commonly eaten grains and steel-cutting and "rolling" do the least damage to the natural nutrients. Oat bran cereal, though lower in protein, is rich in cholesterol-lowering dietary fiber. When you cook hot cereals, use skim milk as part or all of the liquid and you'll greatly improve their nutritional value (see Chapter 4, page 92, for a nutritious oatmeal recipe). You can obtain a free oats cookbook containing more than sixty recipes using this nutritious grain from the Quaker Oats Company. Write to Quaker Oats Wholegrain Cookbook, P.O. Box 14081, Baltimore, Maryland 21268.

Among cold cereals, there's a veritable supermarket of confusing choices, and hardly a month goes by without some company introducing yet another manufactured wonder that's supposed to make breakfast a "total experience" for young and old. Still, among the leaders of the nutritional list are two old-timers: Shredded Wheat, which is made from whole grain with no sugar added, and Cheerios, which (since they're made from oats) contain more protein (4 grams per 1-ounce serving) than nearly all ordinary competitors. There are also a number of newer high-protein products that yield about 6 grams of protein per ounce. Cereals containing bran or whole grains are relatively high in fiber. However, those that contain 100 percent of the daily requirement of a long list of vitamins don't make much sense. Unless you plan to live on nothing but one bowl of dry cereal all day, there's no need to get your whole day's supply of any vitamin at breakfast.

Puffed cereals give you more air than nutrition, though they are low in fat and salt. And the sugar-coated varieties send dollar signs dancing in front of dentists' eyes. Manufacturers introduced sugar-coated cereals in the 1940s to counter a crumbling market for cereal. The gimmick worked—too well from a public-health viewpoint. Many of these cereals contain sugar and other sweeteners as their leading ingredient. A single serving may have as much as 4 teaspoons of sugar on the chewy pieces that stick to teeth and provide banquets for decay-causing bacteria.

Also watch out for granolas. True, they contain lots of nutritious goodies—nuts, seeds, raisins, oat flakes, etc. But they're also high in sugars (remember, honey and molasses are sugars) and fats (from added oil plus the oil in the nuts and seeds) and, ipso facto, high in calories. A 1-ounce serving of granola—¼ cup—contains about 130 calories and hardly covers the bottom of your cereal bowl; most people eat more than the recommended serving size. Many granolas are also made with coconut, which contains highly saturated fat. If granola is a big hit in your household, you'd be better off making your own, leaving out the coconut and cutting back on the oil and sweeteners. Or try sprinkling just a handful of a commercial granola on top of some other unsweetened packaged cereal to add a satisfying crunch.

RICE, CORN, AND OTHER GRAINS

In the Far East, rice is practically synonymous with food for millions of people. Next to wheat, it's the world's most widely grown food grain. Although whole-grain—brown—rice retains all the original nutrients of the rice kernel, nearly all the rice eaten in non-Western countries is white *polished* rice. Although polishing seems to render the protein in rice more digestible, it has the unfortunate disadvantage of stripping the rice of some of its protein and many of its valuable vitamins and minerals, especially the B vitamins. Polished rice has only 60 percent of the riboflavin, less than half the B_6, a third of the niacin, and only 20 percent of the thiamin of the original rice kernel.

Parboiled or *converted* white rice retains more of the original nutrients because the process of parboiling "pushes" some of the vitamins from the bran into the white endosperm. Instant and "minute" rices are the lowest in nutrient content. The length of the rice grain influences its cooked consistency (the shorter the grain, the stickier the cooked rice) but has little nutritional significance.

Rice is considered a good source of carbohydrates for diabetics since tests have shown that, calorie for calorie, less insulin is required to assimilate the starches in rice than the starches, for example, in potatoes.

A cup of cooked brown rice has 230 calories; white rice 220; and instant rice 180.

I often eat some version of the following for breakfast or lunch.

Leftover Fried Rice

1 tablespoon oil
½ cup chopped onion
½ cup chopped or thinly sliced celery
3 cups cooked rice (white or brown)
½ cup cooked meat (ham, pork, beef) or poultry, cut into bits
½ cup leftover cooked vegetable (e.g., carrots, peas, sliced broccoli, green beans, etc.)
Imported soy sauce, to taste (optional)

Heat the oil in a skillet. Sauté the onion and celery for a few minutes. Add the rice, and stir to separate the kernels. Add the meat and vegetables and cook, stirring, just enough to heat through. Sprinkle with soy sauce if desired. Yield: 3 to 4 servings.

Note: You can substitute cooked bulgur or kasha (buckwheat groats) for all or part of the rice.

In contrast to rice, corn is primarily a New World staple, first cultivated by the Indians of South, Central, and North America. When combined with dried beans and green vegetables, corn provided sound nutrition for the Indians, as it can for us. In fact, corn bread and beans are the main sources of protein and carbohydrates in traditional Mexican diets.

What Americans commonly eat today is *sweet corn,* in which about 20 percent of the kernel is natural sugars. *Field corn,* which has more starch and much less sugar, is used to make corn meal and hominy grits. In the late 1800s, when field corn was a staple in the diet of our ancestors, it was served as a cereal or made into breads and muffins, and Americans ate 117 pounds of corn each year. Today, we feed most of our home-grown corn (America's largest crop) to cattle, which convert the vegetable protein and starch to animal protein and fat. Corn starch, which we do eat, is just that—purified starch. It has none of the valuable nutrients found in the whole corn kernel.

Perhaps the most familiar form of corn to Americans is popcorn. Without butter or oil and with just a gentle sprinkling of salt, popcorn makes an excellent low-calorie, high-fiber nibble food. A cup of fat-free popcorn has only 29 calories, so that even if you ate *2 quarts* of the stuff, you wouldn't exceed the calories in 25 potato chips!

A cup of sweet corn kernels has 137 calories, a cup of corn grits (coarsely ground corn that is dried and cooked) has 125. Corn meal, which can be purchased either as the whole ground kernel or degermed and enriched, yields 120 calories per cooked cup.

Another grain worth knowing about is *bulgur* (sometimes called burghul), a favorite in Arab nations. Bulgur is wheat that has been parboiled, dried, and cracked. Sometimes, however, it is refined and the bran removed, so before you buy it, if you can, check the irregular grains to see if the dark bran covering is still there. It can be purchased in bulk in groceries that cater to a Middle Eastern trade, or packaged in health food stores, specialty stores, and supermarkets. (Check the counter where rice or hot cereals are sold.)

Cous-cous, from North Africa, is also a cracked wheat grain, but it is usually quite refined (and thus less nutritious) and light in color. *Pearled barley* has been milled to remove the nutrient-laden outer covering. *Millet,* a popular staple grain in much of Africa, India, and China, is primarily used for bird feed in the United States. While not remarkable in nutritional qualities, it is good food for people, too.

Then there's *buckwheat,* one of the first crops grown in America by European settlers and a staple in the Soviet Union, though little known in most of the world. Buckwheat is really not a grain, though it is used as one. The edible kernels, called groats, are known as kasha and are actually the fruits of the plant. Buckwheat is rich in high-quality protein, containing about half the amount of protein in an equivalent weight of beef. One serving—about ¾ cup of cooked groats —provides a quarter of the recommended daily allowance for protein for the average adult. Buckwheat is also a good source of thiamin, niacin, riboflavin, potassium, and iron.

Buckwheat is usually consumed as flour or grits, with all its natural nutrients intact. The grainlike, nutty-flavored groats can be used as a cereal, vegetable, or main course. It is usually found in the supermarket near the rice or among specialty food items. For further information about buckwheat, including recipes (see one below) and where to buy it, write to The Birkett Mills, P.O. Box 440A, Penn Yan, New York 14527.

Among some of my favorite "grain" recipes are the following:

Basic Bulgur

1 tablespoon margarine	2 cups broth, bouillon, or water
1 small onion, chopped	Salt and freshly ground black
1 cup uncooked bulgur	pepper, to taste

Melt the margarine in a saucepan. Add the onion, and sauté until translucent. Add the bulgur and stir to coat, cooking for a minute or two.

Add the broth, salt, and pepper, bring to a boil, lower the flame to a simmer, and cover. Cook about 15 minutes or until all the liquid is absorbed. Yield: 4 servings.

Tabbouli (Middle Eastern Salad)

1 cup uncooked bulgur
2 cups boiling water
2 tomatoes, finely diced
1 bunch scallions with tops, finely chopped
1 cup parsley, finely chopped
3 tablespoons chopped fresh

mint, or 2 teaspoons dry mint flakes
¼ cup vegetable oil
¼ cup lemon juice
1 teaspoon salt
¼ teaspoon cumin
¼ teaspoon orégano (powdered)
Freshly ground pepper, to taste

Put the bulgur in a bowl, and pour the boiling water over it. Let this stand for about 1 hour. Drain well, squeezing out as much water as possible. Add the remaining ingredients. Chill. Serve on a bed of lettuce. (Can be eaten using lettuce leaves as a scoop or with pieces of pita bread.) Yield: 6 to 8 servings as a salad, 12 as hors d'oeuvres.

Buckwheat and Bows

1 tablespoon margarine
1 medium onion, chopped
1 egg, slightly beaten
1 cup buckwheat groats (kasha), coarse or whole

2 cups boiling broth, bouillon, or water
Salt and freshly ground pepper, to taste
¼ pound macaroni bows, cooked and drained

In a skillet that has a cover, melt the margarine and sauté the onion until it is translucent. Mix the egg with the buckwheat groats and add to the skillet. Cook, stirring, until the grains are dry and separate. Add the liquid, salt, and pepper, cover, and simmer for 15 minutes or until all the liquid is absorbed. Stir in the macaroni. Yield: 4 servings.

PASTA

If one food had to be chosen to please all the world's children, pasta in any or all of its many sizes, shapes, and forms would undoubtedly be the hands-down winner. Pasta is made from a hard spring wheat called durum, which is totally unsuitable for breads and cakes because it won't rise. The durum wheat is refined into a white flour called *semolina*, which is mixed with water and other ingredients to make a dough that can be cut into the desired shape. Semolina is about 13 percent protein, with a good balance of essential amino acids.

While a cup of plain cooked spaghetti is not exactly brimming with vital nutrients, it does have a fair amount of protein (6½ grams), potassium, phosphorus, and calcium, and very little fat. Cooked al dente, the cup yields 192 calories; cooked to a softer stage, a cup would contain 155 calories because it holds more water. Be sure to buy enriched products. Many forms of pasta are now available in high-protein varieties, in which high-protein soy flour has partly replaced the semolina. You should also be able to get whole-wheat spaghetti, made from whole durum flour mixed with other wheat flours. Some noodles (for example, spinach or "green" noodles) have vegetable powder added, and others are made with egg. Both of these would be more nourishing than plain pasta.

DRIED BEANS AND PEAS

In vegetables like soybeans, kidney beans, pinto beans, navy beans, lentils, and black-eyed peas, the carbohydrates come packaged with a nutritional bonus—lots of high-quality protein. Dried legumes are the richest sources of protein in the vegetable kingdom. A cup of cooked soybeans contains 20 grams of protein, just a little bit less than a cup of ground beef. But the soybeans have half the calories—230 compared to 470 for the beef—and none of the saturated fat and cholesterol. A cup of cooked kidney beans or lentils has about 15 grams of protein and 215 calories. Beans and peas also contain a number of essential minerals, including potassium and phosphorus. Fresh beans and peas, however, are not rich in protein because they are not mature seeds.

Peanuts (a legume), nuts, and seeds are also good sources of protein as well as carbohydrates, but these foods contain considerable amounts of fat (albeit polyunsaturated vegetable oils) and therefore lots of calories. Ten large walnuts have more than 300 calories; ten large peanuts, 105. A tablespoon of sesame or sunflower seeds has about 50 calories. See Chapter 24 for a further discussion of legumes and seeds.

OTHER FRUITS AND VEGETABLES

Most fruits and vegetables are good sources, not only of starch, but of natural sugars. I say "good" because in this case the sugars come in a low-calorie package along with healthy supplies of vitamins, minerals, and trace nutrients and indigestible fiber. Many vegetables contain small but significant amounts of protein as well. The fiber and water content of fruits and vegetables add satisfying bulk and volume to your diet and help prevent overeating. A type of fiber called *pectin* that is found in many fruits and vegetables, including apples and carrots, can help to lower blood levels of cholesterol. Fruits can satisfy that end-of-the-meal sweet craving in a nutritious, nonfattening way.

Fresh fruits and vegetables are richer sources of vitamins, minerals, and trace nutrients than fruits and vegetables that have been canned, since vital nutrients are lost during processing and storage. Frozen fruits and vegetables are almost as nourishing as fresh. But there's no point in relying on fresh produce if what you ultimately consume is first cooked in ways that destroy the natural goodness or preserved with lots of sugar or salt. If, instead of boiling them in water, vegetables are steamed, baked, or stir-fried (cooked tender-crisp in a small amount of oil) or consumed along with the liquid they're cooked in (as in soups or stews), you—not the sink drain—get most of their natural nutrients.

Steamed Vegetable Pot

New potatoes	Broccoli, florets and sliced stems
Herbs, as desired	Zucchini, thickly sliced
Salt and freshly ground black	Onions, sliced
pepper, to taste	Peas
Carrots, sliced	Margarine (optional)
Turnips, cut in chunks	Sesame oil (optional)
Green beans, whole or halved	Grated Parmesan cheese (optional)

In a large kettle fitted with a deep steamer basket, add several inches of water (but keep the water level below the bottom of the basket) and place the potatoes in the basket. Sprinkle with herbs (for example, dill weed and thyme), salt, and pepper, cover the pot, and bring to a boil. Lower flame and about 5 minutes later, add carrots and turnips plus desired seasonings. In another 10 minutes, add onions, beans and peas, and 5 minutes later, add the zucchini and broccoli, seasoning the layers as desired. Keep an eye on the water level, and if it drops too low add some more. Steam until desired degree of doneness is reached (small new potatoes take about 25 to 30 minutes to cook after the water boils). Remove vegetables by lifting out the steamer basket. Save the water at the bottom of the pot for soups or bread baking. Serve the vegetables with melted margarine or a dash of sesame oil, or sprinkled with grated Parmesan cheese.

Note: The vegetables used can be varied according to taste. Steaming vegetables involves a certain amount of trial and error at first until you learn how long each takes to reach desired doneness. The basic rule is to put the longest-cooking vegetables in the steamer first, and add the rest according to their projected cooking times. But take it from one who eats them often, they're well worth the effort.

Super Chicken-Vegetable Soup

1 frying chicken, about 3 pounds
Water
2 potatoes, peeled and diced
2 large carrots, sliced
2 stalks celery, chopped
1 white turnip, diced
1 large onion, chopped

Salt and pepper to taste
Herbs, to taste (for example, basil, thyme, orégano, dill weed)
½ cup orzo or other small pasta
Grated Parmesan, to taste

Put the whole chicken in a kettle with water to cover and bring to a boil. Reduce the heat and let simmer 15 minutes. Remove the chicken, saving the liquid, and when cool enough to handle, discard the skin and remove all the chicken from the bones. Set aside about half the chicken for other uses (such as in a stir-fried dish with vegetables or a casserole). Use the rest for the soup. If possible, refrigerate the stock and discard the fat that hardens on the top.

Add the vegetables to 6 to 8 cups of stock (i.e., the water in which the chicken was poached) and bring this to a boil. Add salt, pepper, and herbs (add extra water, vegetable water, or chicken bouillon if a thinner soup is desired) and boil for 10 minutes. Then add the reserved chicken pieces and orzo. Return to a boil, reduce the flame, and let the soup simmer for 10 minutes. Serve sprinkled with grated Parmesan cheese. Yield: 8 to 10 servings.

The most nutritious way to eat fruits and vegetables is raw. Fresh fruit salads and green salads are well known to Americans. And in recent years, many people have discovered that vegetables other than the traditional tomatoes, cucumbers, carrots, green peppers, and celery are delicious raw. Much to our nutritional benefit, it's now not so unusual to find salad bars and appetizer trays replete with raw zucchini, broccoli, cauliflower, turnips, and mushrooms as well as the traditional fare. (See pages 179–180 for how to preserve the nutrients in cooked vegetables.)

MILK PRODUCTS

Skim milk and many products made with skim or partially skimmed milk are nutrient-laden foods in which simple carbohydrates provide the bulk of calories. In skim milk, for example, 57 percent of the calories come from carbohydrates—namely, the milk sugar lactose —but only 2 percent come from fat (a cup of skim milk has about 0.2 gram of fat). The same is true for buttermilk, which—despite its "fatty" name—is really made from low-fat or skim milk. Plain yogurt prepared from partially skimmed milk (usually 1 or 1½ percent butterfat) is about 40 percent carbohydrate calories and 30 percent fat calories. All these foods are excellent sources of protein, vitamins, and minerals (see Chapter 13).

However, in whole milk and products like cheese that are made from whole milk and cream, fats provide the majority of calories. Your protein, vitamins, and minerals may be the same, but you're paying a high-calorie price for them.

Here's one of my favorite low-cal, low-cost milk recipes:

Blender Buttermilk Fruit Shake

1 cup buttermilk
1 banana
½ teaspoon vanilla extract

1 teaspoon sugar (optional)
4 ice cubes, crushed

Place all ingredients into a blender. Cover and blend a minute or two at high speed until smooth. This nutritious, 185-calorie drink can be a cooling breakfast or snack on a hot summer day. You can use other fruits, such as strawberries, in place of the banana.

----

6 ❧ SUGAR: IS OUR SWEET TOOTH KILLING US?

SUGAR IS, hands down, the nation's most popular food additive. We consume ten times more sugar than all the other 2,600 or so food additives combined, except for salt, a distant second. Next time you open your pantry or go marketing, take a few minutes to check the ingredients listed on the processed foods you buy and see how many of them contain sugar—ketchup, crackers, bread, soups, cereals, peanut butter, nondairy coffee creamers, breading mixes, bouillon cubes, cured meats, salad dressings, spaghetti sauce, not to mention the more obvious sweet puddings, pies, jams and jellies, soft drinks, ice cream, candy, and cake.

The average American eats about 128 pounds of sugar a year. That's a shocking third of a pound—600 calories of sweetening—a day. Even those who "don't eat sweets" probably consume far more sugar than they realize because so much of it is "hidden" in processed foods. For example, a tablespoon of ketchup contains a teaspoon of sugar. More than two-thirds of the sugar our society uses goes into factory-made foods; only a quarter is added in the home. (The rest is used in institutional settings.) Processors use sugar not just for sweetening, but also to help foods retain moisture, to prevent spoilage, and to improve texture and appearance.

Since sugar comes in many different forms, and not all are called "sugar," they can easily be overlooked in a cursory check of a package label. As mentioned in the previous chapter, there are two basic types of sugars: *monosaccharides,* composed of single molecules, and *disaccharides,* or double molecules. They all have the suffix *-ose.* (See Table 6.1.)

By far, our most widely used sugar is the disaccharide sucrose, extracted from sugar cane and beets (see Chart 8). As a food additive, sucrose is "generally recognized as safe" (see Chapter 25), which means it can be added to foods in any amount a manufacturer desires. One molecule of sucrose is made up of a molecule each of glucose and fructose, and these are readily split apart in the small intestine by the

Chart 8 • PER CAPITA TABLE SUGAR CONSUMPTION

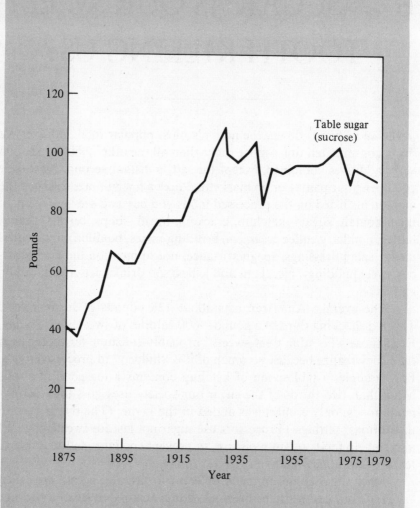

Source: 1875–1909: U.S. Bureau of Census, *Historical Statistics of U.S.—Colonial Times to 1959* (1960), p. 187. 1910–1965: USDA Rep. #138 (1968), p. 84. 1966–76: Sugar and Sweetener Report (May, 1977), p. 31. 1976–preliminary figure.

Table 6.1 • KINDS OF SUGARS

Monosaccharides

Glucose (blood sugar), also known as dextrose
Fructose (fruit sugar), also known as levulose
Galactose

Disaccharides

Sucrose (table sugar)—fructose and glucose
Lactose (milk sugar)—glucose and galactose
Maltose (malt sugar)—two glucose units

---

enzyme sucrase. Sucrose is synonymous with white, refined table sugar. It is also the sugar of raw (unrefined) sugar, turbinado (partially refined sugar), brown sugar, and confectioners' (powdered) sugar.

But while sucrose is our most popular sweetener, it's hardly the only one. In addition to the pure monosaccharides and disaccharides, others include corn syrup and corn sugar, maple syrup and maple sugar, honey, invert sugar, and molasses. Each of these may be listed separately on a product label, leaving you in the dark as to how much added sweetener the product really contains.

Sugar accounts for a total of 24 percent of the calories consumed each day by the average American—14 percent from refined sugars, 4 percent from processed sugars like corn syrup, honey, and molasses, and only 6 percent from natural sources like fruits, vegetables, and milk products. Fully one-fifth of the refined sugar we consume comes in sweetened soft drinks. Since these drinks rarely contain anything of nutritional value other than sugar and water, they are truly the emptiest of calories.

As far as nutrition is concerned, the only benefit of any significance provided by the various forms of sugars is calories, 4 per gram. Some sugars are sweeter than others and thus give you more sweet taste for fewer calories. *Fructose*—fruit sugar, the sweetest of the commonly used sweeteners—is about 70 percent sweeter than sucrose. Glucose, on the other hand, is only two-thirds as sweet as sucrose; maltose is one-third as sweet; and lactose (milk sugar) is only one-seventh as sweet as table sugar.

As for vitamins and minerals, with the possible exception of molasses, there's no inherent advantage of one type of sugar over another. *Brown sugar,* which is sucrose colored with a little molasses, and *raw sugar,* which is unrefined, are no more nourishing than white sugar.

They're all just "pure energy"—calories but no other nutrients of any significance.

Honey, which contains slightly more fructose than glucose and smaller amounts of other sugars (plus water), has small quantities of minerals, mainly potassium, calcium, and phosphorus. But these nutrients are present in such tiny amounts that they have little significance to human nutrition. Consumers Union has calculated that you'd have to eat 91 tablespoons of honey to meet the body's daily requirement for potassium, 200 for calcium, and 267 for phosphorus! In addition, the amounts of these nutrients in honey vary with the type and batch. Although some honeys give you as much as 40 percent more sweetening power than the same number of calories of sucrose, other honeys are less sweet than table sugar. Honey also rots teeth faster than sucrose, and a study at Oregon State University showed that some honeys may contain cancer-causing substances that the bees extract from the flowers they feed on. Various honeys have also been linked to cases of botulism, an often-fatal form of food poisoning, in infants. Some of the poisoned infants had been thought to have died a mysterious "crib death," researchers from the California Department of Health Services report.

Molasses is the liquid that remains after the crystals of sucrose are removed from sugar cane or beet juice. It contains a variety of sugars and small but potentially useful amounts of calcium, iron, potassium, and B vitamins, plus water. The darker molasses are nutritionally superior, and blackstrap molasses is best. As with honey, the nutrients in molasses can vary greatly from batch to batch.

The newest fad in sugar is *fructose,* the monosaccharide that naturally predominates in most fruits. Since fructose is sweeter than sucrose, you can get more sweetening power from fewer calories if fructose is used as the sweetener. A number of manufacturers have decided to cash in on this fact and are substituting fructose for sucrose in their products so they can advertise them as "lower in calories." The calories contributed by sugar in these products may be a third lower than the equivalent product sweetened with sucrose. This may help those with an undeniable sweet tooth and a tendency toward overweight, but large amounts of fructose can cause abdominal pain and diarrhea.

Fructose has a greater advantage for diabetics because, unlike other sugars, it doesn't require insulin to get into the liver and body cells. Thus, when you eat fructose, there's no sudden demand for insulin, which diabetics cannot produce in adequate amounts. Fructose is also a useful sweetener for persons with reactive hypoglycemia (low blood sugar that follows the consumption of sweets), who tend to produce too much insulin when ordinary sugars are consumed.

The sweet alcohols *sorbitol* and *mannitol,* which are used in diabetic products in place of sugar, can cause diarrhea if eaten in large quantities.

Is Sugar Bad for You?

Sugar has been attacked from all sides. Both degree-bearing nutrition specialists and self-styled health-food advocates have been blaming sugar for a wide variety of common health problems. While the guns have been pointed primarily at sucrose (white table sugar), as you've just seen, sugar is sugar.

TOOTH DECAY

The connection between sweets and dental caries is probably better known to Americans than any other presumed health hazard of sugar. In school, at home, or in the dentist's office, it's been drummed into the heads of most people since early childhood that eating sweets will rot their teeth. What effect these admonitions have had on youthful cookie and candy monsters is hard to discern. But a better understanding of the true relationship between sugar and tooth decay will show you how sweets might be consumed with relatively little harm to the pearls in your mouth.

While there is little question that sugar in the diet promotes tooth decay, it's more a matter of *how* the sugar is consumed than *how much* is consumed. Sweets that are eaten between meals are far more damaging to teeth than those consumed with meals. Sweet foods, like dry cereals, raisins, and cookies, that stick on and between teeth and are hard to remove even by a diligent brusher are more damaging than those that are easily rinsed out of the mouth, like soft drinks and ice cream. Furthermore, good dental hygiene—proper brushing techniques and daily use of dental floss—to remove the decay-causing bacteria that live on teeth can largely mitigate the damage caused by eating sweets.

Sugar causes tooth decay because the bacteria in your mouth use this nutrient to produce three substances: a gummy material called glucan that helps the bacteria stick to the teeth; acids that corrode the protective enamel coating on teeth; and a storage carbohydrate that the bacteria can ferment to acids at some later time. When food that is fermentable by these bacteria is eaten, acid is produced at the surfaces of teeth. Little by little the enamel is worn away by the acid, and you end up with a cavity.

Many studies have shown that the amount of tooth decay in populations is directly related to the frequency of sugar consumption. Native populations whose carbohydrate intake was almost exclusively unrefined starches, including the Australian aborigines, Eskimos, and Ghanaians, had little tooth decay before being exposed to sugar-laden refined European-type diets. During wartime in Europe, when sugar was hard to get, the incidence of dental caries dropped dramatically, only to soar after the war when sweets were again readily accessible. And in a study in a Swedish mental institution, where diets could be strictly controlled, researchers clearly demonstrated that the more sugar-containing foods that were eaten between meals, the greater the number of cavities that formed. Sticky, sweet foods were the worst in terms of tooth decay, whereas sweets eaten with meals had little influence on decay, possibly because other foods counter their effects.

Unfortunately for the dental health of Americans, dietary trends are to eat sweets *between* instead of *with* meals. In recent years, there's been a considerable drop in the percentage of meals that are concluded with dessert, and an increase in foods consumed as snacks. Between-meal snacks now account for 15 percent of the typical American's daily calories. If you're interested in protecting your teeth, have your dessert with your meal, don't eat again until the next meal, and brush and floss your teeth after each meal. Sweets should be brushed from your teeth within fifteen minutes after they are eaten. At the very least, rinse your mouth by drinking a glass of water.

There is, incidentally, little difference in the decay-causing ability of sucrose, glucose, and fructose. Interestingly, though, a decay-inhibiting property has been found in chocolate. When chocolate was added to an otherwise decay-producing diet fed to experimental animals, the incidence of tooth decay dropped. And a study in people at the Forsyth Dental Center in Boston showed that chocolate liquor (a constituent of chocolate candy), when mixed with sucrose, neutralized the effect of sucrose on decay-causing bacteria and interfered with their ability to produce acids from the sugar. It would appear from these and other related studies that if you find you can't resist sweets now and again, the least evils are chocolate milk and plain chocolate bars, preferably consumed with meals rather than as between-meal snacks.

Sugars also seem to cause more damage to teeth when the diet is deficient in iron. When iron was added to the diet of rats fed half their calories as sugar, the rate of tooth decay was reduced by 75 percent. Yet, many American children do not have enough iron in their diets. This is particularly true of children from poor families, who also are the largest consumers of sweet foods.

The damage caused by sugar can start in infancy, long before parents are likely to give much thought to tooth decay. Large numbers of young children from all social classes are being seen in dentists' offices with what is called "nursing-bottle syndrome"—a set of badly rotted front teeth (see also Chapter 13). It happens because the baby is repeatedly allowed to go to sleep with a bottle. It matters little whether the bottle contains milk or juice (water is harmless, though). The bacteria produce acids from the sugars in the little pools of liquid that lie against the sleeping child's teeth. The syndrome can even occur in a breast-fed baby who is allowed to linger too long at the breast. To prevent nursing-bottle syndrome, babies should be fed and the bottle taken away before they are put to bed.

OVERWEIGHT

Sugar, per se, doesn't make you fat. Sugar is no more fattening than starch or protein and less than half as fattening as edible fats. *What does make you fat is eating more calories than your body uses up.* It matters not to the body whether extra calories come from sugar, starch, protein, or fats. Excess calories are stored as body fat, and the needle on the scale creeps up, up, up. Why, then, are sweets said to be fattening? The answer harks back to the question of caloric density. In the food processing plant and in kitchens everywhere, a lot of sugar calories can get packed into a rather small quantity of food. By eating sweets, you're likely to overconsume calories long before your stomach is full. In one study, volunteers who ate all their carbohydrates as refined sugar often felt hungry, but those fed a similar number of carbohydrate calories as vegetables and cereals complained of being "stuffed." You can easily down your whole day's calorie quota by eating one candy bar, one wedge of pecan pie, and one dish of ice cream—hardly a satisfying quantity of food.

One pound of apples contains 263 calories, whereas 1 pound of Tootsie Rolls has 1,792. A 2-ounce piece of a chocolate bar has the same number of calories as 3 medium-sized bananas that together weigh more than a pound. It's easy to see that the fruit would satisfy your appetite a lot faster than the candy. In other words, you'd be likely to eat fewer calories worth of fruit than candy. In addition to fewer unwanted calories, the fruit provides far more essential nutrients and dietary fiber than the candy. It stands to reason, then, that fruit (preferably fresh, not packed in heavily sweetened syrup) is a much healthier dessert and snack than candy (see Table 6.2).

For most people there's a limit on how sweet they like their foods and how much sweet food they can eat at any one time. But some people seem to have a propensity for becoming "sugarholics." Triggered usually by some psychological stress, they go on binges, devouring large quantities of sweets (a whole box of candy, a bag of cookies, a quart of ice cream) in quick succession. The eventual result is usually obesity —and malnutrition. Sugar, it seems, is like an opiate for some people. Some of those who finally break out of the binge-eating pattern are able to do so only by refraining from eating sweets.

DIABETES AND HYPOGLYCEMIA

The cause or causes of diabetes are unknown. However, there does seem to be a genetic factor involved that predisposes certain people to developing the disease. And there is a relationship to diet, particularly a diet too high in calories.

Diabetes is a failure of the pancreas to produce adequate amounts of insulin in response to a rise in blood sugar. Blood sugar rises when food is eaten and absorbed through the intestinal tract. Concentrated amounts of sugar can cause a precipitous rise in blood sugar, stimulating the pancreas to release insulin. Insulin is a hormone that is supposed to clear the blood of excess sugar by delivering it to body cells where it is used for energy or converted to fat for storage. When a person is obese, the fat cells may eventually become insensitive to insulin and fail to remove excess sugar from the blood.

In laboratory experiments, when rats genetically prone to diabetes are fed a high-sugar diet, they become obese and develop the disease. But rats on a sugar-free diet do not. It is not known, however, whether some people have a genetic predisposition to developing diabetes on a high-sugar diet comparable to that of the specially bred rats.

Dr. Aharon M. Cohen of the Hebrew University, Hadassah Medical College in Israel, studied the effects of dietary sugar on 16,000 people, including 5,000 who emigrated from Yemen to Israel. None of the newly arrived immigrants had diabetes, although the disease was common among Yemenites long settled in Israel. An examination of the diet revealed that while little sugar was consumed in Yemen, once in Israel the Yemenites quickly adopted a more Westernized diet that

Table 6.2 • SWEETS: "EMPTY" CALORIES VERSUS FULL

Item	Weight	Calories	Protein (g)	Fat (g)	Carbohydrate (g)	Calcium (mg)	Iron (mg)	Potassium (mg)	Vit. A (IU)*	Thiamin (mg)	Riboflavin (mg)	Niacin (mg)	Vit. C (mg)	Sodium (mg)
Chocolate fudge	1 ounce	113	0.8	3.5	21.3	22	0.30	42	Trace	.01	.03	0.10	Trace	54
Banana, large	7 ounces	116	1.5	0.3	30.2	11	1.00	503	260	.07	.08	1.00	14	1
Sandwich cookies (2)	1.4 ounces	99	0.9	4.5	13.8	5	0.15	8	0	.01	.01	0.01	0	96
Applesauce (1 cup)	9 ounces	100	0.5	0.5	26.4	10	1.20	190	100	.05	.02	0.10	2	5

*IU = international unit (5 IUs equal 1 retinol equivalent).

Note: By comparing the items in each pair listed above (based on analyses in Agriculture Handbook No. 456), you'll see that for approximately the same number of calories, you get a much larger quantity of food, considerably more essential vitamins and minerals, and considerably less potentially harmful ingredients (like fat and sodium) if you choose the banana over the chocolate fudge or the applesauce over the sandwich cookies. Not shown in the above analysis of nutritional content is the further advantage of more dietary fiber in the banana and the applesauce.

included lots of sugar. Many, for example, drank numerous cups of coffee each day, stirring in five or six spoonfuls of sugar into each cup! Dr. Cohen showed that those who developed diabetes while living in Israel came from a similar genetic background to those who remained in Yemen free of diabetes. Nor was there any age difference between the Yemenites in Israel with diabetes and those who remained healthy in Yemen that could account for the findings of diabetes among the émigrés.

However, many experts believe that obesity is far more important a factor in diabetes than sugar consumption. Many people with incipient diabetes can prevent its development by losing weight. Of course, excess sugar consumption is often a part of the overweight problem and thus indirectly a cause of the diabetes.

Once diabetes develops, if insulin treatment is required to control the disease, consumption of sweets must be greatly restricted. Diabetics who crave a sweet taste must rely on artificial sweeteners and certain sweet-tasting substances such as sorbitol and mannitol that are very slowly absorbed and therefore don't produce a rapid rise in blood sugar. However, most diabetics can handle diets containing relatively large amounts of starchy foods since these foods do not place urgent demands on the body's insulin factory.

Eating sweets has also been blamed for another relatively rare blood-sugar disorder known as hypoglycemia, or low blood sugar. In certain people (*far fewer* than some books and articles would lead you to believe), the body overreacts to a rise in blood sugar and produces far too much insulin to clear it. This sends the blood sugar plummeting downward, causing any of a number of distressing symptoms including shakiness, weakness, faintness, headache, mental dullness, and confusion. Similar symptoms can be caused by a number of other health problems, including an attack of anxiety.

Insulin overshoot, as doctors call the overproduction of insulin in response to a sugar load, happens to some extent to everyone who consumes a concentrated dose of sugar, especially between meals. It's probably an evolutionary hangover from our early days as a species when the only sources of sugar in the human diet were fruits and vegetables, which come into the body diluted by other digestible nutrients plus water and fiber.

The body was not designed to handle sugar in concentrated forms, such as in a piece of cake or candy bar. When it "sees" that amount of sugar, it "thinks" a lot of other food is coming in along with it and enough insulin is released to handle the whole load. For concentrated sweets, that turns out to be too much insulin, and too much sugar is cleared from the blood. The result is low blood sugar, which in some people can produce very distressing symptoms.

A correct diagnosis of hypoglycemia is generally based on a special test in which the patient is given a concentrated glucose solution to drink. The changing level of blood sugar is then monitored for five hours. A diagnosis of hypoglycemia is made if at some point during the test the patient's blood sugar drops considerably below normal and *at the same time* the patient experiences symptoms typical of hypoglycemia. Without the accompanying symptoms, the patient cannot be said to have hypoglycemia, since many perfectly healthy people also develop considerable drops in blood sugar following a glucose challenge.

In an even better test for hypoglycemia, the patient's blood sugar level is measured when in the course of normal living symptoms appear that are believed to be related to low blood sugar. If a person's blood sugar is really low when symptoms are present, then hypoglycemia is said to be the cause.

Those rare individuals with true hypoglycemia (the disorder is only one-tenth to one-twentieth as common as diabetes) are treated with a sugar-restricted diet that includes many high-protein minimeals throughout the day. Recent studies by Dr. James W. Anderson at the Veterans Administration Hospital in Lexington, Kentucky, showed that a diet high in starchy carbohydrates and fiber also helps. Although sugar cannot be said to cause hypoglycemia, the disturbing symptoms can often be avoided by dietary habits that help to maintain a more or less constant blood-sugar level.

HEART DISEASE

A few specialists, most notably Dr. John Yudkin of London, author of *Sweet and Dangerous,* claim that a diet high in sugar is the most important dietary cause of clogged arteries and heart disease. However, the evidence that has been gathered to support this theory is meager compared to that which relates heart disease to dietary fats and cholesterol. True, looking at a number of countries throughout the world, there does seem to be a relationship between the incidence of heart disease and the amount of sugar in the diet. But, in those countries where lots of sugar is consumed, the diets are also very high in animal fats. Most heart-disease experts believe that fats are by far the more important factor (see Chapter 3).

If dietary sugar is related to heart disease, it may do its dirty work through insulin. Insulin directs the conversion of blood glucose into fatty acids and triglycerides. Triglycerides are a kind of blood fat that can promote the development of atherosclerosis. In a study at Brookhaven National Laboratory in Upton, New York, 12 people were first fed a high-starch, low-sugar diet and then switched to a low-starch, high-sugar diet containing the same number of calories. The high-sugar regimen resulted in 2 to 5 times more conversion of sugar into triglycerides. In another study, conducted by researchers at the U.S. Department of Agriculture's nutrition institute in Beltsville, Maryland, and at the University of Maryland in College Park, volunteers were placed on a six-week diet in which 30 percent of the calories came from sugar. This is only slightly more sugar than the typical American diet contains. Other volunteers were fed a similar diet, but wheat starch was substituted for the sugar. Those on the sugar diet developed significantly higher levels of fats (cholesterol and triglycerides) in their blood.

About 20 million Americans have a genetic tendency to develop high blood levels of triglycerides when on diets containing sucrose. These so-called carbohydrate-sensitive individuals face a higher-than-normal risk of developing heart disease on the typical American diet, and are usually advised by their physicians to greatly restrict their intake of sugar. Sugar may also contribute to heart disease by increasing the blood pressure-raising effects of a high-salt diet, according to a study of monkeys at Louisiana State University.

Was Life Always So Sweet?

Humankind has coveted sweeteners throughout history. Honey was popular with Neanderthal man. The sweet extract from sugar cane was an important product in India around 5000 B.C. Honey, figs, and dates were consumed in ancient Egypt, primarily by the upper classes. (These wealthy Egyptians, incidentally, were the ones with worst tooth decay, studies of mummies have shown.) Certainly, people have always valued sweetness and equated it with goodness—witness "sweet mystery of life," "sweet smell of success," "sweetheart," etc.

But, the records suggest that at no time in history have people eaten more sweeteners than Americans do today. In 1875, the average American consumed just slightly more than 40 pounds of sweeteners a year. By 1910, the annual total had already risen to more than 70 pounds a person. And now it's about 128 pounds. Added sweeteners furnished 11.5 percent of our total calories in 1909; now they provide 18 percent. Sugars have displaced the more nutritious complex carbohydrates that used to form the bulk of our carbohydrate calories. In 1909, only 32 percent of total carbohydrates eaten were sugars; by 1980, the proportion that was sugar had risen to 53 percent.

Even the enormous growth in the use of noncaloric artificial sweeteners in the past two decades has done little or nothing to curb the American appetite for sugar. And when the price of sugar quadrupled in 1974, consumers screamed but they still bought sugar. Sugar consumption that year dropped a whole 3 percent!

Sugar can be the ace up a food company's sleeve. When processors want to create a market for a new product or stimulate sales of an old product, they're likely to succeed by making the products sweet or sweeter. Witness the sugar-coated cereals, which put ready-to-eat breakfasts back in the running, and the sweet adulteration that turned already-sugary granola into cookies (granola bars) and candy (chewy granola bars). More than half the weight of some breakfast cereals is sugar, making them more sugary than chocolate candy (see Table 6.3). In June, 1980, the Department of Agriculture released a second analysis of ready-to-eat breakfast cereals—this time of fourteen nationally sold granolas, which ranged from 22 to 32 percent sugar by weight. Table 6.4 shows what the department found.

Under consumer pressure, most baby-food manufacturers stopped sweetening their jars of puréed fruit. But the sugar content of the fruit hasn't necessarily dropped because the manufacturers now use riper fruit with a higher sugar content.

Actually, from a nutritional standpoint, we needn't eat any sugar at all. Sugar is a cheap source of energy that's easy to digest. But so is starch. The body can readily convert starches into sugar (individual molecules of glucose) and use them for energy. Metabolically speaking, this is the better way to stoke the body's furnace, because it results in a more even blood-sugar level (see the section on diabetes, pages 126–129).

Cutting back on sugar will require, among other things, many of us to terminate our love affair with the sweet taste. Evidence suggests that while we have an innate preference for sweets, we spend much of our lives cultivating that preference into a passion. Some, in fact, call it an addiction, since the more sweets people eat, the more sweets people seem to want.

If saccharin (the noncaloric sweetener) is injected into the womb, a five-month-old fetus will increase the rate at which it swallows the

Table 6.3 • HOW SWEET IS BREAKFAST?
THE SUGAR CONTENT OF READY-TO-EAT CEREALS

Product	*Manufacturer*	*Total sugar (% dry weight)*
Honey Smacks	Kellogg	56.0
Apple Jacks	Kellogg	54.6
Froot Loops	Kellogg	48.0
Sugar Corn Pops	Kellogg	46.0
Super Sugar Crisp	General Foods	46.0
Crazy Cow (chocolate)	General Mills	45.6
Corny Snaps	Kellogg	45.5
Frosted Rice Krinkles	General Foods	44.0
Frankenberry	General Mills	43.7
Cookie-Crisp, Vanilla	Ralston-Purina	43.5
Cap'n Crunch's Crunch Berries	Quaker Oats	43.3
Cocoa Krispies	Kellogg	43.0
Cocoa Pebbles	General Foods	42.6
Fruity Pebbles	General Foods	42.5
Lucky Charms	General Mills	42.2
Cookie-Crisp, Chocolate	Ralston-Purina	41.0
Frosted Flakes	Kellogg	41.0
Quisp	Quaker Oats	40.7
Crazy Cow (strawberry)	General Mills	40.1
Cookie-Crisp, Oatmeal	Ralston-Purina	40.1
Cap'n Crunch	Quaker Oats	40.0
Count Chocula	General Mills	39.5
Alpha-Bits	General Foods	38.0
Honey Comb	General Foods	37.2
Frosted Rice	Kellogg	37.0
Trix	General Mills	35.9
Cocoa Puffs	General Mills	33.3
Cap'n Crunch, Peanut butter	Quaker Oats	32.2
Post Raisin Bran	General Foods	30.4
Golden Grahams	General Mills	30.0
Cracklin' Bran	Kellogg	29.0
Raisin Bran	Kellogg	29.0
C.W. Post, Raisin	General Foods	29.0
C.W. Post	General Foods	28.7
Frosted Mini-Wheats	Kellogg	26.0
Country Crisp	General Foods	22.0
Life, Cinnamon Flavor	Quaker Oats	21.0
100% Bran	Nabisco	21.0
All-Bran	Kellogg	19.0
Fortified Oat Flakes	General Foods	18.5
Life	Quaker Oats	16.0
Team	Nabisco	14.1

Table 6.3 continued

Product	Manufacturer	Total sugar (% dry weight)
Grape-Nuts Flakes	General Foods	13.3
40% Bran Flakes	General Foods	13.0
Buc Wheat	General Mills	12.2
Product 19	Kellogg	9.9
Concentrate	Kellogg	9.3
Total	General Mills	8.3
Wheaties	General Mills	8.2
Rice Krispies	Kellogg	7.8
Grape-Nuts	General Foods	7.0
Special K	Kellogg	5.4
Corn Flakes	Kellogg	5.3
Post Toasties	General Foods	5.0
Kix	General Mills	4.8
Rice Chex	Ralston-Purina	4.4
Corn Chex	Ralston-Purina	4.0
Wheat Chex	Ralston-Purina	3.5
Cheerios	General Mills	3.0
Shredded Wheat	Nabisco	0.6
Puffed Wheat	Quaker Oats	0.5
Puffed Rice	Quaker Oats	0.1

Source: Based on an analysis published in 1979 by the U.S. Department of Agriculture of cereals that account for 90 percent of those purchased by Americans.
Note: For a more reasonable balance of nutrients, concentrate on those cereals that contain less than 10 percent sugar. Note that most of these are the brands you grew up with, in contrast to the sugar-laden brands introduced during recent decades. If additional sweetening is desired, garnish your cereal with fresh fruit.

sweetened amniotic fluid. Given the chance, newborn rats will consume sugar water in preference to a nutritious diet, even to the point of malnutrition and death. Experiments with newborn infants show a similar preference for sweetened drinks. As increasing amounts of sucrose are added to the baby's bottle, the rate of sucking increases—up to the sugar concentration of a Coke!

Gary Beauchamp, a biopsychologist from the Monell Chemical Senses Center at the University of Pennsylvania, points out that our sweet taste served us well in the course of evolution. It helped us to know when foods like fruits and berries were ripe and ready to eat. But, he adds, in recent times "we've separated the good taste from the good food," and our sweet taste is no longer working to our advantage.

During the first two years of life, Dr. Beauchamp reports, the taste

Table 6.4 • THE SUGAR CONTENT OF GRANOLAS

Product	Manufacturer	Total sugar (% dry weight)
Country Morning	Kellogg	30.5
Nature Valley Granola (Fruit and Nut)	General Mills	29.0
Quaker 100% Natural (Raisin and Dates)	Quaker Oats	28.4
C. W. Post—Raisin	General Foods	27.8
Vita Crunch—Almond	Organic Milling	27.6
Vita Crunch—Raisin	Organic Milling	26.7
Heartland—Raisin	Pet	26.0
Nature Valley Granola (Cinnamon and Raisin)	General Mills	25.2
Quaker 100% Natural (Apple and Cinnamon)	Quaker Oats	25.2
C. W. Post—Plain	General Foods	24.8
Vita Crunch—Regular	Organic Milling	23.7
Familia	Bio-Familia	23.4
Heartland—Coconut	Pet	22.3
Quaker 100% Natural (Brown Sugar and Honey)	Quaker Oats	21.6

Source: Analysis published in 1980 by the U.S. Department of Agriculture, Nutrient Composition Laboratory, Beltsville, Maryland.

for sugar stays pretty much the same. But older children—between the ages of nine and fifteen—like highly sweetened foods better than younger children do. This does not prove that early exposure to sweets gets children "hooked" on them, but it doesn't disprove it, either.

"Quick Energy" and Other Sweet Myths

Probably the most prevalent sales pitch for sweets is that they give you "quick energy." The idea, supposedly, is that in addition to helping "the medicine go down," a spoonful of sugar helps to pick you up—an antidote to the midmorning, midafternoon, and early-evening doldrums. The next best thing to caffeine, all predicated on the notion that you're sagging because your blood sugar is low and all you need is a little sweet spurt to get you going again.

Not so. The only ones to benefit from the quick rise in blood sugar a sweet will bring are diabetics in insulin shock (too much insulin resulting in too low a blood sugar) and athletes in the throes of a strenuous workout such as a marathon run or Channel swim. For the rest of us, the sweet-induced euphoria, if there is one, is gone in minutes. That's because the moment your blood sugar rises, your pancreas starts pouring out insulin to bring it down again and you're soon back to normal, if not worse off than when you started.

Eating something sweet before an athletic competition won't do you a particle of good because the sugar will already be in storage by the time you need it in your blood. The only way around this is to consume slugs of sugar periodically throughout the course of the event. But few of us exercise to the point where that should become necessary (see Chapter 23).

The body maintains a small but usually adequate carbohydrate storage depot to call upon when energy output demands it. It is called glycogen, stored in the liver and in the muscles, and it can be readily converted into glucose when the body needs to bring up the blood sugar. The body also can burn fatty acids for fuel along with glucose. But when the glucose supply is exhausted, fats burn inefficiently.

As for the supposed appetite-squelching effects of sugar, dieters who eat a sweet in the hope of curbing their appetite for meals may find that their gimmick backfires. The spurt in blood sugar is followed by a spurt in insulin, which in turn is followed by a fall in blood sugar. You can end up hungrier than when you started out!

How to Cut Down on Sugar

It would make better nutritional sense if sweets were eaten as an occasional treat, rather than as part of the daily diet. Many people find that when they decide to forgo sweets for a while (a week or longer), their craving for them gradually subsides. And as the sweet habit subsides, instead of gorging on sweets to make up for lost time, they are likely to be satisfied with smaller quantities than they used to be. The following tips can help you to reduce your consumption of "empty" or unneeded sugar calories.

• *Don't buy sweet snacks or candy* "to have in the house." Instead, keep a plentiful supply of fresh fruits and vegetables. If you must have a carbohydrate "nibble food," try popcorn without butter—23 calories a cup.

• *Get in the habit of serving fruit*—preferably fresh fruit—for desserts. If you must rely on canned or frozen fruit, look for brands that are packaged in water instead of sweetened syrup. Fruit contains nutritionally useful quantities of vitamins, minerals, and fiber as well as natural sugars. Unlike ice cream or cake, fruits have no fat or cholesterol. However, dried fruits—raisins, dates, figs, dried apples and apricots, etc.—have a high concentration of sugar (because most of the water in the fruit has been removed) and are sticky, making them less desirable for your weight and teeth.

• *Instead of buying cakes, pies, or cookies, make your own* and cut the sugar in the recipe by a third or more. You might try making "dessert" breads that contain relatively little sugar and are loaded with nourishing ingredients like whole-wheat flour, oatmeal, nuts, raisins, and perhaps a fruit or vegetable like pumpkin, zucchini, cranberries, carrots, or peanut butter. The following breads are some of my family's favorites. They can be made in quantity by doubling or tripling the ingredients, and the breads can be stored in the freezer for months.

Cranberry-Nut Bread

1 cup all-purpose unbleached flour
1 cup whole-wheat flour
½–⅔ cup sugar
1½ teaspoons baking powder
½ teaspoon salt
½ teaspoon baking soda
3 tablespoons vegetable oil
4 teaspoons grated orange peel
¾ cup orange juice
1 egg, beaten
1⅓ cup cranberries, sliced in half or coarsely chopped (see note)
½ cup nuts (walnuts or pecans), coarsely chopped

Preheat the oven to 350 degrees. In a bowl sift together the first six ingredients. In another bowl combine the oil, orange peel, orange juice, and egg. Add the liquid ingredients to the dry ingredients, mixing just enough to moisten. Fold in the cranberries and nuts. Pour the batter into a greased 9×5×3-inch baking pan (or two 7×3×2-inch pans). Bake for 50 to 60 minutes (less time if the smaller pans are used) or until a toothpick inserted into the center of the loaf comes out clean. Remove the bread from the pan, cool, and wrap. To avoid crumbling, store overnight before slicing. Yield: 1 large loaf or 2 small loaves.
Note: Fresh cranberries bought in season can be stored whole in the freezer.

Zucchini-Cheese Bread

1½ cups unbleached white flour
1½ cups whole-wheat flour
⅓ cup sugar
3 tablespoons grated Parmesan cheese
5 teaspoons baking powder
1 teaspoon salt
½ teaspoon baking soda
1 cup shredded unpeeled zucchini, squeezed dry in cloth
⅓ cup margarine, melted
1 cup buttermilk
2 eggs
2 tablespoons grated onion

Preheat the oven to 350 degrees. In a bowl combine flours, sugar, cheese, baking powder, salt, and baking soda. Mix in the zucchini. In a separate bowl combine the margarine, buttermilk, eggs, and onion. Add this to the flour-zucchini mixture. Pour the batter into a greased 9×5× 3-inch pan. Bake for 55 to 60 minutes. Remove the bread from the pan and cool. Yield: 1 loaf.

Carrot Cake

4 cups grated carrots
1 cup sugar
1½ sticks (¾ cup) margarine, cut up
½ cup water
1½ cups whole-wheat flour
1 cup unbleached white flour
1 tablespoon cinnamon
1 teaspoon ground cloves

1 teaspoon baking soda
¾ teaspoon ground allspice
½ teaspoon nutmeg
½ teaspoon baking powder
½ teaspoon salt
2 eggs
½ cup raisins
Confectioners' sugar (optional)

Preheat the oven to 350 degrees. In a saucepan combine the carrots, sugar, margarine, and water and bring to boil, stirring. Reduce the heat and simmer the mixture for 5 minutes and let cool. In a bowl sift together the flours, cinnamon, cloves, baking soda, allspice, nutmeg, baking powder, and salt. In a large bowl, beat the eggs until they are lemon-colored and add cooled carrot mixture and then the flour mixture, stirring until just combined. Add the raisins and divide the batter between two greased 9×5×3-inch pans (or four 7×3×2-inch pans). Bake for 35 to 40 minutes, or until a toothpick inserted into the center of the cakes comes out clean. Remove the cakes from the pans. If desired, dust the loaves with sifted confectioners' (powdered) sugar. Yield: 2 large cakes or 4 small cakes.

Apple-Nut Bread

1 cup whole-wheat flour
1 cup unbleached white flour
2 teaspoons baking powder
¼ teaspoon salt
6 tablespoons margarine
½ cup sugar
2 eggs

1 large tart apple, peeled and coarsely shredded (1 cup)
1 cup finely chopped walnuts
½ cup (2 ounces) shredded cheddar cheese
¼ cup skim milk

Preheat the oven to 375 degrees. In a small bowl, combine the flours, baking powder, and salt and set aside. In large bowl cream the margarine and sugar, then beat in the eggs and continue beating until the mixture is fluffy. Stir in the apple, about ¾ cup nuts, and the cheese. Add half the flour mixture, stirring until moist. Stir in the milk, then add the remaining flour mixture and blend well. Pour the batter into a greased 9×5×3-inch pan or two $7 \times 3 \times 2$-inch pans. Sprinkle remaining nuts on top. Bake for 35 to 40 minutes, or until a toothpick inserted into the center of the bread comes out clean. Remove the bread from the pan, cool, and wrap. Best if stored overnight before slicing. Yield: 1 large loaf or 2 small loaves.

• *Don't use sweets as a reward* for children, and ask friends and relatives not to bring them as gifts.

• *Eliminate soft drinks from your diet.* This one measure could bring about half the reduction in sugar consumption that was recommended in the Dietary Goals. And don't switch to artificially sweetened soft drinks before you read about saccharin and aspartame in Chapter 25. Try calorie-free club soda, seltzer, or mineral water (even better because it contains less sodium than club soda; see Chapter 10).

• If you put sugar in your coffee or tea, try gradually reducing the amount you use.

• *Try new combinations of foods to create sweet flavors* without adding sugar. For example, use sweet spices and herbs, such as cardamom, coriander, basil, nutmeg, ginger, or mace. Caramelize the sugar naturally present in fruits and vegetables to make them taste sweeter. You can put grapefruit, bananas, onion, or tomatoes under the broiler or let the water just cook out in a pan of carrots. A little sprinkle of shredded coconut will make fresh fruit taste sweeter.

• *Start reading the labels* on all the processed foods you buy. The ingredients must be listed in order of their prominence in the product, with the ingredient present in the largest quantity listed first. Don't worry about sugar as a minor ingredient in foods like soups or bread or in condiments like ketchup that are eaten in very small quantities. But if sugar or some other sweetener is among the top three ingredients in a major food product, beware.

The consumer who is trying to figure out how much sugar there may be in a particular product can be easily misled. Although ingredients must be listed in order of their relative amounts, by dividing up the various types of sugar added to a product (as is currently required by federal food regulations), manufacturers can hide just how much is really there. Thus, a box of cereal may list "sugar" as the third ingredient, "corn syrup" as the fifth and "honey" as the seventh. But if these were added together, sugar might turn out to be the leading ingredient!

You can also be misled by a listing of sugar as a percentage of the product or as the number of grams of sugar in 100 grams of the foodstuff. These numbers can be greatly reduced merely by adding water to the product, but without lowering the actual amount of sugar by one crystal! Thus, a package of powdered drink mix would contain a much larger *percentage* of sugar than the diluted drink, but the *amount* of sugar in the package and in your glass is exactly the same. A Coke, for example, has a lower *percentage* of sugar than a dry bouillon cube, but the soda contains a far larger *quantity* of sugar.

Listing the amount of sugar in grams rather than in common kitchen measurements is also misleading for most consumers, who are not yet readily conversant with the metric system. Few, for example, would realize that the 11 grams of sugar in a 1-ounce serving of Frosted Flakes actually means the addition of *1 tablespoon* of sugar to your bowl of cereal (see Table 6.5).

Table 6.5 • HOW MUCH SUGAR IS REALLY IN YOUR FOOD?

Food	Serving size	Teaspoons sugar
Candy		
Chocolate bar	1 ounce	7
Chocolate fudge	1½-inch square	4
Chocolate mint	1 medium	3
Marshmallow	1 average	1½
Chewing gum	1 stick	½
Cakes and Cookies		
Chocolate cake, iced	¹⁄₁₂ cake	15
Angel food cake	¹⁄₁₂ cake	6
Sponge cake	¹⁄₁₀ cake	6
Cream puff, iced	1 average	5
Doughnut, plain	3-inch diameter	4
Macaroons	1 large or 2 small	3
Gingersnaps	1 medium	1
Molasses cookies	3½-inch diameter	2
Brownies	2×2×¾-inch piece	3
Ice Cream		
Ice cream	½ cup	5–6
Sherbet	½ cup	6–8
Frozen yogurt	½ cup	7
Thick shake	11 ounces	10

Table continues on next page

Table 6.5 continued

Food	Serving size	Teaspoons sugar
Pies		
Apple	⅙ medium pie	12
Cherry	⅙ medium pie	14
Pumpkin	⅙ medium pie	10
Pecan	⅐ medium pie	12
Drinks		
Sweetened soda	12 ounces	6–9
Chocolate milk	8 ounces	6
Eggnog	8 ounces	8
Orange juice	4 ounces	2½
Pineapple juice, unsweetened	4 ounces	2⅗
Grapefruit juice, unsweetened	4 ounces	2½
Kool-Aid	8 ounces	6
Cooked Fruits		
Peaches, canned in syrup	2 halves, 1 tablespoon syrup	3½
Rhubarb, sweetened	½ cup	8
Apple sauce, unsweetened	½ cup	2
Prunes, sweetened and stewed	4 to 5, 2 tablespoons syrup	8
Fruit cocktail	½ cup	5
Dried Fruits		
Apricots	4 to 6 halves	4
Prunes	3 to 4 medium	4
Dates	3 to 4	4½
Figs	2 small	4
Raisins	¼ cup	4
Spreads and Sauces		
Jam	1 tablespoon	3
Maple syrup	1 tablespoon	2½
Honey	1 tablespoon	3
Chocolate sauce	1 tablespoon	4½
Yogurts		
Lowfat yogurt, plain	1 cup	4
Lowfat yogurt, flavored	1 cup	8½
Lowfat yogurt, fruit	1 cup	13

Sources: The U.S. Department of Agriculture, the American Dental Association, the American Dietetic Association and the Center for Science in the Public Interest, among others.

PART TWO

The Noncaloric Nutrients

7 ❧ THE GREAT FIBER FAD

THE 1970s witnessed a revolution in the dietary habits of millions of Americans—a sudden interest in the undigestible plant materials called fiber. People who previously regarded bran as little more than cattle feed began gobbling it up like their two-stomached, four-legged friends. A host of new "high fiber" cereals and breads crowded in next to the sugar-coated and the white enriched varieties that dominate supermarket shelves. One company successfully marketed a bread that contained wood fiber. And many of the old standbys, like All-Bran, Shredded Wheat, and whole-wheat breads suddenly began selling out. In one year there was a 20-percent increase in sales of breads containing bran. The fiber fad reached such unexpected proportions that by mid-decade, there was actually a shortage of bran in the United States!

The fad started in 1970 with the publication of a medical report by a renowned British physician, Dr. Denis Burkitt. He pointed out that in nations where the diet normally includes large amounts of fiber, there are relatively few cases of cancer of the colon and rectum, diverticulosis and other benign intestinal diseases, hemorrhoids, hiatus hernia, appendicitis, varicose veins, gallstones, and heart disease. All these disorders are common among Americans and in other industrialized Western societies, where the typical diet is low in fiber. Burkitt's observation sparked much criticism—charges, for instance, that he had failed to consider other differences in diet and life style between Western nations and his sample—but also a great deal of new research on the role fiber might play in human health. And the findings were widely summarized and extravagantly championed in books, magazines, and newspaper articles.

In all probability, however, it took just two facts to fan the flames of the fiber fad: one, that increased fiber—our grandparents called it "roughage"—in the diet is a highly effective antidote to constipation; the other, that fiber is a very low calorie way to fill the belly. With half of America fixated on bowel regularity and the other half chronically on a diet, fiber was a shoo-in.

Burkitt was hardly the first to extol fiber. In 1920, Dr. John Harvey Kellogg of the famous Michigan cereal family prescribed a diet of fruits, cereals, and fresh vegetables to counter what he considered an unhealthy state of colonic affairs among many Americans. Dr. Kellogg, who was medical director of a sanitorium in Battle Creek, favored potatoes, dates, carrots, wheat bran, nuts, and steel-cut Scotch oats to reduce problems that might stem from a sluggish gut.

There's no question that fiber was once a far more common constituent of the American diet than when Burkitt's theory struck. Through this century, consumption of fiber has declined at least 25 percent as whole-grain breads and cereals yielded to the refined varieties and as fats and sweets gradually replaced many fibrous starchy foods, fruits, and vegetables.

What Is Fiber?

All fiber comes from plants: from cell walls that give plants their firm structure and from nonstructured substances that are mixed with plant starches. With one exception, the various types of plant fibers are all polysaccharides, or complex carbohydrates. Dietary fiber is defined as those components of food that cannot be broken down by enzymes in the human digestive tract. Except for some "processing" by teeth, fiber passes through our digestive tract into the large intestine pretty much intact. Once in the colon, about half of the fiber is fermented by intestinal bacteria, producing gases that include volatile fatty acids, some of which may then be absorbed into body cells through the intestinal wall.

There are many different kinds of fiber, and each has different properties. Some absorb lots of water, some only a little. Some are completely fermentable by intestinal bacteria, others pass through into the feces mostly untouched. Some, in fact, are not at all "fibrous" in their structure or appearance. The fibers commonly found in human foods are cellulose, hemicelluloses, lignin, pectins, gums, and mucilages. The most common sources of fiber in our diets are whole grains, fruits, and vegetables. In addition, pectins, gums, and mucilages are commonly used as additives in processed foods to improve texture and consistency and as thickening agents.

Different kinds of plants have different types and amounts of fibers. Even within the same plant species, the fiber content may vary according to the plant's variety, growing conditions, the season, and storage conditions, as well as the way the plant might be cooked or processed before consumption.

Until recently, scientists had no good way to analyze the fiber content of foods. They used a crude technique of first soaking the food in solvent, then treating it with hot acid followed by hot alkali. What survived this onslaught was called, not inappropriately, "crude fiber." When the fiber content of food is listed on the package, it is usually crude fiber that is given. However, in analyzing for crude fiber, most of the *dietary* fiber actually present in the food may be lost. Only a portion of the cellulose and hemicelluloses and most of the lignin remain. The pectins, gums, and mucilages—which dissolve in water— are lost. The food you actually eat may contain up to seven times as much dietary fiber as the crude-fiber figure would indicate.

Recently, improved methods of analyzing the fiber content of foods have been developed. While these methods still cannot be said to detect all the dietary fiber in a food, they come closer to the real thing. Table 7.1 shows the fiber content of various common foods as determined by these new techniques.

What Fiber Can Do for You

The health value of the different fibers varies widely. You cannot glean all the possible benefits from fiber by eating only one type of fibrous food. Bran, liberally sprinkled in or on half the foods you eat, is not the total answer. In fact, overconsumption of just one type of fiber may actually be harmful, as you will see later.

Fiber is not considered an essential nutrient. Human beings can survive without any fiber in their diets, and insufficient fiber does not produce a classic deficiency disease. But it is possible that many of the ailments that afflict humankind in developed nations are in one way or another signs of a dietary shortage of fiber. Here's why.

LAXATIVES

The ability of fibrous foods to counter the problem of constipation has long been known to the medical profession and the general public. But only since the advent of the fiber fad have so many had the opportunity to learn this fact firsthand. Fiber can stimulate the smooth, efficient working of the bowel because it is able to absorb many times its weight in water. It acts like a sponge in the large intestine, drawing water into the feces, making the stool larger and softer and easier to pass.

Table 7.1 • DIETARY FIBER IN YOUR FOOD

Food	Serving size	Weight (g)	Fiber (g)
Breads and Crackers			
Graham crackers	2 squares	15	1.5
Rye bread	1 slice	25	2.0
Rye crackers	3 wafers	20	2.3
Whole-wheat bread	1 slice	25	2.4
Cereals			
All-Bran or 100% Bran	1 cup	70	23.0
Bran Buds	¾ cup	60	18.0
Cracked wheat (bulgur), dry	⅓ cup	50	5.6
Grape-Nuts	⅓ cup	45	5.0
Grits, dry	¼ cup	45	4.8
Rolled oats, dry	½ cup	50	4.5
Shredded wheat	2 biscuits	50	6.1
Fruits			
Apple	1 small	90	3.1
Applesauce	½ cup	120	1.7
Banana	1 medium	100	1.8
Cantaloupe, cubes	¾ cup	120	1.4
Cherries, raw	10	70	0.8
Grapefruit	½	200	2.6
Grapes, raw	16	60	0.4
Orange	1 small	90	1.8
Peach, raw	1 medium	100	1.3
Peaches, canned slices	½ cup	120	1.3
Pear, raw	1 medium	120	2.8
Pears, canned	½ cup	125	1.4
Plum, raw	2 small	90	1.6
Strawberries	½ cup	125	2.6
Tangerine	1 medium	100	2.1
Vegetables			
Beans, green	½ cup	50	1.2
Beets, cooked	⅔ cup	100	2.1
Broccoli, cooked	¾ cup	75	1.6
Cabbage, cooked	¾ cup	100	2.2
Cabbage, raw	1 cup	75	2.1
Carrots, cooked	¾ cup	100	2.1
Carrots, raw	1 medium	100	3.7
Cauliflower, cooked	½ cup	100	1.2

Table 7.1 continued

Food	Serving size	Weight (g)	Fiber (g)
Cauliflower, raw	1 cup	100	1.8
Celery, cooked	⅔ cup	100	2.4
Celery, raw	2½ stalks	100	3.0
Corn kernels	⅔ cup	110	4.2
Cucumber	½ of 7-inch cucumber	100	1.5
Kale, cooked	½ cup	100	2.0
Kidney beans, cooked	1 cup	75	3.6
Lentils, cooked	½ cup	100	4.0
Lettuce	1 cup	50	0.8
Parsnips, cooked	¾ cup	120	5.9
Peas, cooked	½ cup	60	3.8
Potatoes, cooked	⅔ cup	90 (raw)	3.1
Rice, brown, cooked	1 cup	65	1.1
Rice, white, cooked	1 cup	65	0.4
Spinach	2 large leaves	50	1.8
Summer squash, cooked	½ cup	100	2.2
Summer squash, raw	1 5-inch squash	100	3.0
Turnips, raw	1 cup	100	2.2

Source: The above fiber analyses were prepared by Dr. James W. Anderson, professor of medicine and clinical nutrition at the University of Kentucky Medical Center in Lexington, Kentucky.

People on high-fiber diets not only have larger stools, but also get rid of their wastes sooner after eating. The time it takes for food to travel from the mouth through the rectum is known as "gut transit time." Gut transit time for African villagers eating a high-fiber diet averaged 36 hours, compared to 77 hours for British men who consumed low-fiber diets like ours. In addition, daily fecal output for the Africans weighed four times as much.

In the United States, more than 700 different laxative preparations are sold over the counter, and 1 percent of all doctors' prescriptions are for laxatives. Many of these drugs act as stimulants to the colon, and their repeated use can lead to a chronic inability of the colon to act on its own. These drugs may also cause cramps, diarrhea, and excessive loss of fluids and essential minerals. Another type of laxative, the stool softener (Colace is a common brand), is less harmful; it increases the water content of the feces, producing a larger and softer stool. Dietary fiber has a similar effect, and for many reasons—including monetary—

it is the preferred approach to bowel regularity for most people. The best sources of natural laxatives are whole-grain (bran-containing) breakfast cereals and breads, whole fruits, leafy vegetables, and raw carrots. However, finely ground wood fiber used in some breads is constipating.

INTESTINAL DISORDERS

It is believed that a number of disorders of the colon and rectum result from the repeated need to exert considerable pressure to pass the stool. One is hemorrhoids, which are varicose veins of the rectum. Another is diverticulosis, the formation of outpouchings, or pockets, in the large intestine that can become painfully inflamed and infected (diverticulitis). Diverticular disease was virtually unknown in this country at the turn of the century. But it has become increasingly common, so that now an estimated 40 percent of middle-aged Americans have this problem.

Although it has not been proved that diets higher in fiber can prevent hemorrhoids and diverticulosis from developing, logic suggests that they may. A study in Oxford, England, showed that diverticular disease was only a third as common among vegetarians as nonvegetarians. Several studies have suggested that high-fiber diets can relieve problems with hemorrhoids and diverticular disease once they develop. Interestingly, until recently it's been common medical practice to place patients with diverticular disease on very low-fiber diets to reduce "irritation" to the large intestine.

A similar practice of treating patients who have irritable bowel syndrome (spastic colon) with low-fiber diets has also been challenged by recent studies of the benefits of fiber. In one study of 26 patients, half of whom were fed 20 grams of wheat fiber a day for six weeks, a significantly greater improvement in symptoms and muscular activity of the colon was noted as a result of the high-fiber diet.

However, *patients with bowel disorders should not start a high-fiber diet without first consulting their physicians.* In certain cases, such as when intestinal obstruction or severe inflammation are present, increased fiber may be harmful.

CANCER

Another potential benefit of fiber relates to cancer of the colon, though more studies are needed to confirm this. Cancer of the colon and rectum is the leading life-threatening cancer in the United States today. It is uncommon, however, among peoples in countries where the diets rely less on meats and other animal proteins and more on vegetable (high-fiber) foods. A number of researchers relate the incidence of colon cancer to our excessive consumption of fats, but Dr. Burkitt and a few others believe lack of fiber is the main culprit. According to the fiber theory, fiber reduces the time that cancer-causing substances reside in the gut and dilutes their concentration. It may also change their rate of formation by gut bacteria. A few studies in laboratory animals have shown that fiber can protect the colon from the cancer-inducing action of certain chemicals, presumably by the ability of fiber to bind with those chemicals and wash them out of the digestive tract. And if fat is the factor responsible for cancer of the colon in man, fibrous foods may indirectly protect the colon by reducing the amount of fatty foods that are eaten.

A high-fiber diet may also help to protect against breast cancer, possibly by reducing the formation of estrogen-like chemicals in the gut. A study of 1,481 healthy women in San Francisco showed that those who were chronically constipated (and therefore no doubt consuming a low-fiber diet) were far more likely to have abnormal cells in their breast fluid than women with regular bowel habits.

WEIGHT CONTROL

Obesity is rare in populations where a lot of starchy carbohydrates, complete with their natural fiber, are consumed. But excess weight is a common problem in nations like ours, where the people consume low-fiber diets. The more fiber your diet contains, the fewer calories you're likely to consume. Fiber itself yields few, if any, calories, and many fibrous foods, especially fruits and vegetables, are themselves low in calories. Also, since it absorbs water as it passes through your digestive tract, fiber is filling, and you're more likely to feel satisfied by a high-fiber meal before you've overstepped your calorie quota. This is why the bread diet, 12 slices a day, helped those 16 young men lose unwanted pounds (see pages 102–103). It's noteworthy that the 8 who were given high-fiber bread lost on the average 6 pounds more than those who ate refined white bread.

Other factors undoubtedly contribute to fiber's success in battling the bulge. It takes a long time to chew most fibrous foods. This slows down the process of eating, allowing time for the signals of satiety to reach your brain before you've overeaten. All that chewing also makes you feel like you've eaten something substantial. And although fiber does contribute some calories (through the fatty acids produced by gut bacteria), it also may reduce the amount of calories your body absorbs from the other foods you eat. Possibly because of the decrease in gut transit time caused by fiber, small amounts of the fat and protein you eat are excreted in the feces instead of being absorbed through the small intestine. Therefore, a few of the calories you eat really "don't count."

HEART DISEASE

One of the most encouraging findings about dietary fiber is the ability of some types of fiber to lower cholesterol levels in the blood. It is not known whether this, in turn, will reduce the risk of heart disease, but it is certainly true that in countries where the diet contains a lot of fiber (and little fat), rates of heart disease are far lower than in the United States.

Here, though, is where the type of fiber consumed is especially important. Bran, which is more than 90 percent cellulose, has *no* beneficial effect on cholesterol levels. But pectins (found in most fruits), guar gum (found in beans), and the fiber in rolled oats and carrots can bring about a significant lowering of cholesterol. In fact, recent studies of oat bran have shown that daily consumption of three ounces a day (as cereal, muffins, or as a thickener in soups, sauces, purées, and the like) can lower cholesterol by nearly 20 percent, which would mean a 40-percent reduction in the risk of a heart attack. Oat bran is now available in many supermarkets and most health food stores.

In one recent study, guar gum reduced the percentage of cholesterol in the blood serum by 36 milligrams and pectin by 29 milligrams, whereas wheat fiber (bran) actually raised the cholesterol level by nearly 7 milligrams. Another study involved 10 patients who were taking drugs to lower their high cholesterol levels. When the patients were given 5 grams of guar gum before each meal, cholesterol dropped an average of 10.6 percent over and above the reduction caused by the drugs. A study conducted at the Veterans Administration Hospital in Lexington, Kentucky, suggests that long-term treatment with a very high-fiber diet reduces the harmful LDL cholesterol fraction and increases the beneficial HDL cholesterol. And Scottish researchers showed that eating 7 ounces of raw carrots at breakfast every day for three weeks could reduce cholesterol levels by 11 percent and increase the amount of fat excreted by 50 percent.

Fiber's cholesterol-lowering effect may result from its ability to increase the excretion of bile acids, which are made from cholesterol. In the Scottish study, bile-acid excretion increased by 50 percent. Cholesterol may also become bound to some fibers and be excreted directly in the feces.

The Kentucky researchers also showed that fiber can reduce the blood levels of triglycerides, which, like cholesterol, are related to heart disease. Normally, triglyceride levels are likely to go up when a diet high in carbohydrates is consumed. However, when the carbohydrate is consumed along with plant fiber, this rise does not occur. Even in patients with abnormally elevated triglyceride levels, a high-fiber, high-carbohydrate diet produced a lowering of triglycerides in their blood.

As a further potential benefit to your heart and blood vessels, physiologists at the University of Southampton in England showed that the kinds of fiber commonly consumed by vegetarians can lower blood pressure.

DIABETES

Another recently demonstrated benefit of dietary fiber is its effect on blood-sugar levels and insulin requirements. By including fiber in their diets, some diabetics under medical supervision have been able to get along without insulin or other antidiabetic medication. Here, too, pectins and guar gum are the most effective plant fibers.

In one study by Dr. James W. Anderson, endocrinologist at the Veterans Administration Hospital in Lexington, Kentucky, diabetics fed diets high in carbohydrates and fiber were able to reduce the amount of insulin they needed by half, and those who initially required relatively low doses of insulin were able to discontinue the hormone treatment entirely. This reduction in insulin requirement probably stems from the fact that when carbohydrates are consumed along with fiber, the blood-sugar levels never get as high as they do when the carbohydrates are eaten alone. The fiber seems to slow the absorption of the carbohydrates, and some carbohydrates may actually pass through the digestive tract unabsorbed.

In a study at England's University of Oxford among 27 diabetics, the disease was much better controlled when the patients were placed on a diet high in complex carbohydrates and fiber (primarily from beans) than when the same patients consumed a more traditional diabetic diet low in carbohydrates and high in animal protein. The researchers concluded that further use of a low-carbohydrate diet to treat diabetics can no longer be justified.

Several studies in both healthy individuals and diabetics have shown that when fiber is consumed along with carbohydrates, blood levels of sugar and insulin don't rise as high as when the carbohydrates are eaten fiber-free.

An experiment done at the University of Bristol in England has a telling message both for those with blood-sugar problems and those concerned about overweight and overeating. Ten healthy people were given test "meals" of either whole apples, puréed apples (applesauce), or apple juice. Each meal contained the same amount of sugars. It took 17 minutes to eat the apples, 6 minutes to down the purée, and 1½ minutes to drink the juice. It should come as no surprise to learn that the individuals reported greater satisfaction after eating the apples than after drinking the juice, with the purée producing an intermediate level of satiety. Blood sugar rose to similar levels after all three "meals," but the insulin level in the blood rose twice as high after the juice than after the whole apples. One to three hours later, the blood-sugar levels dropped—back to normal after the apples, but to a level distinctly below normal after the juice. An intermediate but below-normal blood-sugar level occurred after the purée. These below-normal levels, called rebound hypoglycemia, are usually associated with feelings of hunger. Thus, the fiber in the whole apples reduced the demand for insulin and produced a longer-lasting feeling of satiety.

Some Problems with Fiber

Lest all of this sound too good to be true, it turns out that there is no free lunch after all. An increase in dietary fiber can cause problems for some people and in some cases may even interfere with good nutrition. The most common problem, however, is not a serious one—except, perhaps, from a social point of view—and is usually only temporary. That is the tendency for dietary fiber to stimulate the formation of intestinal gas. This occurs in the large intestine, where the previously undigested fiber gets attacked by bacteria. The bacteria can ferment some of the polysaccharides in various fibers to produce such gases as carbon dioxide, hydrogen, methane, and volatile fatty acids. Problems with excessive intestinal gas are most common when first starting a diet containing more fiber than you're used to eating. The severity of the problem is greatly reduced if you increase your fiber intake gradually (a good idea in any case, since too much fiber too soon can also cause diarrhea and bloating). In most cases, the problem with gassiness subsides in a few weeks when your gut's bacterial population adapts to the new menu.

A more serious hazard of a high-fiber diet stems from the ability of fiber to bind other substances and carry them out of the body as waste. When these other substances are carcinogens or other noxious substances, that's all to the good. But when they're vital nutrients, problems of dietary deficiencies could possibly develop. Fiber has been shown to cause some depletion of calcium, zinc, iron, magnesium, phosphorus, copper, and possibly vitamin B_{12}. It also decreases the absorption of dietary protein.

These decreases are not likely to be a problem for most Americans, whose consumption of protein and other nutrients is already in excess of actual need. In addition, at least for calcium, zinc, and probably other of the affected nutrients, a normal balance of intake and output is restored in a matter of weeks after starting a high-fiber diet.

However, the nutrient depletions could be a problem for people like adolescents, the elderly, and the poorly nourished, whose nutrient intake is borderline to begin with. *For this reason, large increases in dietary fiber are inadvisable for such people.* Also, persons with kidney disease, diabetes, or other serious health problems should not radically alter their diets without first consulting their physicians.

How to Increase Your Fiber Intake

Let's start with the *how-not-tos.* Don't go out and buy a jar of fiber pills or tablets. Dr. Peter Van Soest, professor of animal nutrition at the New York State College of Agriculture and Life Sciences at Cornell University, points out that "considering the fineness and size of these pills, you'd have to eat a whole bottle of them to get any benefits!"

Don't buy boxes of bran and pectin and use them to spruce up your otherwise unhealthy diet. Little good can be gained from adding fiber to a diet overburdened with fats and sweets. The idea is to change the kinds of foods you eat, not to use fiber as a food additive. And don't abruptly purge your diet and your household of all refined carbohydrates and replace them with natural, whole-grain kinds. A slow, gradual substitution of high-fiber for low-fiber foods will wreak the least havoc with your digestive system and is more likely to become a lasting way of eating.

A final warning. Don't focus on one or another type of fiber and neglect the rest. Whole grains may be the perfect cure for a sluggish gut, and any type of fiber should help you control your weight. But pectins and gums are important to how your body handles fats, cholesterol, and carbohydrates.

Now for the *dos.* Do make sure you consume a wide variety of fibrous foods in reasonable amounts. Be certain to drink lots of liquids when you eat fiber; otherwise fiber can be constipating instead of stimulating to your gut. In general, coarse fiber is more effective than the same fiber ground fine. Look for the words "whole grain" or "whole wheat" or "whole oats" when you're buying breads and cereals.

Raw fruits and vegetables have more useful fiber than those that have been peeled, cooked, puréed, or otherwise processed, so include fresh fruits and raw vegetables in your daily diet. Add a "salad a day" to the "apple a day."

As for how much fiber you should eat, no one can yet say. Certainly there are populations that consume five times as much fiber as Americans currently do. Few Americans need to, or would want to, eat that much fiber. But a gradual doubling of current intake—say, to 40 grams a day of *dietary fiber* (not *crude* fiber—see Table 7.1, pages 146–147)—is reasonable. This is about the amount commonly consumed by vegetarians in Western nations, with no evidence of ill effect. The best way to achieve this is to substitute high-fiber complex carbohydrates—whole grains, beans, fruits, and vegetables—for some of the animal fats and processed sugars you're now eating.

Above all, remember that the watchword for fiber, as with all else in good nutrition, is moderation. If a little of something is good, that doesn't necessarily—or even usually—mean that more is better.

***

FOR FURTHER READING

Denis Burkitt, M.D., *Eat Right to Stay Healthy* (New York: Arco, 1979).

8 ❧ VITAMINS: MICRONUTRIENTS OR MIRACLE DRUGS?

FIVE-YEAR-OLD Jason is a fussy eater who won't put anything in his mouth that's green, yellow, or orange. Katie, a ninth grader who wants to look like a gymnast, skips breakfast, has cheese and fruit for lunch, and, except for salad, barely touches her supper. Ben, the high-school athlete, grabs a Danish and milk for breakfast, has hot dogs and a Coke for lunch, and wolfs down his meat, potatoes, and rolls at dinner but skips the other vegetables and salad.

Mother, also dieting, has grapefruit, toast, and coffee for breakfast, no lunch, and a dinner without bread and potatoes. Father's breakfast is no bigger, if he has time to eat at all. His bag lunch is a sandwich, cake, and a Coke or—if he's a white-collar worker—a martini, steak sandwich, and coffee. And his dinner is two beers (or two martinis) plus whatever is served. When mother works late, it's a TV dinner and coffee.

Grandmother eats like 5-year-old Jason, picking at her food and skipping those foods she finds hard to chew or digest. Only, unlike Jason, she drinks no milk.

Does anyone in this family, which is hardly unusual in its dietary habits, consume enough vitamins in his or her daily diet to sustain good nutrition and good health? Probably not.

Most of us "know" that the best way to obtain needed nutrients, including the life-sustaining vitamins and minerals, is to eat a so-called balanced diet—one that contains reasonable portions of a variety of basic foodstuffs. (See the description of the Basic Four in Chapter 1.) But the facts of modern life—the pressures of time, catch-as-catch-can meals, constant dieting, and force of habit—often get in the way of a well-rounded diet that is rich in essential nutrients. While diets don't have to be precisely balanced each day to assure good nutrition, prolonged elimination of one or more food categories or overemphasis of certain foods at the expense of others can lead to shortages that compromise health.

Many of the foods we eat today in abundance bear little resemblance to the vitamin-rich foodstuffs nature produces. Some, like refined grains, are systematically stripped of vital goodness. Others are processed or prepared in ways that destroy fragile micronutrients. The growing dependence on factory-prepared meals and restaurant fare and the decline in consumption of such vitamin-rich foods as fresh fruits and vegetables, whole grains, and dairy products has left many Americans with borderline deficiencies of some essential nutrients. Added to vitamin shortfalls in the overly processed American diet are recently recognized vitamin deficiencies caused by certain diseases, drugs, and habits. The young, the old, and the poor are especially vulnerable.

At the same time, others are taking far too many vitamins—stuffing themselves with megadoses of this or that micronutrient under the false assumption that if some is good, more must be better. They conclude, incorrectly, that if a deficiency of a certain vitamin causes a particular symptom, then the appearance of that symptom for whatever reason is best treated by megadoses of the vitamin. However, as you will soon discover, excesses of many vitamins can pose risks just as serious to health as deficiencies of those vitamins.

What Are Vitamins, and What Do They Do?

Vitamins are organic substances derived from living material—plants and animals. They are required in the diet in such tiny amounts —milligram or microgram quantities—that *all the needed vitamins together add up to about an eighth of a teaspoon a day.*

Vitamins have varied roles. They assist in the processing of other nutrients (proteins, fats, carbohydrates, and minerals), and they participate in the formation of blood cells, hormones, genetic material, and nervous-system chemicals. Most of the vitamins assist enzymes in carrying out these various functions, and thus are called *coenzymes.*

If you are lacking one or another vitamin in your diet, or if you consume it in insufficient quantity, characteristic deficiency symptoms develop. But because vitamins have such diverse roles, the deficiency symptoms of a particular vitamin may touch many different body functions, and different vitamins may produce similar deficiency symptoms.

There are 13 undisputed vitamins, and they fall into one of two categories: *fat soluble* and *water soluble.* The *fat-soluble vitamins*—A, D, E, and K—are absorbed through the intestinal membranes into the body proper with the aid of fats in the diet or bile produced by the liver. Disorders like cystic fibrosis that interfere with the digestion of fats can lead to deficiencies of fat-soluble vitamins. These vitamins are stored in body fat, so it's not essential to consume them daily unless you take in only marginal amounts. You can satisfy your requirement for vitamin A by consuming 2 ounces of beef liver once a week or a cup of spinach every five days, or a cooked carrot every other day (there is more vitamin A in biologically available form in cooked carrots than in raw ones).

Since fat-soluble vitamins are stored in the body, they can build up to toxic levels if too much is consumed. With so many people taking megadoses of vitamins, poisonous excesses of one or another fat-soluble vitamin may become as common a medical problem as deficiencies.

The *water-soluble vitamins*—8 B vitamins and C—do not need fat or bile to be absorbed and, for the most part, are not stored in the body. Therefore, they should be supplied in adequate amounts in your diet each day, since they are constantly being used up or washed out of the body through urine and sweat. The water-soluble vitamins are also more fragile; large proportions of these vitamins naturally present in foods may be washed out or destroyed during food storage, processing, or preparation (see tips for preserving vitamins, pages 177–180). Thus, you may think you're eating a food that's a rich source of vitamin C or one of the B vitamins when in fact the nutrient went down the drain with the cooking water. Even fresh fruits and vegetables may lose large percentages of their initial content of water-soluble vitamins before they reach your table.

The vitamin content of different foods may vary considerably, depending on how and where they are produced (soil, sunlight, temperature, and rainfall all can have an effect), when they are harvested, and how they are stored and shipped. Tomatoes ripened on the vine and then canned may have as much vitamin C as those picked green, shipped to market, and, weeks later, eaten fresh. The same is true for frozen orange juice compared to juice freshly squeezed from oranges that were picked underripe and stored at room temperature.

In addition to the 13 fat- and water-soluble vitamins, there are 1 to 5 other substances—including choline and inositol—that some researchers and many vitamin enthusiasts think of as vitamins. However, the scientists who establish our nutrient requirements do not consider them vitamins since they are produced in the body in adequate amounts and cause no known deficiency symptoms when they're not in the diet. This list does not include a number of "pseudo-vitamins," such as B_{17} (laetrile) and B_{15} (pangamic acid), which have been touted as vitamins by food faddists but have no known biological role that could justify this appellation.

Megadoses

Though self-dosing with vitamins in amounts many times greater than the Recommended Dietary Allowance is usually worthless and, as you can see from Table 8.1, fraught with potential hazards, recent studies have suggested that megadoses of certain vitamins sometimes can have druglike benefits quite apart from their usual role as vitamins. None of what follows, however, should be taken as license for self-treatment. All treatment with megadoses of micronutrients should be administered only by physicians who are fully conversant with the risks as well as the possible benefits.

VITAMIN A

Through its role in maintaining healthy skin and mucous membranes, vitamin A is believed to help prevent cancers that arise in epithelial (skin and lining) tissues, such as lung and bladder cancers. In a study conducted at the State University of New York at Buffalo, heavy smokers who consumed low levels of vitamin A were four times as likely to get lung cancer as those who ingested adequate amounts of the vitamin.

But because massive doses of vitamin A are toxic, it cannot be used as such as a cancer preventive. Instead, studies are currently under way testing nontoxic chemical cousins of vitamin A as possible cancer suppressors. These chemicals are not currently available for purchase, and the first results of the tests won't be known for several years.

Megadoses of vitamin A have also been touted as a treatment for hyperactivity in children, learning disabilities, and schizophrenia. However, there is no scientific support for these notions, and the hazards of the therapy are severe. Yale researchers recently described a 4-year-old boy with learning problems who developed fever, irritability, inability to walk, and pain when touched after his grandmother had fed him megadoses of vitamin A.

Table 8.1 • VITAMINS: WHERE YOU GET THEM AND WHAT THEY DO

Best sources	Main roles	Deficiency symptoms	Risks of megadoses
	Fat soluble		
		A	
Liver; eggs; cheese; butter; fortified margarine and milk; yellow, orange, and dark-green vegetables and fruits (e.g., carrots, broccoli, spinach, cantaloupe). Vitamin A is preformed in animal foods. In plants, the yellow-orange "provitamin," called carotene, is converted to an active vitamin in the body.	Assists in the formation and maintenance of healthy skin, hair, and mucous membranes; aids in the ability to see in dim light (night vision); needed for proper bone growth, teeth development, and reproduction.	Night blindness; rough skin and mucous membranes; infection of mucous membranes; drying of the eyes; impaired bone growth and tooth enamel.	Blurred vision, loss of appetite, headaches, skin rashes, nausea, diarrhea, hair loss, menstrual irregularities, extreme fatigue, joint pain, liver damage, insomnia, abnormal bone growth, injury to brain and nervous system. Excessive consumption of carotene-containing foods, while not poisonous, can cause yellowing of skin.
		D	
Fortified milk; egg yolk; liver; tuna; salmon; cod liver oil. Made on skin in sunlight, but required in diet by dark-skinned persons in cold climates, babies, and those confined indoors.	Aids in the formation and maintenance of bones and teeth; assists in the absorption and use of calcium and phosphorus.	In children, rickets: stunted bone growth, bowed legs, malformed teeth, protruding abdomen. In adults, osteomalacia: softening of the bones leading to shortening and fractures, muscle spasms, and twitching.	In infants, calcium deposits in kidneys and excessive calcium in blood; in adults, calcium deposits throughout body (may be mistaken for cancer), deafness, nausea, loss of appetite, kidney stones, fragile bones, high blood pressure, high blood cholesterol, increased lead absorption.

Table continues on next page

Table 8.1 continued

Fat soluble

Best sources	Main roles	Deficiency symptoms	Risks of megadoses
E (alpha tocopherol)			
Vegetable oils; margarine; wheat germ; whole-grain cereals and bread; liver; dried beans; green leafy vegetables.	Aids in the formation of red blood cells, muscles, and other tissues; protects vitamin A and essential fatty acids from oxidation.	Not seen in human beings except after prolonged impairment of fat absorption. Deficiency symptoms in laboratory animals (e.g., reproductive failure, liver degeneration, heart damage, muscular dystrophy) not seen in people, not even those getting very little vitamin E for six years.	None definitely known. Reports of headache, blurred vision, extreme fatigue, muscle weakness. Can destroy some vitamin K made in the gut.
K			
Green leafy vegetables; cabbage; cauliflower; peas; potatoes; liver; cereals. Except in newborns, made by bacteria in human intestine.	Aids in the synthesis of substances needed for the blood to clot; helps maintain normal bone metabolism.	Hemorrhage, especially in newborn infants. In adults, loss of calcium from bones (however, this deficiency is extremely rare). Extra K needed by persons on prolonged antibiotic therapy and those with impaired fat absorption, cancer, or kidney disease.	Jaundice in babies; anemia in laboratory animals.

Water soluble

	Function	Deficiency	Excess	Sources
Thiamin (B₁)	Helps release energy from carbohydrates; aids in the synthesis of an important nervous-system chemical.	Beriberi: mental confusion, muscular weakness, swelling of the heart, leg cramps. Need for thiamin is increased if calories consumed increase.	None known. However, since B vitamins are interdependent, excess of one may produce deficiency of others.	Pork (especially ham); liver; oysters; whole-grain and enriched cereals, pasta, and bread; wheat germ; oatmeal; peas; lima beans. May also be made by intestinal microbes.
Riboflavin (B₂)	Helps release energy from carbohydrates, proteins, and fats; aids in the maintenance of mucous membranes.	Skin disorders, especially around nose and lips; cracks at corners of mouth; sensitivity of eyes to light.	None known. See thiamin.	Liver; milk; meat; dark-green vegetables; eggs; whole-grain and enriched cereals, pasta, and bread; mushrooms; dried beans and peas.
Niacin (B₃, nicotinamide, nicotinic acid)	Participates with thiamin and riboflavin in facilitating energy production in cells.	Pellagra: skin disorders (especially on parts of body exposed to sun), diarrhea, mental confusion, irritability, mouth swelling, smooth tongue.	Duodenal ulcer, abnormal liver function, elevated blood sugar, excessive uric acid in blood, possibly leading to gout. See thiamin.	Liver; poultry; meat; tuna; eggs; whole-grain and enriched cereals, pasta, and bread; nuts; dried peas and beans. Body can convert tryptophan into niacin.

Table continues on next page

Table 8.1 continued

Best sources	Main roles	Deficiency symptoms	Risks of megadoses
		Water soluble	
	B_6 (includes pyridoxine, pyridoxal, and pyridoxamine)		
Whole-grain (but not enriched) cereals and bread; liver; avocados; spinach; green beans; bananas; fish; poultry; meats; nuts; potatoes; green leafy vegetables.	Aids in the absorption and metabolism of proteins; helps the body use fats; assists in the formation of red blood cells.	Skin disorders; cracks at corners of mouth; smooth tongue; convulsions; dizziness; nausea; anemia; kidney stones. Mild deficiency caused by oral contraceptives may cause depression. Otherwise, deficiencies rare. Need for B_6 is increased by increased protein in diet.	Dependency on high dose, leading to deficiency symptoms when one returns to normal amounts.
	B_{12} (cobalamin)		
Only in animal foods: liver; kidneys; meat; fish; eggs; milk; oysters; nutritional yeast.	Aids in the formation of red blood cells; assists in the building of genetic material; helps the functioning of the nervous system.	Pernicious anemia: anemia, pale skin and mucous membranes, numbness and tingling in fingers and toes that may progress to loss of balance and weakness and pain in arms and legs. At risk: strict vegetarians who eat no animal foods; persons who have had part of their stomach removed; those with a genetic inability to absorb B_{12}.	None known. See thiamin.

	Sources	Function	Deficiency	Excess
Folacin (folic acid)	Liver; kidneys; dark-green leafy vegetables; wheat germ; dried beans and peas. Stored in the body so that daily consumption is not crucial.	Acts with B_{12} in synthesizing genetic material; aids in the formation of hemoglobin in red blood cells.	Megaloblastic anemia: enlarged red blood cells, smooth tongue, diarrhea; during pregnancy, deficiency may cause loss of the fetus or fetal abnormalities. Women on oral contraceptives may need extra folacin.	None identified. But body stores it, so it is potentially hazardous. Can mask a B_{12} deficiency.
Pantothenic acid	In all plants and animals, especially liver; kidneys; whole-grain cereal and bread; nuts; eggs; dark-green vegetables. Also made by intestinal bacteria. Lost in refined and heavily processed foods.	Helps in the metabolism of carbohydrates, proteins, and fats; aids in the formation of hormones and nerve-regulating substances.	Not known except experimentally in human beings: severe abdominal cramps, vomiting, fatigue, difficulty sleeping, tingling in hands and feet.	Increased need for thiamin, possibly causing thiamin deficiency symptoms.
Biotin	Egg yolk; liver; kidneys; dark-green vegetables; green beans. Made by microorganisms in the intestinal tract.	Aids in the formation of fatty acids; helps release energy from carbohydrates.	Not known under natural circumstances. Large amounts of raw egg white can destroy biotin, causing loss of appetite, nausea, vomiting, pallor, depression, fatigue, and muscle pain. (Cooked egg white has no harmful effect.)	None known. See thiamin.

Table continues on next page

Table 8.1 continued

Best sources	Main roles	Deficiency symptoms	Risks of megadoses
Water soluble			
C (ascorbic acid)			
Citrus fruits; tomatoes; strawberries; melon; green peppers; potatoes; dark-green vegetables.	Aids in the formation of collagen; helps maintain capillaries, bones, and teeth; helps protect other vitamins from oxidation; may block formation of cancer-causing nitrosamines.	Scurvy: bleeding gums, degenerating muscles, wounds that don't heal, loose teeth, brown, dry, rough skin. Early symptoms include loss of appetite, irritability, weight loss.	Dependency on high doses, possibly precipitating symptoms of scurvy when withdrawn (especially in infants if megadoses taken during pregnancy); kidney and bladder stones; diarrhea; urinary-tract irritation; increased tendency for blood to clot; breakdown of red blood cells in persons with certain common genetic disorders (such as glucose-6-phosphate dehydrogenase deficiency, common in blacks); may induce B_{12} deficiency.

VITAMIN E

Because of its preservative properties (it prevents substances from reacting with oxygen), vitamin E is believed by many to delay the ravages of age by slowing the deterioration of cells. Currently, there is evidence only in laboratory animals and in human tissues growing in laboratory dishes to support this belief. However, several specialists on aging take a vitamin E supplement "just in case" it really works.

There is also some evidence that vitamin E can block the formation of nitrosamines, potent chemicals that induce cancer in laboratory animals. Nitrosamines are produced in the saliva and gastrointestinal tract from the combination of nitrites and amines in foods. Studies of mice suggest that in large doses vitamin E may protect lung tissue from the damaging effects of oxidants in polluted air. The vitamin has proved useful in treating some patients who have intermittent claudication, a circulatory problem of the legs which results in painful cramps. And E is being studied as a preventive for an eye disorder called retrolental fibroplasia, which can cause blindness in premature infants, and as a treatment for fibrocystic disease of the breast, a benign but painful disorder.

But there are as yet no scientific data to support the belief of some doctors that vitamin E supplements can counter some of the annoying symptoms of menopause, including hot flashes and vaginal dryness. Nor is there any convincing evidence for the purported ability of vitamin E to restore or to help in maintaining sexual potency or fertility in people or to prevent heart attacks.

THE B VITAMINS

Studies at the Oregon Health Sciences University School of Medicine suggest that a rare eye disorder called gyrate atrophy, caused by an inherited enzyme deficiency, can be treated with high doses of vitamin B_6. Success with B_6 therapy has been reported in children with another rare genetic disease, homocystinuria, who have a related enzyme defect. However, people who self-treat with large megadoses of B_6 risk severe nerve damage.

Other claims for megadoses of B vitamins have not been substantiated by proper research. Thiamin (B_1) is not an effective mosquito repellant, and niacin (nicotinic acid or nicotinamide) is no cure for schizophrenia, hyperactivity, childhood autism, alcoholism, arthritis, high blood cholesterol, neurosis, or depression. And B_{12} shots, used like a ritual by some physicians to treat patients who are tired, depressed, or "run down," are at best a placebo. They leave you with nothing more than a sore butt, a diminished purse, and, possibly, failure to diagnose the true cause of your symptoms.

Vitamin C

Two-time Nobel laureate Dr. Linus Pauling gave the megadose mania a rousing kickoff in 1970 by proclaiming that vitamin C might "ameliorate" and prevent that peskiest of human ailments, the common cold. Colds always seem to happen when you can least afford them—on vacations, during the preholiday rush, while preparing for exams, generally times of stress when the body is most susceptible to illness. It's little wonder, then, that millions of Americans would latch onto a readily available, inexpensive, and purportedly harmless means to show the cold virus the door. Instead of taking 60 milligrams of vitamin C a day (the amount in 4 ounces of orange juice), millions started taking tablets that totaled 500 milligrams or more, with some people consuming as much as 6,000 to 10,000 milligrams a day (6 to 10 grams).

Pauling, whose Nobel Prizes were for chemistry and peace, wrote a book called *Vitamin C and the Common Cold,* in which he relates that thanks to C he and his wife "experienced a striking decrease in the number of colds that we caught and in their severity." The book was heavily promoted on radio and television, in newspapers and magazines. Throughout the nation pharmacies and health-food stores moved their stockpiles of vitamin C into plain view.

Since scientific conclusions cannot be drawn from anecdotal reports and individual case histories, the medical profession was challenged to document Dr. Pauling's claims. Researchers set up controlled trials in which some individuals were given vitamin C and others a dummy pill of similar appearance. Then the researchers sat back and waited for cold symptoms to appear in the subjects. Studies of thousands of people of different ages, circumstances, and locations have now been completed and the only reasonable conclusion to be drawn from the studies is that vitamin C has no effect on the number of colds people get, but in some people it lessens the severity of cold symptoms. Occasionally, the cold symptoms might be so mild that the victims don't even realize they have a cold! You may say that this is just splitting hairs, since a cold you hardly notice is almost as good as no cold at all. But as you can see from the risks listed in Table 8.1, there is a price to pay for your relief, and it may not be worth it for most people.

Studies of vitamin C have a long history. In the 1750s, vitamin C (then unknown) was the subject of the first controlled experiment on medical record. A British doctor named James Lind demonstrated what many sea captains had discovered centuries earlier on their own —that citrus fruit alone could cure scurvy among sailors who were at sea for months. The finding that only those sailors given the fruit got well led to the inclusion of limes among the rations on long British voyages; it also gave birth to the nickname "limey" for British sailors and the name ascorbic acid (from antiscorbutic, or antiscurvy) for vitamin C.

Through the course of evolution, human beings and a few other animals seem to have lost their ability to manufacture their own vitamin C. We share a need for dietary vitamin C with many primates, guinea pigs, red-vented bulbuls, and Indian fruit bats. Part of Dr. Pauling's argument for megadoses of vitamin C centers on the fact that the modern gorilla, who consumes mostly fresh vegetation, ingests about 4,500 milligrams (4½ grams) of vitamin C daily and that early man probably subsisted on a similar diet. Thus, Dr. Pauling says, we, too, need to consume vitamin C by the gramful.

In addition to its use as a preventive and treatment for the common cold, vitamin C in megadose formulations has been used—sometimes successfully—to treat a number of disorders. These include disorders of collagen synthesis and osteogenesis imperfecta, an abnormality of bone development. Surgery increases the need for vitamin C, and there is some evidence that wound healing is enhanced by vitamin C supplements.

Dr. Pauling and a co-worker have reported that 10 grams of vitamin C per day prolonged survival in patients with terminal cancer. But a controlled study by Dr. Edward T. Creagan of 60 cancer patients at the Mayo Clinic showed no anticancer effect or improved survival. In fact, the patients who survived longest had been treated with a placebo. British claims that the vitamin could lower blood cholesterol and prevent atherosclerosis (clogging of the arteries) and heart attack have not been confirmed by studies in this country.

Megadoses of vitamin C are currently being studied as weapons to block the formation of cancer-causing chemicals in the digestive tract. Researchers at the Medical College of Wisconsin in Milwaukee report the successful treatment of an inherited precancerous condition with massive doses of vitamin C. The condition, called familial polyposis, eventually leads to cancer of the colon or rectum. Timed-release capsules of vitamin C caused polyps to disappear in some patients.

Drs. J. Roberto Moran and Harry L. Greene, pediatric researchers at Vanderbilt University School of Medicine in Nashville, concluded from a study of the benefits and risks of vitamin C megadoses that "at present no strong evidence can be found to support the routine prophylactic [preventive] use of ascorbic acid in well-nourished people." They pointed out that since body tissues become saturated with vitamin C when it is consumed in amounts of 100 to 150 milligrams per day (the rest is simply washed out with the urine), the use of megadoses up to ten times that amount is not advised.

The RDAs and What They Mean to You

MDR, RDA, USRDA—nothing about micronutrients is more mysterious to the average consumer than these government-promulgated abbreviations. They are supposed to help us determine whether we're eating enough of the right things, but for many people they are at worst meaningless and at best confusing.

First, *MDR,* which stands for Minimal Daily Requirement, is passé. Since it is impossible to state the least amount each person should eat of each nutrient and cover everyone's requirements in the process, MDRs have been replaced by a more flexible concept, the *USRDAs.* This stands for United States Recommended *Daily* Allowances. USRDAs were devised by the Food and Drug Administration for nutritional labeling. These are the lists on processed foods and vitamin products that tell what percentage of each of 19 essential nutrients you get per serving or dose. It is a rough guide because it doesn't differentiate among people of different ages and sex who have different nutrient requirements. But it is better than the MDRs because it goes beyond the minimum requirements and provides a reasonable margin of safety for most people.

The USRDAs, in turn, are based on the *RDAs*—Recommended *Dietary* Allowances—derived by a prestigious group of nutritional scientists who advise the Food and Nutrition Board, a committee of the National Academy of Sciences–National Research Council. Every five years or so, the board reviews and revises its recommendations; the latest set was issued in 1980. As the board defines them, the RDAs are "the levels of intake of essential nutrients considered, in the judgment of the Food and Nutrition Board on the basis of available scientific knowledge, to be adequate to meet the known nutritional needs of practically all healthy persons." (See Table 8.2, pages 172–173.)

There are some caveats regarding the RDAs.

The board that established them admits that scientific knowledge of nutritional requirements is far from complete: that the requirements for many nutrients have not been established; that several essential nutrients have only recently been discovered; and that in all likelihood other nutrients will be found to be essential in years to come. Therefore, to be sure that as yet undefined nutritional needs are met, it's important to eat a varied diet and not depend on pills or processed foods artificially stoked with known micronutrients.

The RDAs should not be confused with nutritional requirements. Requirements differ from individual to individual because of inherent genetic differences, among other factors. Therefore, the RDAs represent estimates that exceed the requirements of most people.

The RDAs do *not* cover individuals who have special nutritional requirements as a result of diseases or other abnormalities or as a result of the use of certain medications. Special vitamin requirements will be discussed in the next section.

The amounts listed in the RDAs are not treatments for disorders (other than nutritional deficiency symptoms). The committee said there is "no convincing evidence of unique health benefits" resulting from large excesses of any particular nutrient.

Persons who regularly consume less than the amounts recommended in the RDAs for some nutrients are not necessarily nutritionally deficient. On the other hand, such levels cannot be assumed to be nutritionally adequate; they will be for some people, but not for others.

Except for vitamins A and D, it's not harmful to consume two to three times the recommended levels of vitamins. Many people regularly do through the foods they eat and especially if they take a multivitamin supplement.

But the biggest problem with the RDAs is how to translate the numbers on the list into the foods you put in your mouth. A diet, after all, is not a bunch of numbers, and the RDAs are not meant to be used as rigid formulas to devise ideal menus. The USRDAs partly cope with this problem. But under current law, for most foods manufacturers need not list the proportion of the USRDA a serving provides. Such lists are required only if vitamins or minerals are added or if a nutritional claim is made for the food, such as "Cereal X provides 100 percent of eight essential vitamins." The government is currently exploring new regulations and legislation that would extend nutritional labeling requirements to all processed foods (see Chapter 27). Meanwhile, a wise consumer will eat a varied diet rich in fresh foods. The more limited your menu and the more processed the foods you eat, the more likely your diet will be deficient in one or more essential nutrients. The Food and Nutrition Board suggests that rather than try to meet the daily standard for each nutrient every day, you should average your intake of nutrients over a five- to eight-day period.

Table 8.2 reproduces the RDAs for vitamins (as of 1980). Unless you're a special case, there's no reason to consume more than 100 percent of the RDA for each vitamin. To help you make maximum use of the information in the RDA chart, you should also consult Table 8.3, a list of the approximate vitamin content in portions of common vitamin-in-rich foods. You cannot assume that cooked versions of foods have the same amount of water-soluble vitamins as "fresh" (uncooked and unprocessed) versions of foods.

Do You Need a Vitamin Supplement?

For hundreds of thousands of years, people got all the vitamins and minerals they needed from the foods they ate. The human species evolved in a world devoid of the multivitamin preparations so eagerly swallowed by millions of Americans today. But our ancestors also lacked the processed foods, drugs, cigarettes, and steady supply of alcoholic beverages that could interfere with adequate nutrition.

Today, haphazard eaters, especially those who rely on a limited menu, are likely to shortchange their bodies in needed micronutrients. And for some people, even a reasonably well-balanced and varied diet cannot supply enough of certain nutrients. For most of these people, increasing their consumption of foods rich in certain vitamins could compensate. But for others, a supplement of one or more vitamins in pill form may be beneficial.

Infants are commonly given vitamin supplements though these supplements are usually not needed. This is done because the typical infant diet is narrow, the amount of vitamins different babies absorb from their foods is uncertain, and the vitamin requirements of infants —who may double in size every few months—are great compared to the infants' body size and food capacity. The RDAs for infants are based primarily on the vitamin content of breast milk, an ideal complete food for infants for the first six months of life. There are some differences in vitamin content between breast milk and cow's milk (since nature designed the latter for calves, not human infants), and, therefore, a vitamin supplement may be particularly important for babies who are not breast fed (see Chapter 19).

Vitamin supplements are also commonly given to women who are pregnant or nursing. Again, in the ideal situation, this should not be necessary (except for extra iron, a mineral), since both pregnancy and lactation increase a woman's need for calories and, in the course of eating extra food, she naturally consumes extra vitamins. But for various reasons—for example, "morning" sickness that may extend beyond morning, diets for weight control, inability to tolerate some foods— pregnant women often have reduced blood levels of vitamins A, C, B_6, B_{12}, and folacin. Therefore, a vitamin supplement may be prescribed as a form of nutritional insurance. Obstetricians, preferring to err on the side of excess to assure a healthy mother and baby, generally prescribe a multivitamin and mineral supplement to all their patients who are pregnant and nursing.

But such women should *never* take megadoses of any vitamin or mineral without their doctor's approval. Megadoses of certain vitamins can be poisonous or cause dangerous side effects, and no one is more vulnerable to these effects than the developing fetus and young infant.

Other people who are likely to fall short on essential vitamins from their regular diet include the following:

Heavy smokers. A two-year study by the Canadian government of 4,600 persons showed that those who smoke one and a half packs of cigarettes a day have 30 percent to 40 percent less vitamin C in their blood than nonsmokers. Perhaps more vitamin C is used up by smokers when their body attempts to repair damage to cells caused by toxic elements in tobacco smoke. The vitamin C deficit caused by smoking can be made up by consuming an 8-ounce glass of orange juice each day —approximately 100 milligrams of vitamin C (nearly double the RDA for an adult). A vitamin supplement should not be necessary if each day you eat plenty of fresh fruits and vegetables rich in vitamin C.

Women on oral contraceptives. The birth control pill produces a number of metabolic effects, among them shortages of several water-soluble vitamins. Women on the pill are often found to have reduced blood levels of thiamin, riboflavin, B_6, B_{12}, folacin, and vitamin C. In several cases, particularly that of B_6, dietary additions may not be adequate to compensate for the deficit, and a vitamin supplement is needed. B_6 deficiency while on the pill has been associated with mental depression.

Heavy drinkers. No matter how good their diets, persons who consume a great quantity of alcoholic beverages require more thiamin, niacin, B_6, and folacin than persons who drink only socially or not at

Table 8.2 • VITAMINS: RECOMMENDED DIETARY ALLOWANCES (RDAS)
AND ESTIMATED SAFE AND ADEQUATE INTAKES

Ages	A (RE)*	D (μg)**	E (mg)	C (mg)	Thia-min (mg)	Ribo-flavin (mg)	Niacin (mg)	B_6 (mg)	Folacin (μg)**	B_{12} (μg)**	K (μg)**	Biotin (μg)**	Pantothenic acid (mg)
Infants													
To 6 months	420	10	3	35	0.3	0.4	6	0.3	30	0.5	12	35	2
6 months–1 year	400	10	4	35	0.5	0.6	8	0.6	45	1.5	10–20	50	3
Children													
1–3	400	10	5	45	0.7	0.8	9	0.9	100	2.0	15–30	65	3
4–6	500	10	6	45	0.9	1.0	11	1.3	200	2.5	20–40	85	3–4
7–10	700	10	7	45	1.2	1.4	16	1.6	300	3.0	30–60	120	4–5
Males													
11–14	1,000	10	8	50	1.4	1.6	18	1.8	400	3.0	50–100	100–200	4–7
15–18	1,000	10	10	60	1.4	1.7	18	2.0	400	3.0	50–100	100–200	4–7
19–22	1,000	7.5	10	60	1.5	1.7	19	2.2	400	3.0	70–140	100–200	4–7
23–50	1,000	5	10	60	1.4	1.6	18	2.2	400	3.0	70–140	100–200	4–7
51 and over	1,000	5	10	60	1.2	1.4	16	2.2	400	3.0	70–140	100–200	4–7

Table continues on next page

Table 8.2 continued

Ages	A (RE)*	D (µg)**	E (mg)	C (mg)	Thia-min (mg)	Ribo-flavin (mg)	Niacin (mg)	B_6 (mg)	Folacin (µg)**	B_{12} (µg)**	K (µg)**	Biotin (µg)**	Pantothenic acid (mg)
Females													
11–14	800	10	8	50	1.1	1.3	15	1.8	400	3.0	50–100	100–200	4–7
15–18	800	10	8	60	1.1	1.3	14	2.0	400	3.0	50–100	100–200	4–7
19–22	800	7.5	8	60	1.1	1.3	14	2.0	400	3.0	70–140	100–200	4–7
23–50	800	5	8	60	1.0	1.2	13	2.0	400	3.0	70–140	100–200	4–7
51 and over	800	5	8	60	1.0	1.2	13	2.0	400	3.0	70–140	100–200	4–7
Pregnant	+200	+5	+2	+20	+0.4	+0.3	+2	+0.6	+400	+1	70–140	100–200	4–7
Nursing	+400	+5	+3	+40	+0.5	+0.5	+5	+0.5	+100	+1	70–140	100–200	4–7

Note: These figures were established in 1980 by the Food and Nutrition Board of the National Academy of Sciences–National Research Council to meet the needs of healthy persons. The values listed for vitamin K, biotin, and panto-thenic acid represented estimated safe and adequate daily dietary intakes. All other values are Recommended Dietary Allowances (RDAs).

*RE = retinol equivalent
**µg = micrograms.

Table 8.3 • GOOD SOURCES OF VITAMINS AMONG COMMON FOODS

Food	*Amount*	*A (IU)**	*Thiamin (mg)*	*Ribo-flavin (mg)*	*Niacin (mg)*	*C (mg)*
Bread and Cereals						
Bread, enriched white	2 slices	trace	.07	0.06	0.7	trace
Bread, whole-wheat	2 slices	trace	.09	0.03	0.8	trace
Oatmeal	1 cup cooked	0	.19	0.05	0.2	0
40% Bran Flakes	1 cup	1,650	.41	0.49	4.1	12
Dairy Products						
Milk, whole	1 cup	350	.07	0.41	0.2	2
Yogurt, low-fat plain	1 cup	170	.10	0.44	0.2	2
American cheese	1 ounce	350	.01	0.12	trace	0
Cottage cheese, creamed	½ cup	180	.03	0.26	0.1	0
Fruits						
Apple	1 (6 ounces)	150	.05	0.03	0.2	7
Banana	1 (6 ounces)	230	.06	0.07	0.8	12
Grapes, seedless	10	50	.03	0.02	0.2	2
Orange	1 (6 ounces)	260	.13	0.05	0.5	66
Orange juice	½ cup	250	.11	0.04	0.5	62
Cantaloupe	¼ melon (8 ounces)	4,620	.06	0.04	0.8	45
Vegetables						
Broccoli	1 cup cooked	3,880	.14	0.31	1.2	140
Beets	1 cup sliced	30	.05	0.07	0.5	10
Carrots	1 raw (3 ounces)	7,930	.04	0.04	0.4	6
Beans, green	1 cup boiled	680	.09	0.11	0.6	15
Cabbage	1 cup raw shredded	120	.05	0.05	0.3	42
Peas, green	1 cup cooked	860	.45	0.18	3.7	32
Potato, baked	1 (7 ounces)	trace	.15	0.07	2.7	31
Soybean sprouts	½ cup raw	40	.12	0.11	0.4	7
Spinach	2 ounces raw	4,592	.06	0.11	0.3	29
Tomato	1 (3½ ounces)	820	.05	0.04	0.6	21
Tomato juice	6 ounces	1,460	.09	0.05	1.5	29
Turnip greens	1 cup cooked	9,140	.22	0.35	0.9	100
Meat Group						
Beef, ground	3 ounces cooked	20	.08	0.20	5.1	—**
Chicken, white meat	3 ounces boneless	50	.03	0.08	9.7	—**
Egg	1 large	590	.05	0.15	trace	0
Ham, baked	3 ounces lean	—**	.54	0.25	4.8	—**
Kidney beans	1 cup cooked	10	.20	0.11	1.3	—**

Table 8.3 continued

Food	Amount	A (IU)*	Thiamin (mg)	Ribo-flavin (mg)	Niacin (mg)	C (mg)
Lentils	1 cup cooked	40	.14	0.12	1.2	0
Liver, beef	3 ounces fried	45,390	.22	3.56	14.0	23
Peanut butter	2 tablespoons	—**	.04	0.04	4.8	0
Tuna fish	3 ounces drained	70	.04	0.10	10.0	—**

Source: Based on Agriculture Handbook No. 456. Data for other nutrients in these foods are listed in a series of publications that update Agricultural Handbook No. 8.
*IU = international unit: 5 IUs equal 1 retinol equivalent (RE).
**— = data not available.

all. Alcohol damages the liver and interferes with its ability to store needed vitamins, especially folacin, and to convert the vitamins to their active chemical forms. Alcohol consumption also leads to poor absorption of vitamins from foods, and it increases the requirement for vitamins by using some to metabolize the alcohol and to repair the tissue damage it causes. Furthermore, many heavy drinkers do not eat adequately—they substitute nutrient-deficient alcohol calories for nutrient-rich food calories—and thus further compromise their vitamin intake. Therefore, if you drink the equivalent of four or more shots of alcohol a day, you may need a daily multivitamin supplement. (A shot is ½ ounce of pure alcohol; see Chapter 14.)

Users of certain drugs. In addition to oral contraceptives, use of certain prescription and over-the-counter drugs can result in a vitamin deficiency. Prolonged use of antibiotics can destroy the intestinal bacteria that produce vitamin K and several B vitamins—biotin, pantothenic acid, and possibly thiamin. Dr. Daphne A. Roe, nutrition specialist at Cornell University who is an expert on drug-induced vitamin deficiencies, reports that deficiencies in folacin can result when anticonvulsants used to treat epilepsy are taken, when the cell-killing drug Methotrexate is taken, and when antimalarial drugs are taken. Researchers at the Universiy of California, Davis, showed that the drug sulfasalazine (trade-named Azulfidine), widely used to treat chronic inflammatory bowel diseases, also depletes the body of folacin. The psychiatric drugs chlorpromazine, imipramine, and any triptyline can cause riboflavin deficiency. Use of certain diabetes drugs (metformin and phenformin) can interfere with the absorption of B_{12}. Use of the tuberculosis drug INH, the hydrazide diuretics used to treat high blood pressure, and penicillamine, used in some severe cases of arthritis, can produce a B_6

deficiency. The use of INH may also result in pellagralike symptoms from a niacin shortage. Prolonged use of antacids can destroy needed vitamin C.

Not only can certain drugs interfere with the action of certain vitamins, certain vitamins taken to excess can interfere with the action of certain drugs. If you are under treatment for a medical problem and are taking megadoses of one or more vitamins, be sure to tell your doctor about your vitamin intake.

Persons with certain disorders. Persons with chronic infections, cancer, or chronic loss of red blood cells require additional folacin. Those with obstructive jaundice or chronic intestinal disorders that interfere with the absorption of fats are likely to be deficient in the fat-soluble vitamins, A, D, E, and K. Persons who have had part of the stomach removed, or who have Crohn's disease (regional enteritis) or chronic pancreatic insufficiency, are likely to be short on B_{12}. The parasitic infection giardiasis can also interfere with B_{12} absorption.

Some inherited disorders—for example, familial vitamin-D-resistant rickets—can lead to vitamin deficiencies that cannot be corrected by ordinary vitamin supplements. In such cases, a very large dose, usually administered in a way that bypasses the gastrointestinal tract (or, in this case, use of an activated form of vitamin D), is required for prevention and treatment of severe vitamin-deficiency symptoms.

Surgical and other patients. Extra amounts of vitamin C may be needed to promote healing following surgery, injuries, fractures, and burns.

Elderly persons. Old people tend to absorb less of the B vitamins, especially thiamin, and vitamin C than younger persons and, therefore, may need to consume more than the usual amounts of these vitamins. Also, many old people eat a limited choice of foods that may not supply their full nutritional needs (see Chapter 22). Such persons may benefit from a daily multivitamin and mineral supplement.

Dieters. The wisest way to diet is to continue to eat the full variety of foods in the Basic Four—including bread and cereal products—and cut down only on portion size. With this approach to weight loss, you're unlikely to be short on essential micronutrients. However, persons on extended weight-loss programs, those who have made major cutbacks in their caloric intake (50 percent or more), and those consuming only a limited variety of foods should take a daily multivitamin and mineral supplement.

Athletic women. Studies by Dr. Daphne Roe of Cornell University indicate that physically active women need about double the amount of riboflavin currently recommended.

* * *

If you fall into one of the above categories (except persons with inherited disorders that require extreme therapy), your vitamin supplements should not exceed 100 percent of the RDA for someone your age and sex. The label on the bottle, which lists percentage of the USRDA for each vitamin, can serve as an adequate guide under most circumstances.

Despite the propaganda of some health-food enthusiasts, it makes no difference to anything except your pocketbook whether you take so-called natural vitamins or ones that were synthesized in laboratories. Linus Pauling states, as do most nutrition specialists, that the body cannot distinguish between natural and synthetic forms of a given chemical. As far as your body chemistry is concerned, a chemical is the same regardless of its source. Ascorbic acid—vitamin C—is the same to your cells whether it originated in a rose hip or a test tube. Among the "natural" and synthetic vitamins that are commonly sold, one exception to this principle is vitamin E, but only because the natural forms of E are slightly different in chemical structure and more effective than the manufactured vitamin.

How to Keep the Natural Goodness in Your Food*

By choosing carefully from among the various forms in which the same food may be sold, and by proper storage and preparation of the food at home, you can do a great deal to up the nutritional ante of your diet.

BUYING

• Choose whole-grain cereals and breads rather than refined ones. The greatest concentration of B vitamins and minerals is in the wheat germ and outer layers of the grain. The entire germ and most of the outer layers are removed during milling to refine, or "whiten," the grain.

Some, but not all, of the essential nutrients that are lost during milling are restored when flour or cereals are enriched. In other words, enriched foods are much better than unenriched refined products, but whole-grain products are best. Rice and pasta as well as breads and cereals are readily available in enriched forms. Brown rice contains

---

*Most of this section is based on the findings of detailed analytic studies described in *Nutritional Evaluation of Food Processing,* ed. Robert S. Harris and Endel Karmas (Westport, Conn.: Avi, 1975). Additional facts were gleaned from "Conserving the Nutritive Values in Foods," United States Department of Agriculture Home and Garden Bulletin No. 90.

more vitamins than white, and parboiled ("converted") white rice has more than polished rice.

• If you buy skim milk or nonfat dry milk, be sure it has been fortified with vitamins A and D. These vitamins are lost when fat is removed from the milk. Margarine should also be fortified with A and D.

• Buy fresh or frozen fruits and vegetables rather than canned ones. Many vitamins are soluble in water (all the B vitamins and C) and many are destroyed by the high temperatures involved in canning. As a result, canned foods may retain half or less of the original content of many vitamins; additional vitamins are lost during storage. The losses of B_6 and pantothenic acid can be as high as 91 percent in canned foods. You can't expect to meet the RDA for these vitamins if you subsist on a menu of refined, processed, and canned foods.

Freezing is the least damaging method of food preservation. The main losses through freezing are of vitamin C and thiamin during the blanching (quick, partial cooking in boiling water) of vegetables before they are frozen. However, blanching helps to reduce losses of C, thiamin, riboflavin, and the vitamin A precursor carotene that would otherwise occur during frozen storage.

If you can afford them, boil-in-the-bag frozen vegetables are preferred for their vitamin content. Frozen meats, fish, and poultry, if they are well wrapped, compare favorably to the fresh in vitamin content.

• Shop often for fresh produce, and, if possible, pick fruits and vegetables that have been ripened on the vine. Storage in your refrigerator for one or more days can lead to significant vitamin losses. If you can't shop frequently, you may be better off with frozen fruits and vegetables. Foods that are frozen are picked ripe, usually when vitamin content is at its peak, and then rapidly processed, whereas days or weeks may elapse before fresh produce reaches your table.

• Choose bright-orange carrots, deep-orange sweet potatoes, and dark leaf lettuce (as opposed to a pale head of lettuce) for maximum vitamin A content. When they are tender, cook and eat beet tops and broccoli leaves; both are rich in vitamin A.

STORING

• To minimize vitamin losses during frozen storage, your freezer should be kept at 0 degrees F or below. Even then, frozen beans, broccoli, cauliflower, and spinach can lose from one-third to three-fourths of their vitamin C during a year in the freezer. Such prolonged storage is not recommended. At higher temperatures, losses are even greater. However, frozen orange juice retains its vitamin C well even at 32 degrees F. The longer frozen foods are stored, the greater their vitamin loss. Try to use them within a month or two.

• Canned foods also lose vitamins during storage. They should be kept at about 65 degrees to keep vitamin losses to a minimum. Your pantry should not be near the stove. Vitamin losses after canning are doubled when canned foods are kept at 80 degrees.

• Vegetables like kale, spinach, broccoli, turnip greens, chard, and salad greens should be promptly refrigerated in the vegetable crisper or in moisture-proof bags. They keep their nutrients best when stored at low temperatures (near freezing) and high humidity. Green peas should be kept in their pods until you're ready to use them; if shelled ahead, store them in closed plastic bags. Carrots, sweet potatoes, potatoes, and other roots and tubers keep their vitamins best if kept cool and moist enough to prevent withering.

• Tomatoes, if they are picked underripe, should be ripened at home *away from the sun* at temperatures of 60 degrees to 75 degrees. They lose more nutrients if ripened on a hot, sunny windowsill or in the refrigerator.

• Orange juice, whether freshly squeezed, canned, or reconstituted from frozen concentrate, can be kept in the refrigerator for several days before any vitamin C is lost. There's no harm in keeping fruit juices in the can after opening.

• Milk and bread should be kept in opaque containers away from sun and strong light, which readily destroy their riboflavin.

• Wrap all cut-up and cooked foods well and keep them in the refrigerator.

COOKING

• To preserve water-soluble vitamins, avoid prolonged soaking of fresh vegetables and don't wash rice before cooking. You'll wash B vitamins and C down the drain.

• Prepare salads just before they are to be served. Also delay cutting up and cooking vegetables until the last minute. This reduces the loss of vitamin C.

• Boil vegetables until just tender in the least amount of water possible, using a pot with a tight-fitting lid. Lots of water and prolonged cooking time mean greater vitamin losses. Frozen vegetables should not be thawed or washed before cooking. Baking soda should not be added to the cooking water since it destroys thiamin.

• Pressure cooking is the least damaging cooking technique as far as vitamins are concerned. Steaming is second best, though significant amounts of thiamin, niacin, and folacin can be lost when vegetables are steamed. On average, steamed vegetables lose a third of their vitamin C. Boiling is least desirable, with an average of only 45 percent of the vitamin C preserved. Frying also leads to some loss of vitamin C, but a more serious disadvantage is that the fat significantly increases the ratio of calories to nutrients.

• Meats that are broiled, fried, or roasted retain more B vitamins than meats that are braised or stewed. But in braised meats and stews, you can recapture lost vitamins by consuming the broth. Meats cooked rare retain more heat-sensitive thiamin than well-done meats.

• Potatoes boiled or baked in the skin retain nearly all their vitamins. A whole baked sweet potato retains 89 percent of its vitamin C. If you cut it in half first, only 31 percent of the vitamin is left when it's done. In general, the smaller the pieces into which you cut vegetables before cooking them in water, the greater the vitamin loss.

• Foods that are cooked ahead, stored in the refrigerator or freezer, and later reheated can lose significant amounts of vitamins, especially vitamin C. However, for the sake of convenience this is not of major significance as long as you have other, more reliable sources of vitamin C in your diet.

• When it comes to preserving vitamins, it really doesn't matter whether you cook in pots made of glass, stainless steel, aluminum, or enamel. If you use copper pots, be sure they are well lined. Copper can destroy vitamins C, E, and folacin. Pots made of iron (an advantage if you need extra iron in your diet), brass, or Monel (a nickel alloy) also destroy some of the vitamin C in foods.

• Use the cooking water from vegetables and the drippings from meats (after skimming off the fat) to prepare soup and gravy. That way you recapture many of the lost vitamins. You can also use the vitamin-rich syrup or juice from canned fruits to prepare your own gelatin desserts or fruit-flavored beverages.

FOR FURTHER READING

Editors of *Consumer Guide, The Vitamin Book* (New York: Simon and Schuster, 1979).

Joseph V. Levy and Paul Bach-y-Rita, *Vitamins: Their Use and Abuse* (New York: Liveright, 1976).

9 ⟐ MINERALS: MICRONUTRIENTS OR MEGADOSES?

THE FIELD of vitamins having been so fertile, it was only natural that people would turn to large doses of minerals for the miracles *they* might offer. The shelves of health-food stores these days are well stocked with fat bottles of calcium, magnesium, dolomite (a rock that contains calcium and magnesium), bone meal, zinc, iron, manganese, kelp, liver tablets, and potassium chloride, among other mineral concentrates. Although in small doses minerals are essential to life, with rare exceptions there's little scientific merit—and real and serious risks—associated with megadoses of minerals.

Minerals are inorganic substances that perform a wide range of vital functions throughout the body. Many are part of critical enzyme systems. Although not as fragile as vitamins, some minerals are water soluble and can be cooked out of foods. Minerals can also be bound up by substances in the diet that decrease the body's ability to absorb them.

Essential minerals come in two forms: the *macrominerals,* needed in relatively large (but not megadose) amounts, and the *trace*—or *microminerals,* needed in only very tiny amounts. The macrominerals are calcium, phosphorus, magnesium, potassium, sulfur, sodium, and chloride. (Sodium, which enters our diet primarily as salt, or sodium chloride, is discussed in the next chapter.) The trace minerals (also called trace elements) include iron, zinc, selenium, manganese, molybdenum, copper, iodine, chromium, and fluorine (consumed as fluoride). Animal evidence suggests that one day cobalt, nickel, vanadium, silicon, tin, arsenic, and/or cadmium might be added to the list of minerals that are essential to health in trace amounts, but there is as yet no direct evidence they are needed by human beings. Altogether, minerals make up about 4 percent of your body weight, and the long list of trace minerals adds up to only .01 percent of your total weight.

The best way to get your daily requirement of essential minerals is through the foods you eat. Except for iron and possibly zinc, a reasonably well-structured diet will give your body what it needs for good health without distorting the proper balance and amounts of the various minerals. Table 9.1 shows common sources of the essential minerals, as well as minerals' roles, the deficiency symptoms that may result from their lack, and the risks of overabundance. Table 9.2 and Table 9.3 show the Recommended Dietary Allowances (RDAs) for the various minerals as established in 1980 by the Food and Nutrition Board of the National Academy of Sciences–National Research Council. The levels listed were determined by a specially appointed group of experts, the Committee on Dietary Allowances. For sodium, potassium, chloride, and six trace elements, the committee was unable to determine precise allowances from available data, listing instead "estimated safe and adequate intakes" for these essential nutrients. For substances (like nickel) that you might think are essential minerals but are *not* on the list, the committee could find no evidence that they are required in the diets of human beings.

Calcium

While all the mineral nutrients are essential for life, for several reasons calcium might be said to lead the pack in importance. It's the body's most abundant mineral, amounting to 2 percent of body weight —half the total of all the minerals put together. And it's the macromineral most likely to be in short supply in the diets of many Americans. Calcium is also a favorite of megadosers, some of whom have suffered serious toxic reactions as a result of their self-treatment.

Ninety-eight percent of your body's calcium supply is in your bones, which act as a calcium storage depot; 1 percent is in your teeth; and the remaining 1 percent is scattered in soft tissues throughout your body, where this mineral performs a host of important functions. Calcium helps to build bones and teeth and maintain their strength. Although you probably think of your bones as solid objects of fixed composition, in fact calcium is constantly moving in and out of them. In the course of a year, about a fifth of the calcium in your bones is removed and replaced. Your body has a network of hormones to keep a constant level of calcium in your blood and in other body fluids. This assures a steady supply to all the tissues that need calcium—especially nerve and muscle cells. If your diet contains inadequate amounts of calcium, these hormones remove some from your bones so that the

Table 9.1 • MINERALS: WHERE YOU GET THEM AND WHAT THEY DO

Best sources	Main roles	Deficiency symptoms	Risks of megadoses
Macrominerals*			
Calcium			
Milk and milk products; sardines; canned salmon eaten with bones; dark-green, leafy vegetables; citrus fruits; dried beans and peas.	Building bones and teeth and maintaining bone strength; muscle contraction; maintaining cell membranes; blood clotting; absorption of B_{12}; activation of enzymes.	Children: distorted bone growth (rickets). Adults: loss of bone (osteoporosis) and increased susceptibility to fractures.	Drowsiness; extreme lethargy; impaired absorption of iron, zinc, and manganese; calcium deposits in tissues throughout body, mimicking cancer on X-ray.
Phosphorus			
Meat; poultry; fish; eggs; dried beans and peas; milk and milk products; phosphates in processed foods, especially soft drinks.	Building bones and teeth; release of energy from carbohydrates, proteins, and fats; formation of genetic material, cell membranes, and many enzymes.	Weakness, loss of appetite, malaise, bone pain. Dietary shortages uncommon, but prolonged use of antacids can cause deficiency.	Distortion of calcium-to-phosphorus ratio, creating relative deficiency of calcium.
Magnesium			
Leafy, green vegetables (eaten raw); nuts (especially almonds and cashews); soybeans; seeds; whole grains.	Building bones; manufacture of proteins; release of energy from muscle glycogen; conduction of nerve impulse to muscles; adjustment to cold.	Muscular twitching and tremors; irregular heart beat; insomnia; muscle weakness; leg and foot cramps; shaky hands. Deficiency may occur in persons with prolonged diarrhea, kidney disease, diabetes, epilepsy, or alcoholism, and in those who take diuretics.	Disturbed nervous-system function because the calcium-to-magnesium ratio is unbalanced; catharsis; hazard to persons with poor kidney function.

Mineral	Food Sources	Functions	Deficiency	Toxicity/Excess
Potassium	Orange juice; bananas; dried fruits; meats; bran; peanut butter; dried beans and peas; potatoes; coffee; tea; cocoa.	Muscle contraction; maintenance of fluid and electrolyte balance in cells; transmission of nerve impulses; release of energy from carbohydrates, proteins, and fats.	Abnormal heart rhythm; muscular weakness; lethargy; kidney and lung failure. Deficiency may occur among heavy laborers and athletes who work hard in heat, persons taking diuretics and purgatives, and those with prolonged diarrhea.	Excessive potassium in blood, causing muscular paralysis and abnormal heart rhythms.
Sulfur	Beef; wheat germ; dried beans and peas; peanuts; clams.	In every cell as part of sulfur-containing amino acids; forms bridges between molecules to create firm proteins of hair, nails, and skin.	Not known in humans.	Unknown.
Chloride	Table salt and other naturally occurring salts.	Regulates balance of body fluids and acids and bases; activates enzyme in saliva; part of stomach acid.	Disturbed acid-base balance in body fluids (very rare).	Disturbed acid-base balance.

Table continues on next page

*Sodium, a macromineral, is discussed fully in Chapter 10.

Table 9.1 continued

Best sources	Main roles	Deficiency symptoms	Risks of megadoses
Trace minerals			
Iron			
Liver (especially pork, followed by calf, beef, and chicken); kidneys; red meats; egg yolk; green, leafy vegetables; dried fruits (raisins, apricots, and prunes); dried beans and peas; potatoes; blackstrap molasses; enriched and whole-grain cereals.	Formation of hemoglobin in blood and myoglobin in muscles, which supply oxygen to cells; part of several enzymes and proteins.	Anemia, with fatigue, weakness, pallor, and shortness of breath.	Toxic build-up in liver, pancreas, and heart.
Copper			
Oysters; nuts; cocoa powder; beef and pork liver; kidneys; dried beans; corn-oil margarine.	Formation of red blood cells; part of several respiratory enzymes.	Animals: anemia; faulty development of bone and nervous tissue; loss of elasticity in tendons and major arteries; abnormal lung development; abnormal structure and pigmentation of hair.	Violent vomiting and diarrhea. Cooking acid foods in unlined copper pots can lead to toxic accumulation of copper.

Mineral	Sources	Function	Deficiency	Excess
Zinc	Meat; liver; eggs; poultry; seafood; followed by milk and whole grains.	Constituent of about 100 enzymes.	Delayed wound healing; diminished taste sensation; loss of appetite. In children: failure to grow and mature sexually. Prenatally: abnormal brain development.	Nausea, vomiting; anemia; bleeding in stomach; premature birth and stillbirth; abdominal pain; fever. Can aggravate marginal copper deficiency. May produce atherosclerosis.
Iodine	Seafood; saltwater fish; seaweed; iodized salt; sea salt.	Part of thyroid hormones; essential for normal reproduction.	Goiter (enlarged thyroid with low hormone production). Newborns: cretinism, with retarded growth, protruding abdomen, swollen-looking features, thick lips, enlarged tongue. Persons living far from sea coast should use iodized salt to prevent deficiency.	Not known to be a problem, but could cause iodine poisoning or sensitivity reaction.
Fluorine	Fish; tea; most animal foods; fluoridated water; foods grown with or cooked in fluoridated water.	Formation of strong, decay-resistant teeth; maintenance of bone strength.	Excessive dental decay; possibly osteoporosis.	Mottling of teeth and bones; in larger doses, a deadly poison.
Chromium	Meat; cheese; whole-grain breads and cereals; dried beans; peanuts; brewer's yeast.	Metabolism of glucose.	Possibly, abnormal sugar metabolism (chemical diabetes) and adult-onset diabetes.	Not known.

Table continues on next page

Table 9.1 continued

Best sources	Main roles	Deficiency symptoms	Risks of megadoses
Trace minerals			
Selenium			
Seafood; whole-grain cereals; meat; egg yolk; chicken; milk; garlic.	Antioxidant, preventing break-down of fats and other body chemicals; interacts with vitamin E.	Not known in human beings. Animals: degeneration of pancreas. Parts of country where selenium is low have higher cancer rates and more deaths from high blood pressure.	Animals: "blind staggers"—stiffness, lameness, hair loss, blindness, death.
Manganese			
Nuts; whole grains; vegetables and fruits; tea; instant coffee; cocoa powder.	Functioning of central nervous system; normal bone structure; reproduction; part of important enzymes.	Not known in human beings. Animals: poor reproduction; retarded growth; birth defects; abnormal bone development.	Masklike facial expression; blurred speech; involuntary laughing; spastic gait; hand tremors.
Molybdenum			
Legumes; cereal grains; liver; kidney; some dark-green vegetables.	Part of the enzyme xanthine oxidase.	Not known in human beings. Animals: decreased weight gain; shortened life span.	Goutlike syndrome; loss of copper.

Table 9.2 • MINERALS AND TRACE ELEMENTS:
RECOMMENDED DAILY DIETARY ALLOWANCES (RDAS)

Ages	Calcium (mg)	Phosphorus (mg)	Magnesium (mg)	Iron (mg)	Zinc (mg)	Iodine (μg)*
Infants						
To 6 months	360	240	50	10	3	40
6 months–1 year	540	360	70	15	5	50
Children						
1–3	800	800	150	15	10	70
4–6	800	800	200	10	10	90
7–10	800	800	250	10	10	120
Males						
11–14	1,200	1,200	350	18	15	150
15–18	1,200	1,200	400	18	15	150
19 and over	800	800	350	10	15	150
Females						
11–18	1,200	1,200	300	18	15	150
19–50	1,000**	800	300	18	15	150
51 and over	1,500**	800	300	10	15	150
Pregnant	+400	+400	+150	S***	+5	+25
Nursing	+400	+400	+150	S***	+10	+50

Note: These values were established in 1980 by the Food and Nutrition Board, National Academy of Sciences–National Research Council, to meet the needs of healthy people.
*μg = microgram.
**Although new RDAs were not published in 1985, Board members recommend increasing calcium intake from the 800 milligrams established in 1980.
***Since an ordinary diet cannot meet the iron needs of a pregnant or nursing woman, a daily supplement of 30 to 60 milligrams of iron is recommended.

life-sustaining roles of calcium can continue. Thus, the popular belief that a calcium deficiency can cause a wide range of constitutional symptoms, from muscle cramps to bleeding problems, is simply untrue.

What does happen when your diet is consistently short of calcium is that your bones deteriorate, causing rickets in children and osteoporosis in adults. In fact, the chronic calcium shortage, especially in the diets of women, who get only about one-third the recommended daily amount of calcium from their diets, has resulted in an epidemic of osteoporosis in older Americans. Gradually, starting in the 20s for women and somewhat later for men, calcium is lost from the bones. This loss accelerates in women after menopause, resulting in a shortening and weakening of the long bones and greatly increasing their sus-

Table 9.3 • MINERALS AND TRACE ELEMENTS:
ESTIMATED SAFE AND ADEQUATE DAILY DIETARY INTAKES

Ages	Copper (mg)	Man-ganese (mg)	Fluoride (mg)	Chromium (mg)	Selenium (mg)	Molyb-denum (mg)	Sodium (mg)	Potassium (mg)	Chloride (mg)
Infants									
To 6 months	0.5–0.7	0.5–0.7	0.1–0.5	.01–.04	.01–.04	.03–.06	115–350	350–925	275–700
6 months–1 year	0.7–1.00	0.7–1.0	0.2–1.0	.02–.06	.02–.06	.04–.08	250–750	425–1,275	400–1,200
Children and Adolescents									
1–3	1.0–1.5	1.0–1.5	0.5–1.5	.02–.08	.02–.08	.05–.10	325–975	550–1,650	500–1,500
4–6	1.5–2	1.5–2.0	1.0–2.5	.03–.12	.03–.12	.06–.15	450–1,350	775–2,325	700–2,100
7–10	2.0–2.5	2.0–3.0	1.5–2.5	.05–.20	.05–.20	.10–.30	600–1,800	1,000–3,000	925–2,775
11 and over	2.0–3.0	2.5–5.0	1.5–2.5	.05–.20	.05–.20	.15–.50	900–2,700	1,525–4,575	1,400–4,200
Adults									
	2.0–3.0	2.5–5.0	1.5–4.0	.05–.20	.05–.20	.15–.50	1,100–3,300	1,875–5,625	1,700–5,100

Note: These figures were established in 1980 by the Food and Nutrition Board of the National Academy of Sciences–National Research Council. They represent the range of recommended daily intakes for healthy persons. Lack of adequate data prevented the board from establishing more precise amounts. The board cautions, however, that for many of the substances listed above, toxic levels are only a few times greater than the amount needed for good nutrition. Therefore, the upper levels of the ranges given should not be exceeded on a regular basis.

ceptibility to fractures. Osteoporosis, which afflicts one in four American women past menopause, causes a loss of height with age because spinal vertebrae collapse, producing the not-so-legendary dowager's hump. It is the primary cause of the debilitating hip and wrist fractures that so commonly afflict older women. And it may also be a factor in bone loss in the jaws, which leads ultimately to a loss of teeth through periodontal disease.

Although millions of women are now dosing themselves (sometimes at a doctor's suggestion) with large amounts of calcium supplements, the evidence that such supplements can prevent or stem the progress of osteoporosis is hardly substantial. The supplements do seem to help some, but by no means all, people who take them. Dietary calcium—that is, calcium from foods (see Table 9.4)—is much better absorbed and used by the body than are supplements. Furthermore, no supplement can replace calcium already lost from the bones; at best, it can only slow their further deterioration.

Many factors besides the amount of calcium you consume influence how much of this mineral enters and remains in your body. Vitamin D in an activated form is needed for calcium to be absorbed through the intestinal tract, and older people make less of the active form of this vitamin. Vitamin C improves calcium absorption, as does lactose (milk sugar). But eating too much protein or fat interferes with calcium absorption and greatly increases the amount of calcium your body loses. Inactivity also speeds the loss of calcium. In fact, physical exercise throughout life helps prevent bone loss with age. Some foods contain substances that bind up the calcium these foods contain in a way that prevents the mineral's absorption. These substances include oxalic acid in spinach, chard, beet greens, and rhubarb and phytic acid in the bran of whole grains. However, in an ordinary balanced diet that contains adequate amounts of calcium, such binding is not believed to interfere seriously with the amount of calcium your body obtains. Oxalic and phytic acids do not block absorption of calcium from other foods. Furthermore, the amount of oxalic acid in chocolate is insufficient to significantly affect calcium absorption from milk.

Excess phosphorus, a companion mineral to calcium in your bones, can increase the need for calcium and thus create a shortage even though you may be consuming calcium in adequate amounts. This may be a problem among teenagers who drink too much soda pop (rich in phosphorus) and adults who consume no milk or milk products. A newborn given too much phosphorus relative to the amount of calcium can develop a condition called hypocalcemic tetany. This is more likely to happen if the baby is fed cow's milk, which contains a higher ratio of phosphorus to calcium than breast milk does.

In addition to dietary factors, loss of estrogen at menopause greatly accelerates the loss of calcium from a woman's bones. This rapid loss continues for about three to ten years after menopause, and can be slowed and often halted by estrogen replacement therapy. This hormone treatment, however, can also increase a woman's risk of developing cancer of the endometrium, the lining of the uterus, and any woman who takes postmenopausal hormones is advised to submit to periodic medical examinations to be sure her uterus is not adversely affected. The cancer risk also can be minimized by using a combination of estrogen and progestin, which may result in menstrual-like bleeding once a month.

The need for calcium is greatest during periods of growth—in childhood and adolescence and during pregnancy and lactation. A growing child may need, per unit body weight, two to three times as much calcium as an adult. The percent of calcium absorbed varies with the need, so that children absorb a far greater proportion of the calcium in their diets than adults do. However, you never outgrow your need for calcium.

Consumption of the richest sources of calcium—milk and milk products—has been falling in recent decades. A cup of milk or yogurt or an ounce of hard cheese provides a quarter to a third of the recommended daily amount for adults. (But cottage cheese is only a third as good as milk as a calcium source.) Those who don't like to drink milk might try disguising it in puddings, cereal, baked goods (as the liquid or as nonfat dry-milk solids), ice cream, or ice milk. For those with milk allergy, the enzyme lactase can be used to predigest the lactose in milk, or special milks like soy or acidophilus milk can be substituted (see Chapter 13 for more details). See Table 9.4 for other calcium sources. Keep in mind, however, that typical one-a-day type supplements and fortified food products rarely contain more than a few percent of the USRDA for calcium.

Iron

Between the exhortations of mothers and the persuasion of pharmaceutical advertising, it would be hard not to know about the importance of the trace mineral iron. Who has not heard of "tired blood," with the image (incorrect) it creates of a sluggish stream of vital red fluid barely able to make it through arteries and veins? Iron—or, rather,

Table 9.4 • CALCIUM-RICH FOODS

Item	Serving size	Calcium (mg)
Yogurt, plain lowfat	1 cup	415
Sardines, with bones	3 ounces	372
Ricotta, part skim	½ cup	337
Skim milk	1 cup	302
Whole milk	1 cup	291
Swiss cheese	1 ounce	262
Cheddar cheese	1 ounce	213
American cheese	1 ounce	198
Oysters	¾ cup	170
Salmon, canned with bones	3 ounces	167
Collard greens	½ cup	145
Spinach, cooked	½ cup	106
Mustard greens, cooked	½ cup	97
Corn muffin	2 medium	90
Ice cream	½ cup	88
Cottage cheese, 2% fat	½ cup	77
Kale, cooked	½ cup	74
Broccoli, cooked	½ cup	68
Orange	1 medium	54

Source: Based on data in Agriculture Handbooks Nos. 8 and 456.

lack of iron—is supposed to cause this "slowdown," and Geritol and its iron-containing competitors are just the tonic you're told you need to get that stream flowing again at its normally brisk pace.

Although iron-deficiency anemia (in which your blood is not tired, but *you* are) is the nation's most common nutritional deficiency, self-treatment with iron-containing elixirs and tablets is an unwise course to follow if you suspect you are anemic. As *Consumer Reports* pointed out in its September, 1978, article on iron supplements, "anyone whose blood is not 'normal' should be under a doctor's care, not under the care of commercial pitchmen. Treatment of iron-deficiency anemia requires therapeutic doses of iron, which are larger than the supplemental doses used to offset a marginal diet. Self-diagnosis, moreover, is a tricky business. Weakness, listlessness, and the tendency to tire easily can signal a number of conditions other than anemia. Furthermore, all anemias are not due to iron deficiency."

Popeye's propaganda notwithstanding, spinach is not the best source of iron (walnuts and pistachio nuts have more), and the iron it contains interacts with oxalic acid to form a poorly absorbed compound (see Table 9.1 for other sources). Cooking in cast-iron pots—especially foods, such as tomato sauce, that are acidic—can add significant amounts of iron to your diet.

In general, the iron from animal foods is better absorbed than that from vegetable foods. From 15 to 30 percent of the iron in meats and fish is absorbed, compared to only 5 percent from vegetable sources. Absorption is enhanced by diets containing meat, fish, poultry, and citrus fruits, the latter because of their vitamin C content. Eating a vitamin-C–rich vegetable or fruit along with foods containing iron will increase the iron you get from your meals. Possible combinations include beef and potatoes, pork and tomatoes, and an iron-enriched cereal and orange juice. On the other hand, eggs or tea consumed at the same meal can prevent much of vegetable-derived iron from being absorbed. (However, a new study by the U.S. Department of Agriculture showed that contrary to common belief, wheat bran does not interfere with iron absorption.)

Since only a small percentage of the iron consumed is absorbed, your diet must contain substantially more iron than your body actually needs. The typical diet consumed by adult Americans provides about 6 milligrams of iron for every 1,000 calories. Thus, someone eating 2,000 to 3,000 calories a day would take in 12 to 18 milligrams of iron, more than enough to meet the needs of an adult male. But the average woman eats only 1,500 calories a day, which adds up to only 9 milligrams of iron, half the amount recommended for menstruating women.

The body can store a fair amount of iron in the liver, bone marrow, spleen, and other organs. But when the diet is chronically short of needed iron, these stores are eventually used up. Infants, young children, adolescents, and women of childbearing age are most likely to be short on dietary iron. The need for iron is increased by growth, pregnancy, lactation, and menstruation, and such individuals may not eat enough iron-rich food to fulfill their greater need. As a result, about 5 percent of American women have mild iron-deficiency anemia.

Iron deficiency may also develop in strict vegetarians, who derive all their iron from vegetable sources; in dieters who drastically reduce their caloric intake; and in persons who subsist largely on foods that are high in fats, sugar, and calories but low in nutrients. Otherwise, anemia in men and in women past menopause is rarely related to an iron deficiency. More likely it's the result of an internal bleeding problem that demands prompt medical attention. It may take months or years for symptoms of iron deficiency to develop, but as anemia worsens the symptoms may include easy fatigue, weakness, pallor, and shortness of breath. A blood test will reveal small, pale red blood cells. Adults with iron deficiency are not able to work as hard as they normally would, and children may have a decreased attention span and decreased learning ability which disappear when proper levels of iron are restored.

Iron supplements are commonly prescribed for infants, very young children, and women who are pregnant or nursing. Women with heavy menstrual periods and men and women who are frequent blood donors may also need an iron supplement. This need is best determined by a physician on the basis of a blood test. It is generally advisable for all women who menstruate to have a routine blood test every few years.

Other than through bleeding, the body has no way to get rid of significant amounts of excess iron. Periodic overdoses are stored for future needs, but when overdoses are chronic, the extra iron can build up to toxic levels. The result may be a condition called methemo-chromatosis that can damage the liver, pancreas, and heart. Excess iron may also increase the likelihood of developing bacterial and fungal infections, and it can make such infections more severe because it provides the iron these organisms need to grow.

The body tries to protect itself from an iron overdose by reducing the amount absorbed through the intestinal tract when its needs are satisfied. But this regulatory mechanism is far from perfect, and more iron can be absorbed than is needed. Thus, self-treatment with potent iron supplements can cause more harm than good. See a doctor before you decide to take extra iron.

Mineral Megadoses

A 46-year-old actress had suffered for three years from weird, debilitating symptoms, including muscular weakness, weight loss, and severe abdominal pain. Her career was destroyed and she could barely walk before doctors realized she was suffering from lead poisoning as a result of taking bone meal, prescribed by her doctor for menstrual cramps. Her myth-driven effort to preserve her health by taking mega-doses of calcium and other minerals in the form of bone meal had backfired completely. She hadn't known—and none of the twenty-two doctors she saw thought to ask—that bone meal could be hazardous. However, since bones help to protect the body from toxic substances like lead by removing them from the blood and storing them, bone meal can be a source of dangerous substances.

Many minerals themselves are toxic in large doses. For some, the body insists on a critical balance among them to function effectively. If this balance is disrupted by a megadose of one mineral, a relative shortage of another may be the result. For example, too much phosphorus increases the need for calcium and may produce a calcium deficiency even if you're consuming calcium in recommended amounts. Other minerals, such as iron and magnesium, can be stored in the body and may build up to produce toxic symptoms. And most of the so-called trace minerals, which are needed in only *micro* quantities, are deadly poisons in doses much beyond the amounts essential for good nutritional health (see Table 9.1).

Oddly, the very same people who promote megadoses of essential minerals often condemn one of them—*fluorine*—as a lethal poison even in minute quantities. Yet fluorine is one of the few minerals that, when added to the diet as fluoride in very small amounts, has been proved to promote health by greatly reducing the likelihood of tooth decay. Children living in areas where the water is not fluoridated should be given fluoride supplements, according to the American Dental Association. (But avoid chewable tablets containing sugar since they may partly defeat the purpose.)

Zinc, a mineral that does have established uses in megadose amounts, is usually taken by self-dosers for the wrong reasons. Zinc supplements can benefit persons with vision problems resulting from alcohol-caused cirrhosis of the liver; it can also help men on kidney dialysis machines who become sexually impotent. However, for ordinary cases of impotence, zinc has no known value. Zinc supplements are useful to patients with an inherited disorder called acrodermatitis enteropathica, which can interfere with zinc absorption.

The rest of us really should be worrying, not about megadoses of zinc, but about obtaining enough of this vital trace mineral to avoid a dietary deficiency. Much zinc is lost from foods during processing. Many American infants and children from middle-income as well as low-income families, have marginal zinc deficiencies; for others, zinc intake is only barely adequate. Researchers from the University of Colorado Medical Center have shown that if cereals were fortified with zinc, they could go a long way toward correcting this problem. See Table 9.1 for foods naturally rich in this trace mineral.

Addendum to the Micronutrients: Liver

From the listings of main sources of the various vitamins and minerals, several types of foods stand out as particularly rich in a number of essential micronutrients: dark-green vegetables, whole grains, milk, meat, and—you guessed it—liver.

Liver is like a multivitamin-mineral tablet on your dinner plate (see Table 9.5 for nutrient content). Yet, because it is very high in cholesterol (you may recall that the liver is an animal's main production site for cholesterol), it is not a favorite among nutrition-conscious physicians. And because it's an organ tissue and different in taste and texture from muscle meats, many consumers find it less than appetizing, except perhaps when it's "disguised" in a well-spiced and fatted pâté.

But because of its micronutrient strength, unless you're on a strict low-cholesterol diet, it would be worth your nutritional while to learn to like liver, learn to prepare it well, and eat it, say, once every week or two. You don't need a big serving—2 to 3 ounces provide a healthy supply of iron and other often-needed vitamins and minerals. If you're a menstruating female, liver is most important to you because it's a rich iron source. An iron tablet may upset your stomach, make you constipated, give you diarrhea, or stimulate your appetite. But a piece of liver can be a gourmet delight.

There's no need to pay a fortune for calf's liver, which may cost $3 to $4 a pound. Pork liver is twice as rich in iron as calf's liver and much cheaper. Ordinary beef liver, while a third lower in iron content

Table 9.5 • LIVER: DINING ON A MICRONUTRIENT
"SUPPLEMENT"*

Nutrient	Amount in 3 ounces	% daily intake
Calories	195	10
Protein	22.4 grams	51
Fat	9.0 grams	14
Carbohydrates	4.5 grams	2
Cholesterol	372 milligrams	124
Sodium	156 milligrams	7
Vitamin A	9,078 retinol equivalents	1,134
Thiamin	.22 milligram	22
Riboflavin	3.56 milligrams	296
Niacin	14 milligrams	107
Vitamin C	23 milligrams	38
Iron	7.5 milligrams	42
Phosphorus	405 milligrams	50

*This is a list of the nutrient content of a 3-ounce serving of fried beef liver (according to Agriculture Handbook No. 456) and what proportion of the recommended daily intake of the various nutrients it provides for a woman between the ages of 23 and 50.

than calf's liver, is—at less than $1 a pound—a main-course bargain
that can be almost as delectable when properly cooked. Chicken liver
costs more but some find its texture more pleasing. It rivals beef liver
in nutrient content. Here is one simple suggestion:

Jane's Quick and Easy Smothered Liver

Vegetable oil or margarine
1 medium onion, sliced
Freshly ground black pepper,
  to taste

Herbs and/or spices (optional)
2–3 ounces liver, about ½ inch
  thick
Salt (optional)

Coat the skillet with the oil (I use a brush) or margarine. Sauté the
onion slices, and season with pepper to taste (plus any other herb or spice
you desire). Sprinkle the liver lightly with salt (if desired) and as much
pepper as you please. After a few minutes, when the onions are soft, push
them to one side and add the liver. (You may need to brush the skillet
with oil again before adding the liver.) As the liver fries, flip the onions
so they brown lightly. After the liver browns on one side, turn and cook
a few minutes longer. *Warning:* Liver cooks quickly and is most tender and
tasty when not overdone. To serve, smother the liver with the onions. Yield:
1 serving. Simply multiply quantities for 2 or more. If you are preparing this
dish for people with different desires about doneness, cut the liver into serving
portions before you cook it and leave some pieces in the pan longer than
others.

10 ⚬ SALT: IS THE PILLAR
ABOUT TO COLLAPSE?

S ALT, A CHEMICAL that combines the elements sodium and chlorine, has occupied a premier position in human society since prehistoric times. The Bible speaks approvingly of "the salt of the earth." A good Greek slave was said to be "worth his weight in salt." Salt has been bartered, used for pay, and fought over. A tax on it was sure to bring violent protest. It was once literally worth its weight in gold, traded ounce for ounce. Until early in this century, Ethiopia used salt disks for currency.

According to Dr. Marilyn S. Fregley, behavioral scientist at the University of Florida,* salt was one of our first medicines. It was rubbed on newborn babies in Biblical times to ward off evil spirits, and even now Roman Catholics place salt in the mouth of a child at baptism as a symbol of purity and incorruptibility. Salt has also been a traditional symbol of social status. The most important guests at the dinner table were seated "above the salt." It has truly been the king of seasonings.

In recent years, however, research has linked excessive consumption of salt to *hypertension* (high blood pressure) and its potentially fatal consequences, heart and kidney disease and stroke. Hypertension, one of the nation's most widespread serious diseases, afflicts an estimated 60 million Americans, usually producing no symptoms until one day the signs of permanent organ damage suddenly appear as a chronic illness or death. The main precipitant of hypertension, the weight of evidence indicates, is the mineral sodium, which is 40 percent of the salt molecule by weight. Between 15 and 20 percent of Americans are genetically prone to developing high blood pressure if their diet is rich in sodium, as the typical American diet is.

Hypertension is practically nonexistent in cultures that exist in New Guinea, the Amazon Basin, the Kalahari Desert, and elsewhere, where little or no salt is added to foods. In such cultures—unlike our

*In *Biological and Behavioral Aspects of Salt Intake,* ed. Morley R. Kare (New York: Academic Press, 1980).

own—blood pressure does not "naturally" rise with age; if anything, it drops. Some say it is lack of stress, not lack of salt, that keeps the lid on blood pressure in these cultures. But in a few preindustrial societies, such as the Gashgai nomads of southern Iran, where a lot of salt is consumed, high blood pressure is common despite the lack of societal tensions. On the other hand, in societies where salt and sodium are consumed to great excess, such as in Japan, hypertension is the leading cause of death and disability. Further, the ravages of hypertension are greatest in northern Japan, where salt consumption is highest (see Chart 9).

When 1,346 Americans were grouped according to salt intake, more than 10 percent of those who consumed a lot of salt were found to have high blood pressure, 7 percent of those who consumed an average amount of salt had the condition, but less than 1 percent of those who consumed a small amount of salt had hypertension. A five-year study at the Mayo Clinic showed that sodium restriction alone could lower blood pressure to normal in persons with mild hypertension.

Studies of laboratory rats suggest that excess salt early in life can set the stage for later development of high blood pressure. If rats that are genetically predisposed to hypertension are never given salt, their blood pressure remains normal throughout life. But those that get salt early in life develop hypertension even if the salt is later eliminated from the diet. Unfortunately, it is not possible to determine in advance which people are susceptible to the pressure-raising effects of salt.

What Sodium Does

Of course, sodium is a vital constituent of the human body. Our tissues swim in a salty sea—a vestige, perhaps, of our aquatic evolution. The more salt in that sea, the more water is needed to dilute it to maintain the proper concentration of sodium. Sodium and its equally essential companion chloride (the combining form of chlorine) are the principal regulators of the balance of water and dissolved substances outside cells. You'll recall (from Chapter 9) that this is the job potassium does within cells. These three minerals—called electrolytes—also regulate the balance of acids and bases in body fluids and cells. If the balance of water and electrolytes or acids and bases is disturbed, normal metabolic functions may grind to a near halt.

Eating something salty makes you thirsty because when salt is

Chart 9 • HOW SALT LEADS TO HIGH BLOOD PRESSURE

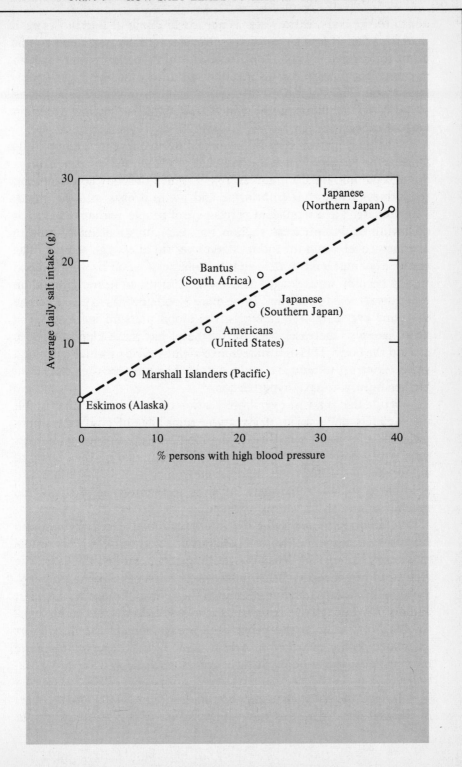

added to the body, extra water is needed to dilute it. Bartenders cash in on this fact of human physiology by offering salty nuts and pretzels gratis to patrons. It's good for business. And if you lose water through sweating, the increased concentration of salt in your blood also stimulates thirst. The "purpose" of thirst is to keep the body functioning properly by maintaining the concentration of salt within a certain narrow range.

The body's machinery for keeping a normal level of sodium in its fluids is the *kidneys*. When the body has too much sodium, the kidneys dump it out into the urine and excrete it. When the body needs sodium, the kidneys reabsorb it from urine and pump it back into the blood. Unfortunately, in a significant percentage of people, perhaps as a result of having to dump excess sodium for years, this machinery fails to operate properly and the kidneys don't get rid of enough sodium. The retained sodium holds water, and the volume of blood rises. The blood vessels become water-logged and more sensitive to nerve stimulation that causes them to contract. Since more blood now has to pass through the same ever-narrower channels, the blood pressure increases. The heart rate also increases because the heart has more blood to pump around the body. This in turn sets up a vicious cycle in which the blood vessels contract to reduce the blood flow. The pressure then rises even further until you have hypertension.

While this is a vast oversimplification of a mechanism that is still incompletely understood, it gives you some idea of how excess consumption of sodium can cause high blood pressure in susceptible persons. Stress adds further to the problem by stimulating the release of an adrenal-gland hormone, aldosterone, which signals the kidneys to hold on to sodium and water. But even in the absence of stress, too much sodium can do serious damage.

In addition to increasing the volume of blood, excess sodium also increases the amount of water in and around body tissues. This results in swelling, or *edema*. When the swelling occurs around the heart, the result can be congestive heart failure—the heart can't pump properly. Swelling in the legs may interfere with the return of blood to the heart and result in difficulty walking and a tendency to form clots in the veins. Swelling of tissues in the pelvic region can increase the discomfort associated with menstruation. And swelling of tissues surrounding the brain may cause emotional disturbances, such as depression and irritability.

In fact, the body's tendency to retain sodium just before the start of the menstrual period is the primary cause of premenstrual weight gain and the distressing symptoms of *premenstrual tension*—bloating, headache, and irritability. Many women find that they crave salt just before their period. If they satisfy that craving, it just makes matters worse because their tissues swell even more than they might otherwise. For women bothered by premenstrual problems and menstrual cramps, doctors recommend a low-salt diet for a week to ten days before the period is due.

It's long been known that pregnant women frequently have salt cravings (witness the infamous desire for pickles in the middle of the night). And it's recently been shown in laboratory rats that oral contraceptives, which mimic the hormonal state of pregnancy, increase the animals' appetite for salt. This, then, may explain the weight gain commonly associated with taking the birth control pill. Without even realizing it, women on the pill may consume more salt, and this in turn holds more water in their bodies. The extra pounds, then, are not fat but water weight.

Too much sodium in body fluids also causes water and potassium to be drawn out of the body's cells. You've undoubtedly noticed what happens when you sprinkle salt on cucumbers or lettuce. They *wilt* because the water in their cells is drawn out by the salt. The same thing happens to your body's cells if the sodium concentration in the fluid that surrounds them is too high. "Wilted" cells simply don't function properly. If they happen to be muscle cells, your muscles can't contract normally and you feel weak and tired (see Chapter 23).

We Eat Too Much Salt

After sugar, salt is our leading food additive, both in factory and home cooking. The average American consumes 10 to 20 grams, or about 2 to 4 teaspoons, of salt a day. That adds up to 15 pounds a year. *But the actual physiological requirement for sodium—220 milligrams a day—is the amount in only a tenth of a teaspoon of salt.* To be on the safe side, the suggested RDA for sodium is many times greater—for adults, 1,100 to 3,300 milligrams of sodium, or 3 to 8 grams of salt (1 teaspoon is about 5 grams). This amount should cover sodium requirements under nearly every circumstance. For youngsters the recommended amount of sodium is much lower (see Table 9.3, on page 190, for the sodium RDA for children).

Yet according to surveys by the Food and Drug Administration, infants in this country consume enough sodium to equal an adult dose of 18 grams of salt a day, and toddlers get the equivalent of a whopping 25 grams. Although food processors recently reduced or eliminated the amount of salt in baby foods, those foods prepared for adults or made at home for baby are still salted to suit an adult's tastes.

In recommending that Americans reduce their daily salt intake to 5 grams, the McGovern committee chose a level at which far fewer persons would develop high blood pressure than currently do. But if you want to get down to the level at which virtually no hypertension occurs, consumption should drop to less than a gram of salt a day.

Dr. Mark Hegsted, head of the Human Nutrition Center of the U.S. Department of Agriculture, notes that the current level of salt intake among Americans is about half the toxic dose. He remarked, "Common sense tells even the uninitiated that it is wise to limit salt intake. Indeed, if salt were a new food additive, it is doubtful that it would be classified as safe and certainly not at the level most of us consume."

When you add up the amount of salt you eat, it's not enough to count only what you add to foods when you cook them or at the table. Some of the sodium in your diet is already in food as it comes from earth and animal, but about two-thirds of it comes from processed "convenience" foods (see pages 206–207 and Tables 10.1 and 10.2).

Enough sodium is naturally present in foods and water to meet the needs of practically everyone. The only exceptions are persons who labor or exercise strenuously for long periods in hot weather. If more than 3 quarts of fluid are lost through sweating (which amounts to about a 6-pound weight loss), then extra salt is needed. According to the recommendations of the Food and Nutrition Board of the National Academy of Sciences, the first 3 quarts of lost sweat should be replaced with plain water. But for each additional quart beyond 3, you'll need an extra 2 grams (about ⅓ teaspoon) to 7 grams of salt, depending on how adapted you are to the climate.

Too much salt can impair athletic performance because it draws water out of your muscle cells and into the spaces outside cells. For optimum muscle function during vigorous exercise, the cells should be filled with water (see Chapter 23).

Failure to replace needed sodium can result in such deficiency symptoms as severe muscle cramps, extreme weakness, nausea, and diarrhea. Sodium deficiency is most likely to occur in persons unaccustomed to exercising hard and long in hot, humid weather. However, when you become adapted to such a climate, your kidneys and sweat glands learn to conserve water and sodium, and the risk of sodium deficiency is greatly reduced.

The Sahara Bedouins consume no salt other than what's in the brackish water they drink. In essence, they are on a low-salt diet, despite their desert environment, and Dr. Claude Paque, a Moroccan physician and anthropologist, found they suffer no ill effects from the heat. Their bodies have learned so well to conserve water and sodium that they hardly sweat at all!

Whether you are adapted or not to the heat, *beware of salt tablets.* They provide too concentrated a dose of salt in relation to the amount of water you're likely to consume. The result is further dehydration of your body's cells. Unless prescribed by a physician for a specific condition, such as heat cramps, salt tablets are dangerous and should not be taken.

Our Salt Appetite Is Acquired

Despite its long and colorful history, salt is a relatively recent addition to the human diet. From what can be determined of the diets of early man and his primate ancestors, we evolved on a diet that was very low in sodium and high in potassium, the latter coming mainly from fruits and vegetables. Our vegetarian ancestors consumed between $2/10$ and $6/10$ gram (200 to 600 milligrams) of salt a day and even heavy meat-eaters reached only about 4 grams of salt on good hunting days. This is no doubt why the human excretory machinery is set up to conserve sodium and to get rid of potassium.

Newborn babies grimace when given something salty to taste, and an infant's consumption of strained foods is certainly not reduced if no salt is added. But young children in this country soon acquire a taste for salt. In one recent study, preschool children selected a salted beef stew over an unsalted one. By adolescence, the taste for salt is firmly established. Note the teenager's tolerance—some would call it a craving —for salty snack foods. Unless intercepted by medical proscription, this early adaptation to highly salted foods continues throughout adulthood.

Dr. Lot B. Page of Newton Lower Falls, Massachusetts, a hypertension specialist who participated in a large and continuing study of salt in the diets of preindustrial peoples, concludes that "it's clear that salt appetite is determined by early dietary habits and has no relationship to salt need." He has found that populations with low blood pressure who have lived for many generations "in desert, arctic and jungle environments use less than two grams per day of sodium. In spite of heavy labor, sweating and breast feeding, they have never suffered from any deficiency state."

Dr. Fregley points out that when the Siriono Indians, a Bolivian hunting tribe, were first introduced to salt by an American cattle rancher, they found it distasteful. But later they developed a craving for it. "This would seem to indicate that once some people are conditioned to salt, they cling to its use stubbornly and may go to great lengths to fulfill an appetite beyond physiological necessity," she concluded.

Hidden Sources of Sodium

When you "want something salty," you may reach for a snack like salted crackers or nuts, pretzels or potato chips. And no one needs to be told that foods like pickles, herring, anchovies, soy sauce, and sauerkraut are loaded with salt. But do you think of cheese, cereals, bread, meat, pudding, pancakes, soups, canned vegetables, tomato juice, and tuna fish as salty foods? Probably not. Yet they're heavily laced with salt and other sources of sodium, including leavening agents, baking powder and baking soda, and such additives as sodium nitrate, sodium phosphate, sodium ascorbate, monosodium glutamate (MSG), and even sodium saccharin, to name but a few.

Sodium levels are naturally high in such *vegetables* as spinach, celery, beets, turnips, kale, and artichokes just as they come from the earth. Dairy products, too, are naturally high in sodium. Half a cup of cottage cheese has as much sodium as 32 potato chips. And your *drinking water* may also be an important hidden source of sodium. In some localities, particularly in the South, sodium levels in water from the tap can be as high as 400 milligrams in an 8-ounce cup. In a Massachusetts town where the water contained 100 parts per million of sodium, high-school students had higher blood-pressure readings than in a comparable town where the drinking water contained only 8 parts per million.

But the heavy use of salt in *processed foods,* which today account for 55 percent of the food Americans eat, is the main cause for concern. The amounts of salt used are large and the pattern of use so pervasive that consumers can't do anything to avoid it short of not eating the products.

Salt as a flavoring agent or flavor enhancer in processed foods is but one of its functions. In *baked goods,* salt is used to help control yeast action, strengthen the gluten, and reduce water absorption to make a better dough. It also improves crust color. Baking soda and baking powder are additional sources of sodium in baked goods. In *processed meats,* all of which contain large amounts of salt (1 to 2 percent by weight), salt is a preservative and it improves texture by making some of the protein soluble. Other sources of sodium in processed meats include food additives, such as phosphates, nitrates, nitrites, MSG, hydrolyzed vegetable protein, and soy isolates, as well as dry skim milk and whey solids.

In *dairy products,* in addition to the sodium naturally present, salt is added to butter as a preservative and to cheese to control ripening, prevent bacterial growth, and enhance flavor development and texture. And, of course, in *fermented foods* like pickles and sauerkraut, salt is the curing agent that preserves the food.

Canned and ready-to-eat foods increase enormously the sodium content of the natural product. Fresh garden peas contain only 2 milligrams of sodium in a 3½-ounce serving, but the same portion of canned peas has 236 milligrams. The same with canned asparagus: there are 4 milligrams of sodium in six fresh spears and 410 milligrams in six canned spears. *And while canning increases the sodium content of vegetables so dramatically, it decreases the amount of potassium in the food.* This is particularly unfortunate because potassium has some protective effect in warding off high blood pressure. Vegetarians, who generally consume a low-sodium, high-potassium diet, tend to have considerably lower blood pressure than other Americans their age.

Some other sodium surprises in processed foods include the following facts, cited recently by *Consumer Reports:*

• 1 ounce of Kellogg's Corn Flakes has nearly twice the amount of sodium as an ounce of Planters Cocktail Peanuts, 260 milligrams versus 132.

• 2 slices of Pepperidge Farm White Bread have more sodium than a 1-ounce bag of Lay's Potato Chips, 234 milligrams versus 191.

• ½ cup of prepared Jell-O Chocolate Flavor Instant Pudding & Pie Filling has more sodium than 3 slices of Oscar Mayer Sugar-cured Bacon, 404 milligrams versus 302.

When salt is added to processed foods, the label has to say so, but it doesn't have to say *how much.* In trying to cut down on salt by avoiding only those foods that taste salty, you may actually be choosing to eat foods that contain even more sodium than the ones you shunned. Table 10.1 and Table 10.2 show the sodium content of common food

Table 10.1 • HOW MUCH SODIUM IS IN PROCESSED FOODS?

Product	Amount	Sodium (mg)
Breads and Cereals		
Pepperidge Farm White Bread	2 slices	234
Wonder Enriched Bread	2 slices	355
Pepperidge Farm Whole Wheat Bread	2 slices	214
Hungry Jack Extra Lights Pancakes	3 (4-inch)	1,150
Kellogg's Corn Flakes	1 ounce	320
Cheerios	1 ounce	330
Kellogg's Special K	1 ounce	227
Kellogg's Sugar Frosted Flakes	1 ounce	186
Soups and Beverages		
Campbell's Tomato Soup	10-ounce serving	1,050
Herb-Ox Instant Broth and Seasoning	1 packet	818
Campbell's Tomato Juice	8 ounces	744
Milk	1 cup	130
Carnation's Instant Hot Cocoa Mix	1 packet (in water)	104
Lipton Vegetable Cup-a-Soup	8 ounces	1,058
Cheeses		
Breakstone's Lowfat Cottage Cheese	½ cup	435
Kraft Processed American Cheese	1 ounce	238
Kraft Cheddar Cheese	1 ounce	190
Meals and Main Courses		
Morton King Size Turkey Dinner	1 dinner	2,567
Swanson Fried Chicken Dinner	1 dinner	1,152
Swanson Turkey Dinner	1 dinner	1,735
Campbell's Beans & Franks	8 ounces	958
Chef Boyardee Frozen Cheese Pizza	6.5 ounces	925
Del Monte Tuna in Oil	3 ounces	430
Oscar Mayer Beef Franks	1 frank	425
Oscar Mayer Bologna	2 slices	450
Oscar Mayer Sugar-cured Bacon	2 slices	285
Skippy Creamy Peanut Butter	2 tablespoons	167
Jif Creamy Peanut Butter	2 tablespoons	155
Chef Boyardee Beefaroni	7.5 ounces	1,186
Vegetables		
B & M Brick Oven Baked Beans	1 cup	810

Table 10.1 continued

Product	Amount	Sodium (mg)
Del Monte Whole Green Beans	1 cup	925
Del Monte Sweet Peas	1 cup	698

Fast Foods

Product	Amount	Sodium (mg)
McDonald's Big Mac	1	962
Burger King Whopper	1	909
Burger Chef Hamburger	1	393
Arthur Treacher's Fish Sandwich	1	836
Kentucky Fried Chicken Dinner; original recipe (3 pieces of chicken)	1	2,285
McDonald's Egg McMuffin	1	914
Dairy Queen Brazier Dog	1	868
Arthur Treacher's Coleslaw	1 serving	266
McDonald's Apple Pie	1 pie	414
Burger King Vanilla Shake	1	159
McDonald's Chocolate Shake	1	329

Snacks and Condiments

Product	Amount	Sodium (mg)
Nabisco Premium Saltines	10 (1 ounce)	430
Ritz Crackers	9 (1 ounce)	285
Nabisco Wheat Thins	16 (1 ounce)	260
Lay's Potato Chips	14 (1 ounce)	230
Mister Salty Very Thin Pretzel Sticks	1 ounce	735
Planters Cocktail Peanuts	1 ounce	132
Heinz Kosher Dill Pickles	1 large	1,137
Wish-Bone Italian Dressing	1 tablespoon	315
Heinz Mustard	1 tablespoon	212
Heinz Tomato Ketchup	1 tablespoon	154

Desserts

Product	Amount	Sodium (mg)
Jell-O Chocolate Flavor Instant Pudding & Pie Filling	½ cup	480
Hostess Twinkies	1	190
Pillsbury Sugar Cookies	3	210
Pillsbury Chocolate Chip Cookies	3	140
Pillsbury Cinnamon Raisin Danish	1 serving (2 rolls)	540
Nabisco Oreo Sandwich Cookies	3	240

Note: Based on analyses by Consumers Union, the Center for Science in the Public Interest, and manufacturers.

items that are high in sodium. Data on the brand-name items were gathered by *Consumer Reports,* the McGovern committee, and the Center for Science in the Public Interest, a consumer group in Washington, D.C. A listing of the sodium content of more than 800 foods, including canned and frozen products (though not by brand name), can be obtained from the Office of Governmental and Public Affairs, Room 507 A, U.S. Department of Agriculture, Washington, D.C. 20250. Ask for the booklet "Sodium Content of Foods."

Another hidden source of sodium is drugs, particularly such over-the-counter medications as antacids. A single dose of Alka-Seltzer, for example, has 567 milligrams of sodium, a dose of Bromo Seltzer contains 762, and Sal Hepatica has 1,000.

Even pet foods are extremely high in salt, which the companies maintain they add to increase "acceptance" by canine and feline consumers. Yet carnivorous animals in the wild eat no salt other than that

Table 10.2 • HIGH-SODIUM VEGETABLES*

Food	*Amount*	*Sodium (mg)*
Artichokes	1	46
Beet greens	1 cup	110
Beets	1 cup diced	81
Carrots	1 cup sliced	51
Celery	1 cup diced	151
Chard	1 cup	125
Collards	1 cup	36
Dandelion greens	1 cup	46
Hominy (corn grits)	1 cup cooked	502
Kale	1 cup	47
Mustard greens	1 cup	25
Olives, green pickled	10 large	926
Olives, ripe	10 extra large	385
Pickles, dill	1 medium	928
Pickles, sour	1 medium	879
Sauerkraut	1 cup	1,755
Spinach	2 ounces raw	40
Spinach	1 cup cooked	90
Turnips	1 cup cubed	53

Source: U.S. Department of Agriculture, Agriculture Handbook No. 456.

*Though most vegetables are very low in sodium (less than 20 milligrams in a 1-cup serving) and thus can be consumed in unlimited quantities on a low-sodium diet, a few are naturally high in sodium and those that are pickled are very high.

which is naturally present in the animals they feed on. The salty diet for domesticated carnivores, however, may be a cause of congestive heart disease, a common problem in "middle-aged" pet dogs.

How to Break the Salt Habit

Craig Claiborne, food writer for the *New York Times* and author of many cookbooks in which the recipes suggest adding "salt to taste," describes himself as a lifelong "salt freak." He recalls as a child snitching pieces of rock salt from the ice-cream maker, and as an adult he has often feasted on whole cans of anchovies, platters of sauerkraut, and pickles. For drinks, he prefers margaritas (a cocktail in which the rim of the glass is dipped in salt), sauerkraut juice on the rocks, and occasionally a concoction of soy sauce and lime juice.

Yet when he found out recently that he had high blood pressure and would have to drastically change his diet, he broke his salt addiction almost overnight with little anguish. Although he admits to occasional lapses (particularly when dining at a friend's home), he also says that he does not suffer without salt. In fact, he has found that his sense of taste became sharper and that gradually the salt-free foods became more enjoyable and palatable.

Here are some tips on how to eat the low-sodium way.

• Start by not adding any salt at the table, and certainly never add salt before you've tasted the food. One salter-before-tasting claimed he could tell if soup needed salt just by smelling it! However, if you cook soup without salt and salt it sparingly at the table, you're likely to end up using less salt, studies show.

• Gradually reduce the amount of salt you use in cooking and baking. Start by cutting the salt in a recipe in half. Then as you get used to less and less salt, cut it in half again and again, until you find you need to add only a tiny fraction of the original amount, if any.

• Experiment with condiments, herbs, and spices, using them in place of salt. Onions, garlic, and peppers are Claiborne's favorites. Dry mustard, lemon juice, and fruits are other possibilities. The list of permissible herbs and spices is nearly endless—from allspice to thyme. Aromatic bitters can add low-sodium zest to soups, salads, vegetables, meat, and fish. (A free recipe folder for seasoning with Angostura Bitters is available from A-W Brands, Inc., 1200 Milik Street, Cartaret,

New Jersey 07008.) But don't use garlic salt, onion salt, celery salt, seasoned salt, soy sauce, MSG, Worcestershire sauce, hydrolyzed vegetable protein, or bouillon cubes since they all contain lots of sodium.

• If you're nervous about experimenting with low-salt cooking on your own, you might pick up a low-salt cookbook or two for recipe guidelines. Among the possibilities are *Craig Claiborne's Gourmet Diet,*

HOW TO SEASON YOUR FOOD WITHOUT SALT*

Meat, Fish, and Poultry

BEEF	Bay leaf, dry mustard powder, green pepper, marjoram, fresh mushrooms, nutmeg, onion, pepper, sage, thyme.
CHICKEN	Green pepper, lemon juice, marjoram, fresh mushrooms, paprika, parsley, poultry seasoning, sage, thyme.
FISH	Bay leaf, curry powder, dry mustard powder, green pepper, lemon juice, marjoram, fresh mushrooms, paprika.
LAMB	Curry powder, garlic, mint, mint jelly, pineapple, rosemary.
PORK	Apple, applesauce, garlic, onion, sage.
VEAL	Apricot, bay leaf, curry powder, ginger, marjoram, orégano.

Vegetables

ASPARAGUS	Garlic, lemon juice, onion, vinegar.
CORN	Green pepper, pimiento, fresh tomato.
CUCUMBERS	Chives, dill, garlic, vinegar.
GREEN BEANS	Dill, lemon juice, marjoram, nutmeg, pimiento.
GREENS	Onion, pepper, vinegar.
PEAS	Green pepper, mint, fresh mushrooms, onion, parsley.
POTATOES	Green pepper, mace, onion, paprika, parsley.
RICE	Chives, green pepper, onion, pimiento, saffron.
SQUASH	Brown sugar, cinnamon, ginger, mace, nutmeg, onion.
TOMATOES	Basil, marjoram, onion, orégano.

Soups

BEAN	Pinch of dry mustard powder.
MILK CHOWDERS	Peppercorns.
PEA	Bay leaf and parsley.
VEGETABLE	Vinegar, dash of sugar.

*From *Cooking without Your Salt Shaker,* by the American Heart Association (available for purchase from local chapters).

by Craig Claiborne (New York: Times Books, 1980); *The Good Age Cookbook,* by Jan Harlow, Irene Liggett, and Evelyn Mandel (Boston: Houghton-Mifflin, 1979) (highly recommended by James Beard, who had to go on a low-salt diet himself); *The Secrets of Salt-Free Cooking,* by Jeanne Jones (San Francisco: 101 Productions, 1979); *Living with High Blood Pressure: The Hypertension Diet Cookbook,* by Joyce Daly Margie and Dr. James C. Hunt (Radnor, Pa.: Chilton, 1979); *Cooking without Your Salt Shaker,* by the American Heart Association, a 145-page spiral-bound cookbook and dining-out guide that can be purchased from your local chapter of the American Heart Association; and *Gourmet Cooking without Salt* by Eleanor Bremer (New York: Doubleday, 1981).

Here's a sprinkling of saltless recipes from the American Heart Association's cookbook.

Beef Bourguignon

¼ cup flour	¼ teaspoon orégano
⅛ teaspoon pepper	⅛ teaspoon rosemary
2 pounds lean beef chuck, well-trimmed and cut into cubes	⅛ teaspoon marjoram
	1 tablespoon chopped parsley
	½ cup dry red table wine
2 tablespoons oil	1 cup water
½ cup chopped onion	2 cups finely chopped fresh tomatoes
1 garlic clove, minced	
¼ teaspoon thyme	2 cups diced raw carrots
¼ teaspoon basil	3 cups diced raw potatoes

Combine the flour and the pepper. Coat the beef with the flour and pepper mixture. Brown the meat in oil. Add the onion and garlic, and cook until tender. Pour off the fat. Add the thyme, basil, orégano, rosemary, marjoram, parsley, wine, and water. Cover and simmer 1 hour, stirring occasionally, adding more water if necessary. Add the tomatoes and simmer 1 additional hour. Add the carrots and potatoes. Simmer 30 minutes. Yield: 9 servings (210 calories per serving).

Chicken Cacciatore

¼ cup oil	4 fresh tomatoes, peeled and chopped
1 garlic clove, minced	
3 chicken breasts, cut in halves and skinned	¼ cup dry white table wine
	¼ teaspoon rosemary
1 medium onion, chopped	1 bay leaf
2 tablespoons chopped green pepper	¼ teaspoon basil
	⅛ teaspoon pepper

Heat the oil and the garlic in a large skillet. Add the chicken and brown. Remove the chicken. Add the onion and green pepper to the skillet, adding more oil if necessary. Cook until tender. Pour off the fat. Return the chicken to the skillet. Add the remaining ingredients. Cover and simmer over low heat 30 minutes, or until the chicken is tender. Remove the bay leaf before serving. May be served over rice. Yield: 6 servings (235 calories per serving).

Tomato Crown Fish

1½ cups water
2 tablespoons lemon juice
1½ pounds cod fillets
⅛ teaspoon pepper
2 large fresh tomatoes, sliced ¼ inch thick

½ medium green pepper, finely chopped
2 tablespoons chopped onion
¼ cup dry bread crumbs
½ teaspoon basil
1 tablespoon oil

Combine the water and lemon juice. Pour over the fish fillets and let them stand for 30 minutes. Drain the fillets. Place the fish in an oiled baking dish. Season with pepper. Place the tomato slices on the fish and sprinkle with green pepper and onion. Combine bread crumbs, basil, and oil, blending well. Spread the seasoned crumb mixture evenly over the tomatoes. Bake uncovered in a 350-degree oven for 25 minutes or until the fish is firm and flakes easily with a fork. Yield: 6 servings (155 calories per serving).

Potato Salad

5 medium red-skinned potatoes, cooked, peeled, and diced
¾ cup chopped celery with leaves
½ cup sliced red radishes
2 green onions (scallions), diced
½ cup mayonnaise

1 teaspoon dry mustard powder
1 tablespoon sugar
¼ teaspoon pepper
¼ teaspoon turmeric
½ teaspoon celery seed (optional)
2½ tablespoons white vinegar
3 tablespoons skim milk

Combine the potatoes, celery, radishes, and onions. In a separate bowl, mix together the mayonnaise, mustard powder, sugar, pepper, turmeric, and celery seed. Add the vinegar and milk and stir until mixed. Combine this with the potato mixture and stir well. Chill before serving. Yield: 6 servings (220 calories per serving).

• Reduce your dependence on processed foods, especially canned soups and vegetables, factory-prepared meals, processed meats, and cheeses. Substitute fresh meats and fresh or frozen vegetables and prepare them with little or no salt. If you use canned vegetables, drain off the liquid, rinse the vegetables, and cook them in fresh tap water (hardly worthwhile since many of the vitamins will be lost this way; better to use fresh or frozen vegetables). Use unsalted butter and margarine (check the frozen-foods department if they are not in the dairy case). Swiss Lorraine is lower in sodium than most other cheeses.

• Check the label on all processed foods. By the time you read this, it's likely that any food that lists "nutrition information" on the label will be required to include the amount of sodium in a serving of the product. Remember, if 2,000 milligrams of sodium is all you should be consuming in a day, 400 milligrams in your morning cereal is a large proportion of your daily total.

• If you're dependent on processed foods, look for those labeled "low sodium" or "low salt." Low-sodium versions are available of such products as processed cheeses, cottage cheese, breads, bouillon cubes, crackers, cereals, canned soups, and canned vegetables. Unfortunately, you have to pay more for the absence of salt than for its presence since these are low-volume products primarily marketed for people with special dietary needs. There is now even a reduced-salt soy sauce.

• Check with your local water district to find out how much sodium comes out of your tap. If it's higher than the 45 parts per million recommended as tops by health officials, you can buy a gadget that attaches to your faucet to filter out the sodium. But *don't use water softeners on your drinking water.* These substitute sodium for the minerals in hard water. (In fact, hard water may be good for you. People who live in areas where the water is soft tend to have a higher rate of heart disease than those living in areas where the water is hard. See Chapter 11.)

• If you are certain you do not have kidney disease, you can use salt substitutes, in which potassium chloride substitutes for sodium chloride. However, food tastes better without it.

• If you have high blood pressure, check with your doctor before taking antacids, cough preparations, laxatives, and vitamin C sold as sodium ascorbate (ascorbic acid is okay). Many of these items are high in sodium.

You may not be able to do much about the salt content of your food when you are at a party or in the home of friends. But in restaurants, you can ask for, and often get, your food prepared without added salt or sodium-containing flavorings. This means, of course, that you must order something that's individually prepared, such as fish or chicken breast or steak. For your salad, order oil and vinegar on the side and add your own dressing. Or bring a small bottle of salt-free home-made dressing with you. Skip the soup since it's nearly always well dosed with salt. Order your potatoes baked, and choose fruit for dessert.

In general, avoid fast-food restaurants. Nearly all their foods are heavily laden with sodium (see Table 10.1, page 208, and Table 21.2, page 397). On airplanes, order a low-sodium meal when you make your reservation. If you travel, you may want to stock up on your own salt-free foods in your hotel room instead of having to contend with restaurants three times a day. For a few dollars a day, most hotels will put a small refrigerator in your room.

The main disadvantage of kicking the salt habit is that the generously salted foods you may encounter when dining out will taste too salty to you. You may even find some of them inedible. But for most people, this is a small price to pay for a healthier diet.

FOR FURTHER READING

Janet James and Lois Goulder, *The Dell Color-coded Low-Salt Living Guide* (New York: Dell, 1980).

PART THREE

What to Drink

II 🌿 IS YOUR WATER FIT TO DRINK?

WATER, it may surprise you to know, is actually our most vital nutrient. It is also our most neglected one. Probably because it provides no calories, it rarely (if ever) appears on charts depicting basic nutrient requirements. Yet, we would all expire a lot sooner without water than without food.

Your insides are an internal sea. As solid as a person may look, the body is actually about two-thirds water—55 to 65 percent water for females, 65 to 75 percent water for males. The difference exists because fat, which makes up a larger proportion of a woman's body than a man's, holds less water than lean tissue does. Newborns of both sexes are about 85 percent water.

Every living cell in your body depends on water to carry out its essential functions. Through the blood and lymphatic system, water carries nutrients and oxygen to cells and removes waste products. The body eliminates these metabolic wastes through the water in sweat and urine. Water is essential to the digestion and absorption of food from the gastrointestinal tract as well as to the elimination of digestive wastes. In fact, the best treatment for constipation is to eat fibrous foods, which increase the water-holding capacity of the stool.

Water lubricates every joint in your body and keeps your soft tissues from sticking together. Water provides a protective cushion for your tissues and for the fetus during pregnancy. And water is the body's natural air-conditioning system. The loss of water through perspiration cools the body and prevents it from building up internal heat. Heat is required for the evaporation of water from your skin, and that heat comes from your body. When you're not sweating noticeably, you're probably losing what is called "insensible," or invisible, perspiration. Even if you're not moving a muscle, your body produces heat through metabolic processes that it may have to get rid of. Some water is also lost insensibly through your lungs (see Chart 10).

All told, the average adult body contains 40 to 50 quarts of water,

Chart 10 • THE INS AND OUTS OF BODY WATER

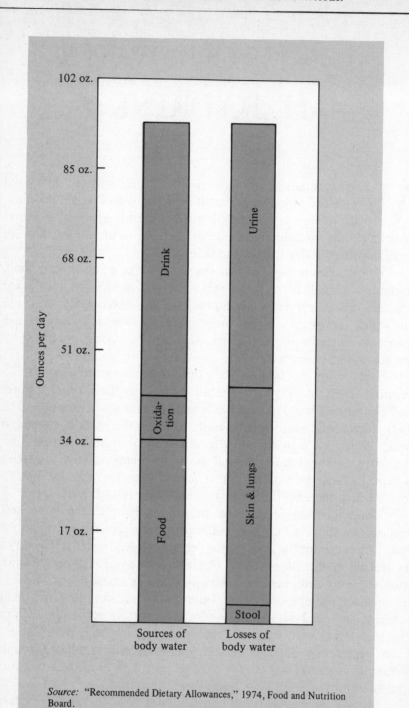

102 oz.

85 oz.

68 oz.

51 oz.

34 oz.

17 oz.

Ounces per day

Drink

Oxida-tion

Food

Urine

Skin & lungs

Stool

Sources of
body water

Losses of
body water

Source: "Recommended Dietary Allowances," 1974, Food and Nutrition Board.

with 40 percent of it inside cells. The percentage of water varies with the tissue: blood, 83 percent; muscle, 75 percent; the brain, 74 percent; and bone, 22 percent.

The water within and outside your cells contains a variety of dissolved salts which regulate the distribution of water. If the concentration of salts outside cells is higher than that inside, water moves out of the cells to try to even things out. One way to visualize this is to think of what happens when you sprinkle salt on lettuce leaves or cucumber slices. The salt draws water from the cells, causing the vegetable to wilt. In the human body, wilted cells are not very effective at carrying out their required tasks, so it's very important to properly balance your intake of water and salts. When your body has more water than it needs, it excretes the excess through the kidneys, and when water is in relatively short supply, the kidneys hold more back. But no matter how little water you may consume, the kidneys must excrete a certain amount—about 10 to 17 ounces—each day to get rid of metabolic wastes.

Thus, neither your kidneys nor your cells can function properly unless you drink enough. You can live a long time without any food (just how long depends in part on how fat you were to begin with), but after two or three days without water, death is usually imminent. With a loss of 5 percent of body water, your skin shrinks and muscles become weak; the loss of just 15 to 20 percent of body water is fatal.

Although it's possible to drink enough water to kill yourself, this only occurs in an extremely rare psychiatric disorder called psychogenic polydipsia, that has as its primary symptom compulsive water drinking. Death results not from the water itself but from the depletion and dilution of sodium in body fluids. The more common problem is *dehydration*—insufficient water intake to compensate for the amount lost. This can be caused by kidney malfunction; the loss of a great deal of blood; repeated bouts of vomiting or diarrhea; high fever; extreme physical exertion; or living in a hot, dry climate without sufficient water to replace what you lose as perspiration.

Your body lets you know when it needs more water through that well-known signal, *thirst.* At least two mechanisms are involved in this warning signal. When the blood becomes too salty, it draws water from the salivary glands. This dries your mouth and makes you feel as if you need a drink. Also, the salty blood signals the brain directly that more liquid is needed. But thirst is an imperfect signal. More than likely, it shuts off before you've drunk enough. Therefore, it's a good idea for everyone—and especially persons who are physically active—to continue drinking beyond the point of quenching thirst. Remember, *extra water can't hurt;* your body will simply get rid of whatever it doesn't need.

Where Body Water Comes From

The average adult consumes and excretes about 2½ to 3 quarts of water a day. For persons living in hot climates or engaging in strenuous physical activity, this amount may exceed 4 quarts. But, you say, "I don't drink ten glasses of liquid a day." No, you probably don't (although it couldn't hurt). More likely, only about 5 or 6 glasses are consumed directly as liquids. Most of the rest comes from the solid foods you eat, and some is derived from metabolic processes within your body.

Just as most of your solid tissues are primarily water, water forms a large percentage of the weight of most solid foods. While milk—a liquid—is 87 percent water, green beans—a solid—are 89 percent water and lettuce is 95 percent water. Even meat is half water and bread is about one-third water by weight. If you eat a lot of fruits and vegetables, you're probably consuming considerably more water than you realize, since most are more than 80 percent water.

It can be tricky trying to figure out if you're getting enough water to meet your body's needs. To be on the safe side, it's a good idea under ordinary circumstances to *drink at least six—and preferably eight— 8-ounce glasses of liquids a day.* These may include juices, soft drinks, milk, coffee, and tea as well as plain water (although coffee and tea may be counterproductive because the caffeine in them acts as a diuretic, causing the kidneys to give up more water than they would otherwise). The more physically active you are at work or at play and the hotter the climate, the more liquids you'll need.

Water and Your Health

While water itself is essential to life, some of the constituents of water can influence the quality of life.

DISEASE-CAUSING MICROORGANISMS

The most notorious of these constituents are microorganisms—. primarily bacteria and viruses. Most of us know not to drink untreated water from streams and rivers lest we ingest disease-causing organisms that were introduced upstream. Thanks to chlorination of water supplies, first introduced in Jersey City, New Jersey, in 1908, epidemics of cholera, typhoid, dysentery, and other water-borne diseases are pretty much a thing of the past in this country. But slips still occur, and experts report that more than 10,000 Americans become ill each year from infectious organisms ingested in drinking water. It is only the unusual outbreak that receives public notice. For example, 16,000 cases of paratyphoid gastroenteritis occurred among residents of Riverside, California, in 1965, apparently caused by bird droppings that fell into open holding tanks of processed city water. More recently, residents of Essex City, Vermont, were struck by an outbreak of giardiasis, an intestinal parasitic infection that was spread through the water supply (which, incidentally, met federal standards for bacterial contamination). In 1978, 32 waterborne disease outbreaks affecting 11,435 Americans were reported to federal health officials.

A national survey made in 1969 revealed that most community water supply systems failed to test their water for bacterial content often enough, and that more than 10 percent exceeded federal limits for bacterial contamination.

Sometimes, even in the best of systems, accidents occur that result in contaminated water reaching consumers. But the public is not always told of such mishaps and properly cautioned to boil all water before using it for drinking or cooking. *If your water should suddenly come out cloudy or discolored from the tap* (harmless cloudiness caused by air bubbles should disperse in a minute or two), *don't drink it.* Consult your local health officials for advice. If you must use potentially contaminated water either from your tap, a mountain stream, or other waterway, boil it first for at least 10 minutes. An alternative is to add liquid chlorine laundry bleach or tincture of iodide. Use 2 drops of bleach per quart of clear water and 4 drops per quart of cloudy water. Mix thoroughly and let stand for 30 minutes. You should detect a slight chlorine odor. If not, repeat the treatment and let stand another 15 minutes. For iodide, use 5 drops per quart of clear water, 10 per quart of cloudy water, mix and let stand for 30 minutes.

But infectious diseases are just part of the drinking-water story. There is mounting evidence that the chemicals and minerals in the water you drink directly affect your health.

TOOTH DECAY AND BONE LOSS

The single, most important measure in preventing tooth decay is drinking water that contains tiny amounts of *fluoride*. Flouride becomes incorporated into the structure of the tooth and fortifies it against decay. Children who, from birth (or before), consume fluoridated water and continue consuming it through the mid-teens have, on the average, two-thirds fewer cavities than those who consume water that lacks fluorides. Whereas a generation ago it was the rare child who reached his or her teens free of cavities, today it's commonplace, thanks to fluoridation. *Fluorides are far more important to decay resistance than heredity.* By the time I reached first grade, I had at least half a dozen cavities. My husband had even more at that age. But both our children, who were exposed to New York City's fluoridated water from the moment of conception, were cavity-free when they started elementary school, and one remains so at age 12.

Fluoride is also important to bone strength. Osteoporosis, the loss of bony tissue with age, is significantly less common in communities serviced by fluoridated water, suggesting that fluoride protects against this disease and the fractures that accompany it. Fluoride combines with the calcium of bone and helps to prevent the loss of calcium common after mid-life. This results in stronger bones.

Yet only 108 million Americans—49.4 percent of the population —were drinking fluoridated water in 1979. For about 10 million people, the water they drink naturally contains enough fluoride to protect teeth and bones. For the other 98 million Americans who drink fluoridated water, fluoride is deliberately added to the water in the treatment plant. On the average, only one part fluoride for every 1 million parts of water is needed (slightly less in hot areas where more water is consumed; slightly more in colder climates).

More than 100 million Americans—including 70 million who live in 6,000 communities with populations of 1,000 or more—are missing out on the benefits of fluoride largely because of scare tactics used by a small but persuasive group of people who oppose fluoridation. Some call it a communist plot to poison our democracy. Others blame fluoridation for a wide range of human ills, including cancer.

Contrary to all claims, fluorides at the levels proposed for water fluoridation do not cause cancer, birth defects, kidney, liver, or heart disease, or any other malady known to modern medicine. Since a claimed link to cancer is the antifluoridationists' most popular and potent weapon, the National Cancer Institute conducted a careful study of cancer rates in communities with and without fluoridated water. Absolutely no relationship was found between the disease and the mineral when factors such as urban living and age of the population were accounted for. Some fluoridated cities do have higher cancer rates than might otherwise be expected, but in most instances this is due to an excess of lung-cancer cases, probably caused by heavy industrial pollution in the area. In other fluoridated cities, the cancer rates were high long before fluoridation was introduced!

In some communities, however, the levels of fluoride naturally present in the water are so high that the tooth enamel develops a mottled appearance. This is not harmful, although it may be unsightly. Obvious mottling does not occur at the levels used in fluoridating water supplies.

If you draw your water from a well, you would have to have it tested for fluoride content. If it lacks fluoride, you may want to give your children fluoride tablets, available where vitamins are sold. If you are interested in having your community's water supply fluoridated, the National Centers for Disease Control, a division of the United States Public Health Service, is prepared to help out with technical advice and dollars for equipment and monitoring. Contact your Water Supply Department, local or state health officer, city council, local dental society, or any community group and urge them to seek federal advice by writing to Dr. Robert C. Faine, Dental Disease Prevention Activity, Bureau of State Services, United States Public Health Service, Centers for Disease Control, Atlanta, Georgia 30333.

HEART DISEASE

Every major component of the diet is somehow implicated in heart disease, and water is certainly among them. Numerous studies—in the United States, Britain, Canada, Sweden, the Netherlands, and South America—have pointed a suspicious finger at *"soft" water*. Although there are some notable exceptions, most studies have found that fatal heart attacks are less common in areas where the water is "hard"—that is, it contains relatively large amounts of dissolved salts.

In one major study directed by Dr. Henry A. Schroeder of Dartmouth Medical School, heart-attack deaths and water hardness were examined for 94 American cities. The researchers found that in cities with soft water, the death rate from heart attacks was significantly higher. In another study by University of Missouri researchers, 23 different characteristics of drinking water and deaths from various causes were compared in 92 metropolitan areas. The researchers found that the more dissolved substances the water contained, the lower were the death rates from heart disease and cancer.

At least two natural "experiments" support the relationship between soft water and heart attacks. In England and Wales, heart-attack death rates dropped in communities where the water became harder, and death rates rose in towns after the water there was deliberately softened. And in Key West, Florida, deaths from heart attacks rose when the city started using soft water from the mainland, and then decreased when Key West switched back to its harder well water.

Hard water is not exactly appreciated by those trying to wash dishes or clothes since it resists sudsing and leaves behind a distinct scum. It also forms a crust of mineral salts in the tea kettle and steam iron. Therefore, some municipalities deliberately soften their water before sending it off to individual consumers. In other cases, however, cities have begun adding substances to their water to harden it. This is done because soft water tends to be highly corrosive. Since it contains few dissolved substances and is somewhat acidic, it dissolves out metals from the pipes it flows through. This damages the pipes and introduces potentially toxic metals into the water that comes out of the tap. One of these contaminants might be cadmium, leached from galvanized pipe. Cadmium is known to be toxic to the heart and has been linked to high blood pressure.

The case against soft water is hardly conclusive. Researchers convinced of a relationship don't know if soft water contains a factor that is toxic to the heart or if hard water contains something protective, such as calcium. But while the jury is still out, certain preventive measures seem wise.

• If your water is soft, let it run for a while before using it first thing in the morning or after it has been unused for several hours. This will clear out the water that's been standing in the pipes and presumably contains the highest levels of leached metals.

• If you feel you must soften your water, soften only the hot water and only use the cold water for drinking and cooking.

• On the community level, water plants could add carbonates to soft water to reduce its corrosiveness. This is now being done in Boston and in Bennington, Vermont, where soft water had been leaching lead into drinking water from old water pipes.

CANCER

In 1974, a startling finding from the Mississippi Delta shook up a nation long-complacent about the safety of its drinking water. The water supply for the city of New Orleans was found to be liberally laced with chemicals that are either known to cause cancer or suspected of doing so. These chemicals—including chloroform, carbon tetrachloride, and others collectively called *trihalomethanes*—were shown to result from a chemical union between organic pollutants in the water and the chlorine added to purify it. The very method that had put an end to epidemics of typhoid, cholera, dysentery, and other water-borne diseases was now creating a new, more insidious hazard. An examination of cancer cases showed, to no one's great surprise, that cancers of the kidney, bladder, and urinary tract were more common in New Orleans than in most other major American cities.

The Environmental Protection Agency, the federal unit responsible for safe drinking water, followed up the New Orleans findings with an 80-city survey which revealed the presence of small amounts of cancer-causing chemicals in water systems throughout the country. Thus far, more than 300 different organic chemicals have been found in drinking water, including 22 known to cause cancer. (Most of the 300 chemicals have not yet been tested for the ability to cause cancer.) Even though they are present in only very tiny amounts, a lifetime of exposure could add up to a considerable risk.

In fact, at least fifteen studies have suggested an association between cancer and chemicals in drinking water. In Ohio, a study of 88 counties revealed higher death rates for cancer of the stomach and bladder among residents serviced by surface water supplies, as opposed to those receiving ground, or well, water. Surface water has been shown to contain higher levels of cancer-causing organic chemicals. More directly, a nationwide survey by National Cancer Institute researchers showed that deaths from cancers of the bladder, kidney, brain, and lymph glands were more common in counties where the levels of trihalomethanes were highest. Other studies have linked trihalomethanes in the drinking water to high rates of colon cancer.

Though none of these associations is proof that the organic chemicals cause cancer, they are certainly worrisome, and the Environmental Protection Agency would like to get these substances out of the drinking water. One way to do that would be to equip water-treatment plants with special filters made of activated carbon granules and run the water through them before it's chlorinated. At the time of this writing, an agency proposal to require such filters in water systems where they're needed was still being debated.

Meanwhile, many consumers have taken matters into their own

hands and have installed *home filtration systems*. According to tests conducted by the EPA, many of these home filters are worthless, especially the inexpensive units that attach to the faucet. However, more costly units—in the $300 range and up—that are attached to the home's main water source can be highly effective. Even the larger, under-the-sink varieties can remove up to 99 percent of potentially carcinogenic trihalomethanes. If you purchase a unit that relies on carbon filters, be sure to change the filters often to reduce the possiblility of bacterial growth that could contaminate your filtered water.

The Environmental Defense Fund, an activist group that has petitioned the EPA for more stringent water safety rules, suggests some interim alternatives that are cheaper and safer than home filtration systems. One is to boil the water you use for drinking and cooking to drive off volatile organic compounds. Bring the water to a boil, reduce the heat, and let it simmer very slowly for 15 to 20 minutes. Then pour it into a jar and store it, covered, in the refrigerator.

Another approach the defense fund suggests is to *construct your own carbon filter*. Granulated activated carbon can be purchased in 1-pound bags from Walnut Acres, Penns Creek, Pennsylvania 17862. In addition to the carbon, you'll need a large funnel and coffee filter papers that fit in the funnel. Start with enough carbon to fill about one-quarter of the funnel. Wash the carbon: Put it into a jar, fill the jar with water, shake and then let the carbon settle. If black particles remain in the water, pour off the water and repeat until the water is clear. Now, with the filter paper in the funnel, pour the water and carbon into the funnel. Set the funnel with the filter and carbon atop a large clean jar and slowly pour your tap water through it. Pour the water from the filled jar into a pan, bring it to a boil and simmer it slowly for 15 to 20 minutes. This will get rid of some organic chemicals and sterilize the water. Then put it back in the jar and refrigerate. Change the carbon every three weeks or after 20 gallons of water have been filtered through it.

OTHER CONTAMINANTS

Toxic heavy metals and cancer-causing organic chemicals are only part of the problem with modern water supplies. Many other substances commonly found in water could present a threat to health, among them:

Sodium. About 17 percent of the population is likely to develop high blood pressure on a sodium-rich diet (see Chapter 10). Some water supplies contain large amounts of sodium naturally; in others, it's a seasonal problem that results from runoff from highways that are salted in winter. The problem is likely to be more serious in areas supplied by surface water. Current regulations do not require seasonal tests for sodium content. Nor is the public informed of test results. Thus, some people on low-sodium diets may unwittingly consume large amounts of sodium in their drinking water.

Nitrates. These chemicals can run off into surface waters from agricultural lands where they're used for fertilizer and seep into ground water from septic tanks and agricultural uses. Nitrates are a direct hazard to infants, and nitrate-laden water has occasionally caused infant deaths. The babies develop a type of anemia called methemoglobinemia, or "blue baby" syndrome, sometimes even when the nitrate level is below the federal limit of 45 parts per million. The dangers of nitrates to older children and adults are still undefined, but a number of scientists believe they can be converted to cancer-causing nitrosamines in the human digestive tract (see Chapter 25, pages 480–482).

Asbestos. The persistent fibers of this pervasive mineral can enter water supplies from many sources: leaching from asbestos-containing pipes, runoff from sanded highways, and industrial pollution. Although the health effects of drinking asbestos are not definitely known, asbestos fibers can cause cancer when inhaled and probably also when ingested. Asbestos workers are prone to cancers of the lung and gastrointestinal tract, as well as an otherwise rare fatal cancer called mesothelioma.

This is by no means an exhaustive list. Other commonly found drinking-water contaminants include arsenic, pesticides (including some suspected of causing birth defects), mercury, lead, radioactive substances, and a host of industrial chemicals. All are potential health hazards.

Most problems with water supplies require community action to correct them. Consumers Union has suggested that concerned citizens form community groups to find out what's in their water and to rally for improvements in water quality. You can start by learning the facts about drinking water. Two publications may be helpful: "Safe Drinking Water for All: What You Can Do," purchased from the League of Women Voters Education Fund, 1730 M Street N.W., Washington, D.C. 20036; and "Manual for Evaluating Public Drinking Water Supplies," available from the Water Supply Division, Environmental Protection Agency, Washington, D.C. 20460.

Then contact your local water superintendent and ask to see the results of recent sanitary surveys and water-sampling tests. Compare these results with the standards set by the Public Health Service, as listed in the EPA manual. If your water meets federal standards, you may want to discuss further improvements. If it doesn't, then an immediate cleanup is in order and the community should be told of lapses through the local media. The media should also be informed if your group gets no cooperation from water-supply officials. What are they hiding?

The Bottled Alternative

Millions of Americans are paying handsomely for a substance they can obtain free (or are already paying for) just by turning on their faucets. The bottled-water business has grown by leaps and bounds in recent years to become nearly a billion-dollar industry. In 1984, Americans consumed 728 gallons of bottled water. But, studies have shown, not all bottled waters are the same, and some may be no better than what comes out of your tap.

There are all kinds of bottled water: some from wells, some from natural springs, some from ordinary tap water that's reprocessed. Some brands of bottled water may have started out as natural spring water, but now that the commercial demand exceeds the spring's supply, other sources—such as tap water—are used. Three-quarters of the bottled water sold in this country is *not* natural mineral water but rather processed water from local taps.

Bottled waters may be "still," naturally carbonated ("effervescent" or "sparkling"), or artificially carbonated with carbon dioxide gas. Some contain considerable amounts of dissolved minerals, either naturally present or artificially added, whereas others are relatively poor in mineral content. Some are alkaline, others neutral. The heavier the mineral content and the more alkaline the water, the stronger its taste.

Although bottled waters have been touted for years as healthy, even therapeutic, all bottled waters are not necessarily good for you. Too many minerals in water can be a health hazard because they may disrupt your body's balance of essential mineral nutrients. Some waters may have high levels of sodium, a potential hazard for persons with heart disease or high blood pressure. Heavy carbonation can be a problem for persons with hiatus hernia and other digestive disorders.

Some waters are processed and bottled under less-than-desirable sanitary conditions and end up with higher bacterial counts than your tap water. An EPA survey in the early 1970s of 25 bottled water plants showed that all had sanitary deficiencies, some bottled-water samples were contaminated with fecal bacteria, and one contained too much lead. Since then, the Food and Drug Administration has set standards for all bottled water sold in interstate commerce. But the standards put no limits on the amounts of pesticides and organic chemicals in the water, and products that are sold within the states they're bottled in are not subject to federal standards.

So before you invest heavily in bottled water, it pays to find out what you're getting. Dr. Robert Harris of the Environmental Defense Fund suggests that you write to the manufacturer and ask where the water comes from, if and how it's processed, the kind and amounts of minerals in it, and the level of carbonation. You might also ask for the results of recent bacterial tests and how often such tests are made. As a general guide, if you're buying processed water, the best treatment would include *filtration* through activated carbon granules (to remove dissolved chemicals and trace metals) and *ozonation* to sterilize it. Some processors first distill the water, which renders it pure and tasteless, and then put back mineral salts. This can also result in an acceptable product.

Bottled *distilled water,* of course, is nothing but pure water, free of chemicals and minerals. The water is first evaporated into steam, which leaves impurities behind, and then recondensed. But it is also tasteless, which makes it undesirable as drinking water for many people.

Dr. Harris says your best bet is unprocessed water that's bottled directly from a spring in a nonindustrial area where few pollutants could reach the water. Such waters would be labeled "natural spring water bottled directly from the source" or with some equivalent statement. Whether it can be called mineral water or not depends on state laws and the amount of minerals the water contains. All bottled water, with or without minerals or carbonation, should be noncaloric.

Here are some further tips to help you through the maze of the more than 500 brands of bottled water now sold in the United States.

• If the label says "spring fresh," spring type," or "spring pure," it's not spring water at all but rather processed tap or well water. The words "naturally carbonated," "naturally effervescent," or "naturally sparkling" indicate that the carbonation was already present in the water; otherwise it was added artificially. But even naturally carbonated water has a processed hitch: as the spring water bubbles to the surface, some of its carbonation escapes; the bottler may capture this runaway carbonation and reintroduce it into the water before sealing the bottles.

• The exact mineral content of *natural spring water* depends on the spring it comes from. Most contain calcium, magnesium, potassium, and sodium (but much less sodium than club soda). Some have lithium, a mineral that's reputed to have a calming effect. (In large doses, lithium is used to treat certain kinds of depression and manic highs.) When minerals are added, it's up to the manufacturer what is put in.

• *Club soda* is processed tap water with heavier carbonation than most spring waters. In addition to forced carbonation, club soda may contain such additives as sodium bicarbonate, sodium chloride, sodium phosphate, and sodium citrate (as well as artificial flavoring with mineral salts), so the sodium content is likely to be higher than plain water or natural spring water.

• *Seltzer,* once known as "two-cents plain" but now a lot more costly and less readily available, is a pure and simple product: thrice-filtered water with added carbonation. No salts, no preservatives, no sugar, and no flavorings are added. It's very low in sodium. It comes in special bottles that are recycled and home-delivered, and it can now be purchased in ordinary soda bottles in supermarkets in some areas. It's reputed to be a digestive aid, although this claim has not been subjected to scientific testing.

Soft Drinks

No beverage in America gives water greater competition than flavored soft drinks. The average American consumes 44 gallons of soft drinks—the same amount as water—and probably no other choice presents a more serious threat to good nutritional health. Soft drinks are the epitome of empty calories. They contain water (with or without carbon dioxide), artificial colorings and flavorings, and sugar—as many as *6 teaspoons of sugar in one 8-ounce serving!* Nothing else. Some noncarbonated drinks add vitamin C, and "fruit" or "fruit-flavored" drinks may even contain some real fruit juice. But for the most part,

Chart 11 • SOFT-DRINK CONSUMPTION

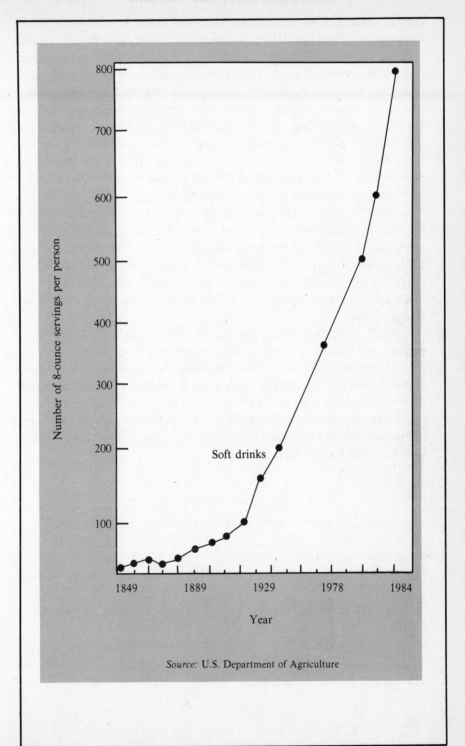

Source: U.S. Department of Agriculture

they are just wet, sweet calories—100 to 120 for 8 ounces of cola, 80 for a cup of ginger ale. Add half that again for the more usual 12-ounce serving. And those that are "low-cal" or "diet" drinks substitute potentially hazardous artificial sweeteners for the empty calories of sugar. Many use a combination of a cancer-promoting food additive, saccharin, and a brain-changing additive, aspartame. Or they rely strictly on aspartame. Either way, it's no nutritional bargain. Yet the sales of soft drinks—especially carbonated soda pop—have skyrocketed in the past half-century. From fewer than 10 8-ounce servings of soft drinks per person in 1899, they climbed to 707 per person in 1984 with no end in sight to their exponential growth (see Chart 11).

Most of the $22-billion market (and that's wholesale only!) is claimed by cola drinks, which accounted for 80 percent of diet-soda sales and 68 percent of regular sodas sold in 1984. (Diet sodas, incidentally, represent only 11 percent of soda sales.) Fully one-fourth of our annual sugar consumption—more than 23 pounds of sucrose per person —comes from drinking soda, and that doesn't even count sugar-laden fruit drinks.

Fruit juices, while not necessarily lower in calories (8 ounces of unsweetened orange juice has 110 calories, grapefruit juice has 90, and grape juice has 170), at least provide essential vitamins and minerals. But let's face it, most people don't drink soda for the sake of nutrition. They drink it because they're hooked on the sweet taste and because they're thirsty. But even here soda is likely to let them down. Sweetened drinks are not the best way to quench your thirst. The sugar actually increases the body's need for water.

FOR FURTHER READING

Carol Keough, *Water Fit to Drink* (Emmaus, Pa.: Rodale, 1980).

12 ~ COFFEE, TEA...

MORE THAN half the world's coffee is consumed in the United States. Only the Swedes drink more coffee per person than we do, and no country comes near to matching our total consumption. Even so, per-capita coffee consumption has been dropping fairly steadily since 1946, when we averaged 20 pounds of coffee a year for every man, woman, and child—or about 1,000 6-ounce cups a person. By 1979, consumption had fallen to less than 9 pounds a person, or 450 cups for the year (see Chart 12).

Why this national craze for a bitter-tasting liquid? A better question might be, "Why not?" for coffee is a socially acceptable, stimulating, and addictive drink that helps to keep you awake and alert at practically no caloric cost—only 5 calories a cup. Coffee, in fact, comes closer than any other part of the typical American diet to giving us something for nothing. The secret of coffee's popularity is the mind-altering drug caffeine, primarily responsible for coffee's stimulating effects. For better or worse, we are a nation of caffeine junkies.

The coffee plant, first cultivated in Arabia (hence the plant's botanical name of *Coffea arabica*), has been recognized as a stimulant for over a thousand years. According to a possibly legendary account, it was discovered by an Arabian goatherd named Kaldi, who had noticed his charges cavorting vigorously about the countryside after dining on little red berries from a certain shrub. Kaldi decided to try some of the berries himself and discovered that they kept him alert during his long vigil.

It wasn't long before some Muslims began advocating coffee consumption to enhance religious diligence (although other religious leaders regarded this as a lapse from faith). Coffee was also used as a medical stimulant, according to an Arabian text written around A.D. 900. Eventually it found its way to Europe, then to North America by the end of the seventeenth century.

The amount of caffeine varies with the type of coffee. On the average, ground roast coffee that is brewed contains 83 milligrams of caffeine per 6-ounce cup. Instant coffee has less—about 60 milligrams in 6 ounces. Decaffeinated coffee that has been treated to remove most of the caffeine has only 3 milligrams of the stimulant per cup. Please

Chart 12 • COFFEE, TEA, AND COCOA CONSUMPTION

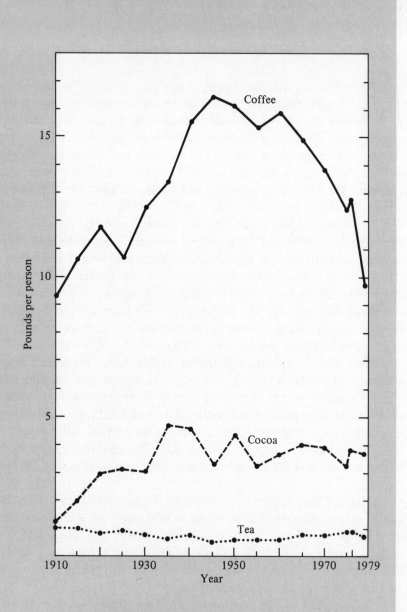

Source: *The Changing American Diet*, Center for Science in the Public Interest and the U.S. Department of Agriculture.

note, however, that if your cup is bigger than 6 ounces (and some coffee mugs are twice that), you'll be consuming proportionately more caffeine. One way to reduce the amount of caffeine in your coffee without switching to decaf is to use a coffee that's been blended with grain or chicory. *Consumer Reports* found these amounts of caffeine in coffee prepared from three such instant blends: Sunrise, 37; Mellow Roast, 30; and Luzianne, 14 milligrams of caffeine per cup.

Caffeine Is in More Than Coffee

By the time coffee was discovered, *tea* was already in use as a stimulant in Asia. Chinese legend relates that Daruma, a Zen Buddhist leader, dozed off during a nine-year meditation. When he awoke, he was filled with remorse. To prevent a recurrence of his "sinful" behavior, he cut off his eyelids and threw them on the ground. Where they landed, a shrub sprouted, and the beverage brewed from its leaves could ward off sleep. It was the tea plant. Tea was harvested in India and Indochina as early as A.D. 700 and was supposedly brought to Europe by early Dutch explorers. To the British today, it remains as much an institution as coffee is in America.

Like coffee, tea contains caffeine—less on average, but still enough to produce a marked stimulating effect. Certain teas contain as much or more caffeine than some regular coffees. The average cup of leaf tea

Table 12.1 • HOW MUCH CAFFEINE DO YOU
CONSUME?

Food or drink	Serving size	Caffeine (mg)
Brewed coffee	6 ounces	83
Instant coffee	6 ounces	60
Coffee-grain blends	6 ounces	14–37
Decaffeinated coffee	6 ounces	3
Leaf tea	6 ounces	41
Instant tea	6 ounces	28
Colas and Dr Pepper	12 ounces	40–72
Cocoa	6 ounces	10
Chocolate	1 ounce	5–10

Sources: Average content, based on data from the Coffee Information Institute, Consumers Union, and Chocolate Manufacturers Association.

contains 41 milligrams of caffeine, about half that of brewed coffee and two-thirds that of instant coffee.

In general, domestic brands of tea have less caffeine than the more expensive imported black teas, and tea brewed from bags has less caffeine than loose tea. An analysis by Daniel S. Groisser of Mountainside Hospital in Montclair, New Jersey, revealed that the caffeine in four domestic brands of tea bags ranged from 18 milligrams for a weak brew of Tetley to 90 milligrams for a strong brew of Red Rose. Among the imported teas, the range was from 26 for a weak brew of English Breakfast in a bag to 107 for the same tea brewed strong. A four-minute steep of a bag of Chinese green tea yielded 36 milligrams of caffeine, whereas the same treatment of Pan Fried loose green tea produced a drink with 81 milligrams of caffeine—as much as in brewed coffee. Two instant teas tested gave 48 milligrams of caffeine for Nestea and 62 for Lipton.

To your body, caffeine is caffeine. Although many people believe that coffee in the evening keeps them awake at night but tea doesn't, it's really all a matter of dose. *If you drink two cups of tea, the effect is the same as one cup of brewed coffee or one and a half cups of instant coffee.*

Tea, however, was never as popular as coffee among Americans. For most of this century, tea consumption has ranged between ½ pound and 1⅕ pounds per person. In 1976, Americans consumed ⅘ pound of tea per person, enough to make about 160 6-ounce cups.

Soft drinks, especially colas, have long been another hugely popular source of caffeine among Americans. The pick-me-up property of caffeine is no doubt a major factor in the overwhelming dominance of colas over other types of sodas. And while the amount of caffeine in soft drinks is much less than in coffee—ranging from 13 to 27 milligrams in 5 ounces—the 12-ounce serving size adds up to 32 to 65 milligrams.

In response to public concern about caffeine, most major producers now sell caffeine-free versions of their leading sodas. For children, at the least, these are better choices. Children are more sensitive to caffeine's effects than adults, and *a young child drinking a can of cola can get approximately the same kick an adult gets from four cups of coffee!* Children are also exposed to the caffeine in *cocoa* and *chocolate.* According to Dr. Philip Keeney of Penn State University, 6 ounces of cocoa contains up to 10 milligrams of caffeine; 8 ounces of chocolate milk mixed as directed also has 10 milligrams of caffeine; and 1 ounce of bittersweet chocolate has 5 to 10 milligrams of caffeine.

When all sources of caffeine are considered, 20 to 30 percent of

American adults consume more than 500 milligrams of caffeine a day —twice what doctors consider a large "drug dose"—and about 10 percent of adults pass the 1,000-milligram mark.

Although caffeine is the strongest stimulant in coffee, tea, and cocoa, these drinks also contain other related "xanthine" compounds —*theophylline* and *theobromine*—that have similar, though less potent, effects. Caffeine is the main xanthine in coffee; but theophylline predominates in tea, and cocoa contains large amounts of theobromine. These chemicals contribute significantly to the stimulant effects of tea and cocoa.

Caffeine's Effects on the Body

The caffeine you consume is absorbed immediately. You notice its effects within half an hour, and peak blood levels are reached about an hour after consumption, tapering off in roughly three and a half hours.

How does caffeine work? First, it has a direct stimulating effect on the brain, both the cerebral cortex, which is concerned with thought, and the medulla, which regulates heart rate, respiration, and muscular coordination. These central-nervous-system effects are responsible for the wakeful state caffeine induces and for "coffee nerves," that jittery, "hyper" feeling associated with drinking too much coffee. Caffeine can also raise the basal metabolic rate and thus increase the number of calories your body burns, a possible aid to weight control. But in doing so it also triggers the release of insulin, which causes blood sugar to drop, producing feelings of hunger.

Third, caffeine stimulates the heart muscle and can make the heart a more efficient pump. (At high doses, however, caffeine can cause a too rapid heart beat.) Under the influence of caffeine, coronary arteries dilate, increasing blood flow to the heart. The effect on blood vessels feeding the brain is just the opposite—they constrict, reducing cerebral blood flow.

Caffeine also relaxes the muscles of the respiratory system and digestive tract. The same happens to the kidneys, causing increased urinary output. Thus, caffeine has a diuretic, or dehydrating, effect on the body. Used as your main source of liquid, then, coffee or tea can be counterproductive. Large amounts of coffee can cause diarrhea while the tannins in tea make that drink constipating, an effect partly countered by adding milk to the tea.

Those who claim they don't function as well without caffeine may

not be imagining things. Caffeine makes voluntary muscles less susceptible to fatigue and enhances the capacity for muscular work. It increases the speed and efficiency of mental and manual tasks and prevents lapses of attention. Small doses of caffeine help to produce a
clearer train of thought, a keener appreciation of sensory stimuli, and
a swifter reaction time. After two cups of coffee, driving skills improve
and typists are faster and more accurate. Even regular consumers of
caffeine-containing beverages do not seem to become immune to these
effects. However, they can easily become dependent on caffeine to
maintain their customary level of work efficiency.

As anyone who has benefited from its stimulating effects can tell
you, caffeine can be a very useful drug. It is used by those who must
do monotonous work or drive long distances, especially at night. It is
frequently used in drug preparations. For example, it might be incorporated into cold and allergy remedies to counteract the sleep-inducing
effects of antihistamines and to relax the bronchial muscles. It is also
included in many headache remedies to constrict blood vessels in the
brain, since dilated blood vessels contribute to migraine-type headaches.

Caffeine can be an alternative to potent and dangerous drugs used
to treat hyperactive children. In some studies two cups of coffee daily
had a paradoxical calming effect on such children, resulting in improved behavior and school performance, although other studies
showed caffeine increased irritability.

Caffeine is also now being used to treat premature babies who have
attacks of apnea, or periodically stop breathing in their sleep. Apnea,
if not corrected in time, can result in sudden infant (crib) death. Caffeine may prevent these episodes of apnea and produces a more regular
breathing pattern in such infants.

Caffeine Hazards

Caffeine is a drug, and no drug lacks unwanted side effects. But
current evidence suggests that the picture is not as bleak as some people
might think, judging from the amount of adverse publicity caffeine
receives. Here are some of the medical problems and controversies that
have surrounded caffeine and coffee drinking in recent years.

Heart disease. Although one study indicated that those who drink
coffee in large amounts are more prone to heart disease than those who

don't drink coffee, several other major studies have not confirmed the risk. Taken at once, large doses of caffeine—200 to 500 milligrams (the amount in two and a half to six cups)—can produce an abnormally fast heart beat, abnormal heart rhythms, or extra heart beats. Caffeine can also increase blood pressure and blood cholesterol. However, there is no convincing evidence that moderate coffee drinking increases the risk of any type of heart disease.

Cancer. Similarly, initial suggestions that coffee drinking can increase the risk of cancers of the bladder and pancreas have not stood the test of further research. In the laboratory, caffeine can cause cancer-like changes in cells at doses twenty to forty times higher than the highest blood level ever measured in a habitual coffee drinker. But at lower doses, caffeine seems to inhibit the cancer-inducing effects of other chemicals. Thus, in ordinary amounts, caffeine may protect against cancer.

Birth defects. Caffeine readily crosses the placenta and so can affect the developing fetus. A number of studies in animals have shown that caffeine can interfere with normal reproduction, causing reduced fertility and such birth defects as cleft palate and bone abnormalities. In a Belgian study, 23 percent of mothers who gave birth to abnormal babies had consumed eight or more cups of coffee a day during pregnancy, whereas only 13 percent of the mothers of normal babies drank that much coffee. Other preliminary studies have linked heavy coffee drinking to a high risk of miscarriage, stillbirth, premature birth, or breech presentation. Although none of these studies is definitive, the Center for Science in the Public Interest and the Food and Drug Administration advise pregnant women and those who wish to become pregnant to avoid caffeine.

Digestive disorders. Caffeine promotes the secretion of acid in the stomach and therefore is not advisable for persons who have ulcers or gastric irritation. However, a carefully designed study showed that both regular *and* decaffeinated coffee can stimulate acid secretion, so ulcer patients may be well advised to avoid coffee in any form.

Coffee is also notorious for its ability to induce heartburn, especially if consumed on an empty stomach. Ohio State University researchers showed this can happen after drinking decaffeinated coffee and acid-neutralized coffee, as well as ordinary roasted ground coffee. All these coffees cause a drop in pressure in the esophagus just above the stomach; the muscle between the stomach and esophagus relaxes and allows some of the acidic stomach contents to come back up, producing the typical burning effects of indigestion. The researchers related this effect not to caffeine, but to the large variety of acids—including tannic, acetic, nicotinic, formic, and citric—found in coffee. Tea also contains acid, in particular tannic acid, that can irritate the digestive tract. However, the effect of tannic acid can be reduced by adding milk to the tea.

Breast disease. In 1979, Dr. John P. Minton, a surgeon at Ohio State University Hospital, reported that breast lumps, pain, and tenderness completely disappeared in 65 percent of 47 women who eliminated all coffee, tea, colas, and chocolate from their diets. In a second study in 1981, he claimed an 83-percent success rate, with some improvement in another 15 percent. One or two other such studies reported similar results in removing all sources of methylxanthines from the diet. All of these studies, unfortunately, are scientifically flawed, and no one has yet done a definitive test of Dr. Minton's theory.

Fever. Caffeine is able to raise body temperature or block the fever-reducing properties of aspirin, according to studies at the University of London. Thus, it may be wise for patients with fever to stay away from tea, coffee, and colas as well as from medications containing caffeine. The warming effect of a hot, caffeine-containing drink is only temporary. Once the caffeine hits your system, it increases the difference between your body temperature and the air (assuming the air temperature is below 98.6 degrees F) and makes you feel cooler or chilled.

Headache. While caffeine helps to relieve headaches in some people, it can trigger them in others. If caffeine seems to cause your headaches or to make them worse, avoid it for a while and see what happens.

Anxiety. Heavy coffee drinking may sometimes bring on symptoms that mimic an "anxiety attack," including headache, jitteriness, upset stomach, and difficulty sleeping that doctors may mistakenly treat with tranquilizers and psychotherapy. Three typical patients with the "anxiety" syndrome, called *caffeinism*, were described by Dr. John F. Greden, a University of Michigan psychiatrist. In one case, a 27-year-old nurse who was drinking ten to twelve cups of strong, black coffee every day (containing a total of more than 1,000 milligrams of caffeine) developed symptoms of lightheadedness, shakiness, breathlessness, headache, and irregular heart beat. All symptoms were gone thirty-six hours after she stopped drinking coffee.

Dr. Greden has also found that psychiatric patients who drink a lot of caffeine-containing beverages tend to be more depressed than other patients, although he is not yet sure which comes first—the depression or the high caffeine consumption.

Curing Your Coffee Nerves

As little as three or four cups of coffee a day can make you psychologically and physically dependent on caffeine, although most caffeine addicts consume considerably more than that. Once hooked, abrupt withdrawal from the drug can provoke such unpleasant symptoms as headache, drowsiness, lethargy, yawning, runny nose, irritability, disinterest in work, nervousness, mental depression, and even nausea and vomiting. The symptoms commonly begin twelve to sixteen hours after the last dose of caffeine. Regular coffee drinkers who abstain from caffeine in the evening may wake up with a headache the next morning.

Dr. Greden suspects that many people who are plagued by so-called tension headaches may really be experiencing the effects of recurrent caffeine withdrawal. These headaches may occur on weekends, when work-related coffee consumption drops off dramatically. If coffee or a pain reliever containing caffeine provides relief but ordinary aspirin does not, then more than likely you're suffering from a caffeine-withdrawal headache.

If you want to break your caffeine habit without knocking your system for a loop, do it gradually. Dr. Morris A. Shorofsky of Beth Israel Hospital in New York recommends a weaning period in which the number of cups of coffee is reduced by one or two a day until you're totally off caffeine.

Alternatives to Caffeine

If you drink a lot of coffee and you'd like to cut down your caffeine intake but not your coffee drinking, then decaf may be your answer. *Decaffeinated coffee* will spare you most—but not all—of the effects of caffeine-containing coffee. You'll recall that with or without caffeine, coffee can stimulate the secretion of stomach acid and provoke heartburn. Although coffee connoisseurs spurn decafs as deficient in flavor and body, many people find them acceptable. Taste tests have given the highest ratings to decafs brewed from ground coffee or prepared from a freeze-dried instant. You may have to try several brands before you find one that pleases you. Substitute it for one or two of your regular cups each day until you're drinking nothing but decaf. Or you can mix decaf and regular coffee in various proportions to reduce your total caffeine intake. This is what I do for my husband, who consumes perhaps eight cups a day. I brew the morning coffee using two scoops of decaf for every one of regular caffeinated coffee. This cuts his caffeine intake by two-thirds.

Some consumers are concerned about the safety of decaffeinated coffee. Several years ago, studies sponsored by the National Cancer Institute revealed that the solvent commonly used to remove caffeine from coffee caused cancer in mice. Since residues of this solvent, called trichloroethylene or TCE, remained in the finished product, its further use was banned. Companies using TCE switched to methylene chloride. In one study mice treated with methylene chloride developed more lung tumors than those that weren't exposed to the chemical, but the difference in tumor development was not statistically significant and could have been due to chance. Industry-sponsored tests have shown no hazard, and studies of workers who have been exposed to the chemical for up to thirty years showed no apparent health effects. More important to the consumer, an analysis by Consumers Union revealed no residue of methylene chloride in the finished coffee.

In some of the more expensive brands of decaffeinated ground coffee and coffee beans, the caffeine is removed through a steam process developed in Switzerland rather than with a chemical. Currently, however, the supply of beans decaffeinated by this method is limited.

Other alternatives to caffeine are the *grain-based beverages,* such as Postum and Pero. These are very low in calories—12 per cup for Postum, which is made from bran, wheat, and molasses, 7 per cup for Cafix, a West German product made from barley, rye, chicory, and beets. If not in your supermarket, such products can usually be found in health-food stores. One—Wilson's Heritage, a 100-percent barley product made in Kansas—can even be brewed like coffee, perhaps mixed with your favorite coffee. However, excessive consumption of such grain products may have a laxative effect or cause flatulence.

Still another choice is caffeine-free *herbal tea.* Herbal teas have enjoyed increasing popularity in recent years and can now be purchased in supermarkets as well as health-food and specialty-food stores. But beware: herbal teas can be a more serious health hazard than has ever been linked to caffeine.

The Herbal-Tea Menace

Three young women looking for an herbal substitute for tea and coffee bought a box of senna leaf tea at a health-food store. They prepared it the usual way, steeping ½ to 1 teaspoon of leaves for each cup of tea. They each drank a cup or two of the resulting brew, and about three hours later all developed severe abdominal cramps and watery diarrhea. Two had palpitations. They received emergency medical treatment and recovered a day later. The women had not realized that senna leaves contain a chemical, anthraquinone, that is a strong cathartic.

A young couple in Denver bought burdock root tea from a local health-food store, then brewed a pot and drank some. Shortly afterward, they experienced blurred vision and dry mouth, but thought nothing of it until two days later when the wife decided to drink half a cup of the tea that was still in the pot. Within five minutes, she again had blurred vision and a dry mouth, but this time her behavior and speech became bizarre. Her husband said she appeared to be hallucinating, and he brought her to the hospital emergency room, where she was found to have been poisoned by an atropinelike chemical in the tea.

A 43-year-old Wisconsin woman developed nausea, vomiting, stomach cramps, and severe diarrhea within half an hour of drinking a cup of poke root tea. She had purchased the tea in a health-food store and prepared it as directed, with ½ teaspoon of powdered poke root in a cup of boiling water. She required extensive treatment at the University of Wisconsin Hospital to counteract the effects of the poisoning.

Many other such mishaps have been reported in the medical literature in the past few years as increasing numbers of Americans have experimented with herbal teas. Most people are unaware that *herbal teas may contain potent chemicals that can disrupt the normal functions of body and mind.* And the product labels rarely contain warnings of possible adverse effects.

Herbal teas come from plants, and plants, after all, are the source of nearly half of our prescription drugs. From plants come chemicals that stimulate the heart, lower the blood pressure, excite the nervous system, induce vomiting, counter constipation, and sedate the brain, among other potent effects.

"Herbal teas are drugs, not foods," says Dr. Ara Der Marderosian, professor of pharmacognosy at the Philadelphia College of Pharmacy and Science. "They are crude complexes containing many impurities and active components with a variety of possible undesirable effects. Some are actually too dangerous to be used at all."

Generally, the active ingredients are present in low concentrations, so moderate consumption of an herbal tea is usually no problem for otherwise healthy persons. But the amounts of the active chemicals in brewed herbal tea can vary greatly depending on how and where the plant was grown, the parts of the plant used, and how the tea is brewed. Also, some teas are sold as mixtures of several herbs, possibly containing chemicals with effects that potentiate one another; the buyer has no way of knowing what the possible hazards of such a mixture may be. And unsuspecting people who think that if some is good more must be better may poison themselves with an overdose.

The Medical Letter, an independent drug advisory for physicians, has outlined the following potential dangers of herbal teas:

Cathartic teas, including those with senna leaves, flowers, and bark, buckthorn bark, dock roots, or aloe leaves, can cause severe diarrhea.

Allergenic teas, such as those from chamomile, goldenrod, marigold, and yarrow, can cause severe allergic reactions—including fatal allergic shock—in persons sensitive to ragweed, asters, chrysanthemums, and related plants. Delayed allergic reactions and sun sensitivity can follow consumption of tea from the leaves of St.-John's-wort.

Cancer-causing substances are present in tea made from sassafras root bark. Tannins in tea, including ordinary tea and peppermint tea, have been linked to high rates of cancer of the esophagus and stomach. Adding milk to the tea binds the tannins and presumably protects the digestive tract from their effects.

Diuretics are present in teas made from buchu, quack grass, and dandelion, but their effect is believed to be no worse than that of the xanthines in coffee and ordinary tea.

Poisons that could cause fatal reactions are found in Indian tobacco, shave grass (horsetail), and mistletoe leaves, sometimes used improperly for making tea.

Nervous-system toxins are found in catnip, juniper, hydrangea, jimson weed, lobelia, nutmeg, and wormwood. These can cause a variety of severe untoward reactions, including hallucinations.

Dr. Varro E. Tyler, dean of pharmacy at Purdue University in West Lafayette, Indiana, notes that comfrey, a very popular herbal tea, contains several alkaloids that are toxic to the liver and one that has produced tumors in the liver and bladder of laboratory animals. And although the root-beer flavor, safrole, from sassafras root bark was banned because it causes cancer, sassafras for making tea can still be purchased in some health-food stores, Dr. Tyler points out. Dr. Tyler is the author of *The Honest Herbal* (Philadelphia: George F. Stickley Co., 1982), a complete guide to what herbs can and cannot do for your health.

Dr. Julia F. Morton, director of the herbarium at the University of Miami in Coral Gables, Florida, warns that alfalfa tea, a favorite among herbal-tea enthusiasts, contains saponins that can disrupt digestion and respiration. She also notes that a tea used safely on occasion for its laxative or diuretic effects could become a health hazard from repeated or prolonged use.

The substances in some herbal teas can interact with or counter the effects of prescribed medications, according to Dr. Alvin B. Segelman, pharmacognosist at Rutgers University in New Brunswick, New Jersey. "I view the growing popularity of so-called 'herb teas' among the American public with serious concern," Dr. Morton says. "What is not fully realized by most consumers is that the majority of the plants being so exploited today formerly appeared in texts on medical botany as possessing active constituents affecting one or more organs of the body. They are not necessarily suitable for daily beverage use."

What should *you* do about herbal teas?

• Read the label. The package should tell you what's in it and caution you about pharmacological effects. It should also say something about caffeine content. (One popular herbal tea, described as an ideal morning tea, has twice as much caffeine as a regular cup of coffee.) If the label is uninformative, don't buy the product. If you're really anxious to try the tea, first write to the manufacturer for the desired information. *If such information is not available, stay away.*

• Don't start with a strong brew or drink several cups at once. Try half a cup of weak tea the first time, and if that goes down without ill effect, you might try a full cup the next time. Brew fresh tea each time, since active chemicals are slowly leached from the plant as it steeps.

• Don't race out into the wilds, guide book or no, and start picking leaves, roots, berries, and flowers to make tea. Sometimes one part of a plant is perfectly safe, whereas another part of the same plant contains a lethal poison. Many plants have dangerous look-alikes that can fool the uninitiated. Such a mix-up, in fact, killed an elderly couple from Chehalis, Washington, who after visiting a health spa that recommended comfrey tea, picked some leaves along the road. But what they thought was comfrey turned out to be foxglove, the source of the highly toxic heart drug digitalis. Don't rely on a book or what you remember from a lecture. *Pick only what a knowledgeable collector tells you is safe.*

• Don't drink herbal teas as if they were water. They are best used as an occasional beverage, not for regular consumption. Remember, herbs contain drugs, and all drugs should be used with caution and discretion.

13 ❧ ...OR MILK?

"YOU NEVER outgrow your need for milk." Or do you? The idea that children need milk to form strong bones and teeth and that adults need milk to maintain them had each American drinking 45 gallons of milk a year in 1950. But recently, as we learned more about possible harmful effects of milk (mostly in adults), as birth rates fell, and as soft drinks shot up in popularity, consumption of fluid milk fell by about a third, to 32 gallons a year. Offsetting this decline, some solid-milk products rose dramatically. Per person, we now eat nearly five times as much hard cheese as we did early in this century, and yogurt consumption increased 18-fold between 1964 and 1984. In any case, milk and milk products are still a major part of American nutritional life.

A Nearly Perfect Food

On an item-by-item basis, cow's milk contains nearly all the nutrients needed to maintain life and support growth. Except for breast milk, diluted cow's milk is, in fact, the ideal food for newborn babies (see Chapter 19), although some nutrients—among them iron, vitamin C, copper, and manganese—are not present in adequate amounts in milk to meet the needs of older children and adults.

Milk is a good source of high-quality *protein*. A cup of milk contains 8 grams of balanced protein—one-fourth of the daily protein needs of a young child and one-eighth to one-sixth that of an adult. Thus, a child who drinks a quart of milk a day gets all the protein he or she needs from that one source. Milk protein is especially good as a complement to proteins from grains and vegetables. Milk contains an abundance of the amino acid lysine, which is not well supplied by grains. Thus milk in your cereal bowl improves the protein value of the cereal.

Milk *fat*, also about 8 grams per cup of whole milk, is easy to digest compared to other animal fats. However, 65 percent of milk fat is saturated fatty acids, and only 4 percent is polyunsaturates. For those concerned about consuming too much fat and too many calories, milk is readily available with much or all of its fat removed, but with its remaining nutrients intact.

Milk contains more *carbohydrates*—11 grams per cup—than either protein or fat, which makes it a more desirable source of protein than, say, meats, which have only fat and protein. However, milk's main carbohydrate—the sugar lactose—cannot be readily digested by many people because they are deficient in the enzyme lactase needed to split lactose into its component sugars before absorption through the intestine. (See pages 254 and 255.)

As for the essential *micronutrients,* milk and milk products are our main source of calcium. Two cups of milk supply three-fourths of the calcium requirement for preteenaged children and for adults. Other minerals plentiful in milk include phosphorus, potassium, and, alas, sodium, a potential problem for persons with high blood pressure. Milk is a good source of many B vitamins. Although it has little vitamin D naturally, nearly all milk is fortified with it, making milk the main dietary source of vitamin D. Vitamin A is also sometimes added to milk. Milk's main micronutritional failing is a shortage of iron.

Types of Milk Products

Many people are confused by the wide array of milk products now available. Among the prevalent myths and mistaken impressions are that buttermilk is rich in butterfat, that whole milk contains 20 percent fat, that nonfat dry milk is deficient in nutrients, that raw milk is better than pasteurized, that sour cream has less fat than sweet cream, and that yogurt is less fattening than milk. Following is a brief description of the more popular "liquid" milk products, based on information from the National Dairy Council.

Whole milk contains not less than 3.25 percent milk fat and 8.25 percent other solids (protein and carbohydrates). Vitamin A (at least 2,000 international units per quart) and vitamin D (at least 400 international units per quart) may be added to it; the label must state the amounts used in *fortification.* Whole fluid milk must be *pasteurized* to destroy harmful microorganisms if it is to be sold in a state other than where it was produced. All *grade A* milk is pasteurized. Some states permit the sale of *raw* (unpasteurized) milk produced within their borders, but it may contain hazardous microorganisms. *Certified* milk may be raw or pasteurized, but the dairies that produce it must conform to precise sanitary regulations that greatly reduce the risks associated with uncertified raw milk. But even certification does not guarantee that the milk is safe. *Homogenization* is a process that disperses the fat globules in milk to keep them from separating out; it has no bearing on the healthfulness of the milk.

Low-fat milk has had some or most of the fat skimmed off. It may contain from 0.5 percent to 2 percent fat, but it must have at least the same amount of nonfat solids (protein and carbohydrates) as whole milk. Thus, except for fat calories, it's nutritionally comparable to whole milk.

Skim or nonfat milk has had nearly all the fat removed, ending up with less than 0.5 percent fat. But it, too, must contain at least 8.25 percent nonfat solids. *Nonfat dry milk* is made by spraying defatted milk into hot air or by spraying hot air into the milk. Because of its low moisture content, nonfat dry milk can keep without spoiling for a very long time. Nearly all nonfat dry milk is fortified with vitamins A and D. When reconstituted with water in the recommended amounts, it is nutritionally comparable to fluid milk, minus fat and calories.

Filled milk has had some or all of the milk fat removed and replaced with any other kind of fat or oil. Some products contain coconut oil, which is more saturated than milk fat. Filled milk is different from *imitation milk,* which may contain such ingredients as corn syrup, vegetable fat, and vegetable or fish protein. Although by legal definition filled milk is considered nutritionally inferior to milk, from the consumer's standpoint it may not be.

Evaporated milk may be whole or skim milk (the label says which) from which about 60 percent of the water has been removed by evaporation. The concentrated milk is then sealed in containers and sterilized. Because most of the water has been removed, it contains a much higher percentage of solids and more calories than ordinary milk.

Buttermilk is made from skim milk or low-fat pasteurized milk to which a bacterial culture is added to ferment the milk sugar. It has a tart flavor and a buttery, thick texture, but unless whole milk, whole-milk solids, or liquid butter has been added to it (resulting in granules or flakes of butter in the cold milk), it is a low-fat product.

Yogurt is also made from milk treated with a bacterial culture. If whole milk is used, the yogurt contains at least 3.25 percent fat; from low-fat milk, 0.5 percent to 2 percent fat; and from nonfat milk, less than 0.5 percent fat. Check the label. If it doesn't say low-fat, it's whole-milk yogurt. It may be plain or flavored, with or without fruit. Nonfat milk solids and various additives may be used to improve the texture and stability of the product. Flavorings generally raise the caloric content of yogurt by 50 to 100 calories a cup, making the yogurt more fattening than plain milk. Plain yogurt made from skim or low-fat milk gives you the most protein for the fewest calories per cup, whereas plain whole-milk yogurt has the least protein, the most fat, and more calories. Because of the amount of sweeteners used in frozen yogurt, it has about the same amount of calories as ice cream—130 to 160 per ½ cup. However, the fat content is only about 2 percent, whereas ice cream is 10 to 16 percent fat.

Sour cream is pasteurized, homogenized cream that has been cultured with bacteria. It contains at least 18 percent milk fat.

Cream also contains not less than 18 percent fat. In addition to milk fat and milk, it may contain concentrated milk, dry milk, or skim milk. Half-and-half is a mixture of milk and cream, containing at least 10.5 percent fat but not more than 18 percent fat. Light cream has between 18 and 30 percent fat; light whipping cream has between 30 and 36 percent fat; and heavy cream (or heavy whipping cream) is at least 36 percent fat.

Special milks. There are also a number of specialty milk products for people with dietary restrictions. These include *lactose-reduced low-fat milk, acidophilus milk* in which much of the lactose has been predigested, and *low-sodium milk* from which 95 percent of the sodium has been removed.

Many Do Outgrow Their Need for Milk

In fact, about two-thirds of the world's people do, starting around the age of two. After infancy, about 70 percent of American blacks, Indians, and Jews, and more than 80 percent of Asian and Middle Eastern populations become increasingly unable to digest the milk sugar lactose. Instead, they get gas, bloating, abdominal cramps, and diarrhea when they consume more than a certain amount of milk and milk products containing lactose. Such people derive relatively few nutritional benefits from milk. In only a few population groups do the vast majority of adults retain their full ability to digest lactose, among them northern Europeans and their American descendants and a few African tribes. Thus, from the standpoint of evolution, it is "normal" to outgrow your need for—and ability to benefit from—milk.

Before lactose can be absorbed through the intestinal tract, it must be broken into its component sugars, glucose and galactose, by an intestinal enzyme called lactase. Except in the case of a rare genetic

Table 13.1 • MILK PRODUCTS AT A GLANCE

Product	% fat	Calories
Milk (1 cup)		
Whole	3.5	160
2%	2.0	120
"99% fat-free"	1.0	100
Skim	0.2	88
Evaporated whole	8.0	345
Buttermilk (from skim milk)	0.2	88
Buttermilk (from low-fat milk)	1.0	100
Chocolate drink	2.0	190
Chocolate (with whole milk)	3.5	213
Cream (1 tablespoon)		
Half-and-half	12.0	20
Light	20.0	32
Light whipping	31.0	45
Heavy whipping	38.0	53
Coffee whitener (nondairy)	14.0	20
Sour	18.0	30
Yogurt (1 cup)		
Low-fat plain	1.7	120
Plain (whole milk)	3.4	150
Low-fat flavored (e.g., vanilla)	2.0	190
Low-fat with fruit preserves	2.0	250
Cottage Cheese (½ cup)		
Uncreamed (dry curd)	0.3	65
Creamed (regular)	4.2	120
Low-fat	1.0	80
Frozen Dessert (1 cup)		
Sherbet	2.0	270
Ice milk	4.3	185
Soft-serve ice milk	2.6	250
Ice cream (regular)	10.0	270
Soft-serve ice cream	13.0	375
Ice cream (rich)	16.0	350
Frozen custard	10.0	335
Frozen yogurt	2.0	290

Sources: U.S. Department of Agriculture and National Heart, Lung and Blood Institute.

disorder, in all population groups lactase levels are high at birth and throughout the first year or two of life. After that, in most people, the lactase level drops with age, and in some it nearly disappears.

Lactose intolerance, as this enzyme deficiency is called, is not an all-or-nothing phenomenon. A person may show lactose intolerance on a standard test (the test involves drinking four glasses of milk on an empty stomach) but may be able to handle small amounts of lactose— the amount, for instance, in a glass of milk—if it is consumed slowly along with other foods. Most people with lactase deficiency have no trouble with the amount of milk that might be added to a cup of coffee. But some must avoid all sources of lactose, including foods to which nonfat milk solids have been added.

Lactose is present in fluid milk (whole, low-fat, and skim), cream, dry milk powder (with or without fat), evaporated milk, filled milk, buttermilk, yogurt, and ice cream. However, in some milk products, lactose levels have been reduced by bacterial cultures that predigest it. These include ripened (hard and soft) cheeses, yogurt, buttermilk, sour cream, and acidophilus milk. In these products, bacteria called lactobacilli have "soured" the milk by breaking down some of the lactose, and in foods containing live cultures—for example, some brands of yogurt—further decomposition of lactose may occur in the digestive tract of the consumer. All these fermented products are suitable fare for many people afflicted with lactose intolerance. (A helpful hint: All products marked "parve" are milk-free.)

Another possibility is *"sweet acidophilus" milk,* which tastes the same as ordinary milk. Instead of having the bacteria predigest the lactose, the organisms are added to the cold milk; they don't grow and break down lactose until the milk is warmed in the human digestive tract. However, cooking with sweet acidophilus milk or adding it to a hot drink destroys the bacteria before they reach the consumer.

A better-tested method, shown to permit symptom-free milk consumption in persons highly sensitive to lactose, involves the *addition of the enzyme lactase* to the milk at home. Lactase-treated milk can be used in cooking. However, since the component sugars in lactose are considerably sweeter than the lactose itself, the enzyme treatment gives the milk a decidedly sweet taste. But the milk actually contains no more carbohydrates or calories than before enzyme treatment. The enzyme is marketed in liquid form as the product LactAid. Four or five drops of the liquid enzyme are added to a quart of milk, which is then left to stand for 24 hours before drinking. About 70 percent of the lactose is converted. LactAid can be purchased in many health-food stores and pharmacies or possibly through your physician. It can also be obtained by mail directly from LactAid, Inc., P.O. Box 111, Pleasantville, N.J.,

08232, or call the company's hotline: 800-257-8650 (in New Jersey, 609-645-7500). You can get a trial size that will convert four quarts of milk. The company also sells LactAid tablets that can be taken just before consuming foods or drugs that contain lactose. Similar "milk digestant" tablets can be purchased in some health-food stores.

Other Black Marks against Milk

Despite its basic excellence as a food for infants and young children, milk can cause a number of problems in the pediatric-aged group, and some of them may interfere with good nutrition.

Milk allergy. Some infants are allergic to one or more of the proteins in cow's milk, which contains nearly three times as much protein as human breast milk. If the infant's immature digestive system can't handle the proteins properly, the baby may become sensitized to them and develop a range of symptoms that are easily confused with other health problems. They include eczema, diarrhea, colic, constipation, irritability, asthma, ear infections, refusal to eat, and excessive fatigue, among others. The best way to diagnose milk allergy is to remove all milk and milk products from the child's diet and see if the symptoms disappear. Because it's so difficult to diagnose, no one knows exactly how common this problem is. Various studies have estimated that it afflicts anywhere from 1 in 14 children to 1 in 300. It is more likely to occur if the baby is fed cow's milk before the age of six months.

Iron deficiency anemia. Children who drink a lot of milk to the exclusion of other foods may not get enough iron in their diets and consequently may become anemic. The problem is aggravated by the fact that cow's milk can cause a chronic loss of microscopic amounts of blood from the gastrointestinal tract. Milk is a poor source of iron, although many commercial infant formulas are now supplemented with iron. The American Academy of Pediatrics has recommended that milk intake be restricted in children with nutritional iron deficiency, children who "won't eat," and children who tend to be constipated. Others have suggested weaning babies to a cup as early as possible as a way of cutting down on excessive milk consumption.

Nursing-bottle syndrome. Many young children today develop severe decay of their front teeth. This can lead to premature loss of the baby teeth and improper growth of the permanent ones that follow. Ironically, milk, which is so important to forming strong, healthy teeth, is the usual cause. Nursing-bottle syndrome, as the problem is called, results from repeated instances in which the child goes to bed with a bottle. The child dozes off and pools of milk collect around the front teeth and provide ideal growing conditions for decay-causing bacteria. Milk is the most common, but not the only, culprit. Fruit juice can have the same effect. So can allowing the baby to linger at the breast. Dentists who treat children recommend two avenues of prevention: either give the child a bottle before putting him or her to bed or put water in the bedtime bottle.

Milk can also cause health problems for adults, even if adults have no difficulty digesting lactose.

Acid stomach. Although milk has long been the traditional salve for ulcer patients, whose condition is aggravated by gastric acid, a recent study showed that milk itself provokes the stomach to release this irritating acid. Researchers at the Veterans Administration Hospital in Los Angeles tested whole, low-fat, and skim milk. All three stimulated gastric-acid secretion, and the ability of the milk to neutralize that acid was short-lived. On the basis of their findings, the authors seriously questioned the wisdom of prescribing frequent milk consumption for ulcer patients.

Cardiovascular disease. When it comes to diseases of the heart and blood vessels, milk has three strikes against it: most of its fat is saturated; it contains a fair amount of cholesterol (33 milligrams per cup); and it's high in sodium (120 milligrams per cup). Two of these potential hazards—the fat and the cholesterol—are greatly reduced in low-fat milk and practically nonexistent in skim milk. But sodium remains high in all milk and milk products except special low-sodium milk and cheeses.

An analysis by a British researcher of deaths in forty-three countries showed a strong correlation between the amount of milk consumed and deaths from heart attacks. The researcher, Dr. Jeffrey Segall, noted that two studies of ulcer patients, who presumably drink a lot of milk, revealed that they were twice as likely as others their age to suffer a heart attack. But this fact may have more to do with how such people respond to stress than to the amount of milk they drink. At the moment, the role that milk plays in heart disease is unclear.

"Milk Factor" and Heart Disease

One of the most intriguing recent findings about milk is that it can lower the level of cholesterol in the blood. Even whole milk, with all its saturated fat and cholesterol, has this effect, as does low-fat and skim milk. The effect was first noted in conjunction with yogurt, which seems to have more of this mysterious milk factor than unfermented milk. In the early 1970s, Dr. George V. Mann, biochemist and nutritionist at Vanderbilt University, was doing some studies with the Masai tribe in Africa and accidentally discovered that something in yogurt lowered serum cholesterol even when the diet contained large amounts of cholesterol.

The Masai have long intrigued heart researchers because their diet is high in cholesterol yet cardiovascular disease is practically nonexistent in their society. A typical Masai tribesman consumes 4 to 5 quarts of fermented whole milk each day plus a fair amount of meat. Yet something seems to protect the Masai from the ravages of heart disease so common among other people on high-cholesterol diets. Dr. Mann was studying the effect of a food additive on cholesterol levels among young Masai men. He found that, with or without the additive, their cholesterol levels dropped despite the fact that all the men in the study consumed very large amounts of the fermented milk and gained significant amounts of weight. Dr. Mann later repeated his experiments with American volunteers and again found a cholesterol-lowering effect from yogurt.

Since then, a number of studies have confirmed this effect in laboratory animals as well as in human volunteers. It has been shown to occur with whole milk, buttermilk, and skim milk as well as yogurt. The effect is greatest with skim milk or with fermented whole or skim milk, consumed in amounts ranging from 2 to 4 quarts a day. However, both butter and cream raise cholesterol levels in people. And it has not yet been shown that the cholesterol-lowering effect of milk does in fact protect against heart disease.

A number of substances in milk have been studied in an attempt to isolate the responsible factor, but as yet the precise substance or group of substances involved is not known. If and when it can be identified, however, it may be possible to use the pure chemical as a dietary supplement to keep cholesterol levels low in persons prone to coronary heart disease. Meanwhile, the consumption of milk, yogurt, and buttermilk may be better for your heart than most nutritionists realize.

FOR FURTHER READING

Jacqueline Hostage, *Living without Milk* (White Hall, Va.: Betterway, 1979). A guide to milk-free shopping and cooking, including recipes.

14 ⚬ ALCOHOL: NUTRIENT OR NEMESIS?

ALCOHOL preceded people here on earth, and judging from the earliest human records, it was a popular item in the prehistoric diet. Ancient civilizations used it, too, in many ways: as an adjunct to feast and celebration; as part of religious rites; as an internal and external medication, and as a food. The list would need little amendment to describe the role of alcohol today for the 95 million Americans who imbibe it and who derive 10 to 20 percent of their calories from it.

Alcohol was the "therapeutic" ingredient in elixirs peddled by medicine men from the rear of stagecoaches, and remains today a major ingredient in many nostrums, including cough medicines, cold cures, diarrhea remedies, pain killers, and vitamin tonics like Geritol and Geriplex taken by the elderly to boost their vitality.

Whether consumed by the glass or teaspoon or directly from the bottle, alcohol is unquestionably the nation's leading mood-altering drug. Some doctors even prescribe it as a tranquilizer or sedative for patients with arthritis, high blood pressure, heart disease, and digestive problems, as well as for convalescents and the elderly. You may think of alcohol as a stimulant because it loosens tongues, aggressions, and inhibitions, but it actually has an anesthetic, or narcotizing, effect. It puts the brain to sleep, starting with the frontal lobe, or reasoning portion. The apparent stimulation associated with a few drinks reflects the fact that this is the part of the brain that normally holds tight rein on your more licentious self. With alcohol, the control is lifted.

As the dose of alcohol increases, the narcosis moves on to the brain's speech and vision centers, and the frontal lobe is further anesthetized. Finally, at still larger doses, alcohol hits the part of the brain that controls the voluntary muscles, producing the staggering gait we associate with being drunk. If enough alcohol is consumed in a very short time, brain function can become so depressed that coma and death follow.

Table 14.1 • HOW ALCOHOL AFFECTS YOU

Amount distilled spirits consumed in two hours	Typical effects on body and brain
3 ounces	Release of tension; carefree sensation; loosening of judgment, thought, and restraint.
4½ ounces	Tensions and inhibitions of everyday life lessened.
6 ounces	Voluntary motor action affected; hand and arm movements, walk, and speech clumsy.
10 ounces	Severe impairment: staggering, loud, incoherent, emotionally unstable, very drunk; 100 times greater than average traffic risk.
14 ounces	Deeper areas of brain affected; parts controlling response to stimuli and understanding stuperous.
18 ounces	Asleep, difficult to arouse; incapable of voluntary action, like surgical anesthesia.
22 ounces	Coma; anesthesia of centers of brain controlling breathing and heartbeat; death.

Source: From information furnished by the National Clearinghouse for Alcohol Information, as reproduced in Morris Chafetz, M.D., *Why Drinking Can Be Good for You* (New York: Stein & Day, 1976).

Fortunately, most drinkers rarely get beyond the relaxing effect induced by low blood levels of alcohol—a drink or two consumed in an hour or more. And, it is a pleasure to know, that amount of alcohol may be good for you.

Alcohol and Your Heart

Most Americans, accustomed to the idea that everything enjoyable is immoral, illegal, fattening, or hazardous to health, are likely to distrust the statement that a drink or two a day can actually improve health. Surely, that idea must emanate from the nation's brewers, winemakers, or distillers. After all, alcohol is a killer in large doses; in small doses, you assume, it must still do its dirty work, if slowly. Maybe it does. But the facts show that when alcohol is consumed in moderate amounts, the benefits usually outweigh the risks.

In 1926, a pioneering study showed that moderate drinkers—those who consumed one or two drinks a day on the average—lived longer than abstainers, heavy drinkers, former drinkers, and occasional drinkers. Several more recent studies have indicated the same thing. The main benefit seems to be to the heart and blood vessels. Nondrinkers and very light drinkers are more likely to suffer heart attacks than those who consume one or two drinks a day. Moderate drinkers also have higher levels of a protective substance in their blood called high-density lipoproteins, or HDLs (see Chapter 3). These proteins are believed to help prevent the accumulation of fatty deposits in the arteries feeding the heart, and thus may reduce the risk of heart attack. Although moderate amounts of alcohol can raise blood levels of triglycerides (fatty substances that promote arterial clogging), the net effect seems to be a beneficial one. It's also possible that moderate doses of alcohol help the heart by relieving stress and relaxing the muscles that squeeze the arteries and narrow the passageways through which blood must flow.

But as with many other aspects of nutrition, just because a little alcohol may be good, more is not necessarily better. In fact, from the standpoint of your heart alone, heavy drinking can be devastating. Drinkers who consume a lot of alcohol are more likely to develop high blood pressure and to die young from heart disease, stroke, and related disorders than those who consume little or no alcohol. Prolonged heavy drinking can cause cardiomyopathy—a disease of the heart muscle—and drinking bouts can provoke abnormal heart rhythms.

Alcohol has been shown to damage heart muscle cells and to diminish the amount of blood the heart can pump. This effect is most pronounced in persons with pre-existing heart disease. Therefore, many cardiologists advise their heart patients to consume no more than one drink a day. And persons with severe heart damage or congestive heart failure are commonly told to abstain completely. "The secret to a long life is to stay busy, get plenty of exercise and don't drink too much. Then again, don't drink too little"—Hermann (Jackrabbit) Smith-Johannson, 103-year-old cross-country skier.

Deadly in Large Doses

Even for healthy people, alcohol can have disastrous effects if they imbibe too heavily, especially if heavy drinking is a practice of long standing. *Alcohol is a toxic drug*—toxic to the brain, the heart, the liver, and the gastrointestinal tract. Here are some effects that have helped to give "demon rum" its notoriety.

Accidents. Alcohol is a factor in nearly half the nation's traffic fatalities—more than 20,000 deaths a year. Drunk driving is the direct cause of 44 percent of driver deaths and 36 percent of adult pedestrian fatalities. Among drivers arrested because they were intoxicated, the average alcohol level found in their blood exceeded 0.2 percent. To reach such a level, a 180-pound man would have to consume ten drinks within an hour on an empty stomach! Alcohol is also an important contributor to home accidents, accounting for one-seventh to one-fifth of accidental deaths in the home.

The increased accident rate among drinkers is a direct result of alcohol's effects on the brain. While tests show that small amounts of alcohol actually improve performance skills involved in driving, larger doses impair reflex responses and muscular coordination, slow reaction time, and interfere with judgment. At the same time, however, the intoxicated driver may actually believe he or she is driving better than usual.

Even moderate drinking can diminish visual skills needed for safe driving. A study at the University of California at Berkeley showed that one or two drinks temporarily reduce the ability to identify and track moving objects, recover from glare, and distinguish certain colors. The effects can last for five or six hours after the last drink.

Liver disease. The liver is the body's sole agent for detoxifying alcohol and converting it to usable energy. More than 95 percent of alcohol consumed is metabolized by the liver; the remainder is excreted unchanged in breath, urine, and sweat. The more you drink, the harder your liver has to work to clear your blood of this cellular poison.

Alcohol "demands" that it be metabolized before the liver performs its normal duty of converting fatty acids to usable energy. A "fatty liver" (accumulations of fat in the liver) can result. This condition is reversible by abstaining from drink. Alcoholic binges—spurts of heavy drinking—can precipitate a more serious inflammation of the liver called alcoholic hepatitis. And prolonged heavy drinking can lead to cirrhosis, a chronic and potentially fatal degeneration of the liver that also increases the risk of liver cancer. Persons with hepatitis or cirrhosis must avoid alcohol completely.

Cancer. As with liver disease, cancer is primarily a risk among those who drink heavily, especially if they also smoke cigarettes. Alcohol seems to act either as a cofactor in causing cancer or as a promoter of cancer growth that is initiated by some other factor. Compared to

Table 14.2 • IS IT SAFE TO DRIVE?

| | *Number of Drinks in an Hour** | | | |
	1 or 2	*3 or 4*	*5 or 6*	*7*
% alcohol in blood**	.01	.05	.10	.15
Are you intoxicated?	Normally not.	You may be.	You very likely are.	You definitely are.
If you "must" drive,	Take it easy.	Use extreme caution.	DON'T.	ABSOLUTELY DO NOT!

Source: Adapted from chart prepared by the U.S. Department of Health, Education, and Welfare.
*One drink equals 1 ounce of 100-proof whiskey or one 12-ounce bottle of beer.
**The approximate level for a 160-pound man.

nondrinkers, those who consume a lot of alcohol are two to six times as likely to develop cancer of the mouth and throat, the exact level of risk depending upon whether they also smoke. The combination of heavy drinking and heavy smoking increases the risk by fifteen times that of nondrinkers and nonsmokers. Cancer of the larynx is ten times as common, and cancer of the esophagus up to twenty-five times as common among those who drink heavily as among those who abstain or drink moderately.

A relationship has also been found between deaths from rectal cancer and the amount of beer consumed in various states and nations. Beer and Scotch whiskey, both made from malt, have recently been shown to contain a potent cancer-causing agent, N-nitrosodimethylamine, or NDMA. This nitrosamine has caused cancer in nearly every kind of laboratory animal tested so far. (See page 480.)

Gastrointestinal injury. Alcohol increases the acidity of the stomach, impairs the stomach's action, and damages the stomach lining. The irritant effects of large doses of alcohol are well known to those whose overindulgence has provoked an abrupt rebellion by the stomach. While alcohol is not thought to cause ulcers, it can certainly make existing ulcers worse. Alcohol can also injure the lining of the small intestine and interfere with the ability of the small intestine to absorb vital nutrients. This is one reason why alcoholics can develop nutritional deficiencies even if they follow a good diet.

Sexual performance. As an aphrodisiac, alcohol leaves something to be desired. For at the same time that it stimulates an *interest* in sexual activity, it can impair *performance*. At least, in men. Alcohol causes the liver to produce excessive amounts of an enzyme that breaks down testosterone, the male sex hormone. The result can be a temporary loss of potency. Prolonged heavy drinking by male alcoholics can result in a chronic undersupply of testosterone with a consequent shrinkage of the testicles and growth of the breasts.

Fetal development. In the mid-1970s, researchers at the University of Washington identified a pattern of growth abnormalities and birth defects common among babies of women who drank heavily during pregnancy. The researchers named it fetal alcohol syndrome. It is characterized by growth retardation before and after birth, small head size, a flattened, blank-looking face, and poor small-muscle function. Heart malformations and mental retardation may also occur.

Following this discovery, many doctors advised their pregnant patients to limit alcohol intake to at most two drinks a day. Some are even more conservative. Noting that a safe level of alcohol has not yet

been defined, they urge total abstinence throughout pregnancy, preferably starting when a woman first tries to conceive.

Other bad effects. Alcohol, commonly used to help people relax
so that they can more easily fall asleep, is ineffective as a sleeping pill
in anything more than the smallest amounts. It diminishes the amount
of REM, or dream, sleep and can actually make *insomnia* worse.

A heavy dose of alcohol can precipitate an attack of *gout*—painful
deposits of uric acid in the joints, especially the big toe—because it
reduces the body's ability to get rid of uric acid. The problem is corrected by abstinence.

Alcohol in large doses can also diminish the body's ability to fight
off *bacterial infections.* And, as you will see in this chapter, alcohol can
interfere with the body's supply of essential nutrients.

Alcohol stimulates the release of insulin, and drinking on an empty
stomach can cause a precipitous drop in blood sugar and the *symptoms
of hypoglycemia* in some people. This is especially true for mixed drinks
in which the mixer contains sugar. The combination of alcohol with
sugar, which also stimulates insulin release, can produce a severe reaction, including headache, nausea, dizziness, and irritability.

What's "a Drink," Anyway?

What you consider "a drink" may be quite different from what "a
drink" means to your wife, your boss, or your mother-in-law. To some,
a drink is a double martini on the rocks, to others it may be a Bloody
Mary, and to still others a glass of sherry. Some people erroneously
think a drink refers only to distilled spirits and not to wine or beer. And
some people mistakenly assume that as long as they stay away from the
"hard stuff," they can't get drunk or develop a drinking problem.

Actually, the definition of a drink depends not on the drink's color,
name, where or how it's served, or what it's mixed with. It depends only
on how much alcohol is contained in a serving of the beverage. If you're
trying to determine how much you drink, your calculation must be
based on the *absolute alcohol content* of the beverages you consume.
The following will guide you through the confusing maze of alcoholic
beverages.

Distilled spirits. Alcohol is made by the fermentation of the sugars
and starches in plants, most commonly grains, fruits, and sugar cane.
In making distilled spirits, the fermented mash is distilled to separate

the alcohol and flavoring chemicals, called congeners, from the unfermented plant residue and water. This concentrates the alcohol.

The alcohol content of distilled spirits is measured as "proof." One degree of proof equals 0.5 percent of alcohol. Thus, a beverage that is 80 proof contains 40 percent alcohol; one that is 90 proof is 45 percent alcohol; and 100 proof equals 50 percent alcohol.

Scotch, gin, whiskey, rum, vodka, brandy, and cognacs are distilled spirits. Most are 80 proof, although higher proofs of some are available. The label should state the proof. Brandy is distilled from the fermented mash of grapes or other fruits and then aged. Cordials and liqueurs (one and the same) are made from distilled spirits that are mixed with fruits, flowers, herbs, or other plant flavorings and are sweetened.

Wines. Wine is produced primarily from the fermentation of grapes. If some other plant, such as rice, is used, the label must say so. Wines are not distilled, so they contain more water and less alcohol than distilled spirits. They also contain unfermented carbohydrates. The alcohol content of wines varies greatly: 8.5 to 10 percent for most French and German wines; 12 to 14 percent for most American wines; 17 percent for sake (Japanese rice wine); and 18 to 21 percent for sherry and port.

Beers. Beers are made from fermented malt beverages. They also have less alcohol and more water than distilled spirits plus some unfermented carbohydrates. They have a lower percentage of alcohol than wine. The most popular light lager beers and ale have 4.5 percent alcohol (in some states, grocery stores are only allowed to sell "3.2 beer," which is beer with 3.2 percent alcohol). The heavier, darker beers like bock, porter, and stout, have about 6 or 7 percent alcohol.

In most studies, *one drink* is taken to mean *0.5 ounce of absolute alcohol.* Based on the most common types of alcoholic beverages sold, then, one drink would be defined as any of the following: one jigger (1½ ounces) of 80 proof distilled spirits; 1 ounce of 110 proof distilled spirits; one 12-ounce glass of lager beer; one 8-ounce glass of stout; one 5-ounce glass of French wine; one 4-ounce glass of American wine; or 3 ounces of sherry.

If you really want to know how much you're drinking, measure the alcoholic beverage before you pour it into your glass. Or measure your glasses so you know how much they hold. One person's wine glass is another's water goblet, so "a glass of wine" can mean a lot of different things unless it's measured.

Alcohol Calories Do Count

As you will see in Chapter 17, you can't ignore the caloric content of the substances you drink. This is especially true for alcoholic beverages. Absolute alcohol measured in a chemistry lab contains 7 calories per gram, more than the same weight of proteins or carbohydrates and slightly less than fats. A half ounce of absolute alcohol—the alcohol content of one drink—contains approximately 100 calories of alcohol.

However, the body doesn't use alcohol calories as efficiently as those contained in other essential foodstuffs. So for practical purposes, you can figure the calorie value of absolute alcohol as being between 5 and 6 calories per gram, or 70 to 85 calories per drink.

Chances are, though, that when you drink, you're consuming more than just the calories from alcohol. If you're drinking beer or wine, you have to add on the caloric value of the unfermented carbohydrates—sugars and starches. Cordials and liqueurs contain sweeteners, which add calories. And if you're consuming mixed drinks, you have to figure on the calories in the mix, unless you use plain water, club soda, mineral or spring water, or seltzer, which contain no calories. Table 14.3 lists the caloric content of typical drinks and mixers.

The liver is the only organ that can use alcohol as a source of energy, and sooner or later the liver burns up all the alcohol you consume. None is left for energy storage as fat. But just because excess alcohol calories are not stored as fat, that doesn't mean you can't get fat from drinking more calories than your body needs. Instead of storing the extra alcohol as fat, your body will simply convert more of the other foods you eat to fat. The calories going in—whether as food or drink—will always equal those going out, with the leftover stored as fat for future energy needs.

The Antinutrient Nutrient

Because alcohol supplies your body with usable energy, it must be considered a nutrient. But more than any other source of calories except sugar, alcohol is *empty calories.* It gives the body nothing but fuel. This is especially true of distilled spirits.

Beer and wine do contain other nutrients—some vitamins and minerals (in addition to carbohydrates)—but these are present in amounts too tiny to be of any nutritional value. According to Dr. Frank L. Iber of Tufts University School of Medicine in Boston, 1 ounce of bread contains more nutrients, including vitamins, than a bottle of beer.

Table 14.3 • THE CALORIES IN YOUR DRINKS

Beverage	Amount	Calories
Alcohol		
Beer and ale	12 ounces	140–150
Light (low calorie) beer	12 ounces	95
Extra-light beer	12 ounces	70
Wine, dry table	3½ ounces	87
Wine, dessert	2 ounces	81
Vermouth, dry	1 ounce	33
Vermouth, sweet	1 ounce	50
Distilled spirits		
(gin, rum, vodka, whiskey)		
80 proof	1½ ounces	97
86 proof	1½ ounces	105
90 proof	1½ ounces	110
94 proof	1½ ounces	116
100 proof	1½ ounces	124
Cordials and liqueurs	1 ounce	70–115
Brandy and cognac	1 ounce	65
Mixers		
Club soda	8 ounces	0
Cola	8 ounces	96
Ginger ale	8 ounces	72
Mineral water	8 ounces	0
Quinine water (tonic)	8 ounces	72
Seltzer	8 ounces	0
Tom Collins mixer	8 ounces	112

Dr. Janet B. McDonald of the U.S. Public Health Service Hospital in San Francisco points out that although most of the vitamins in grapes are lost in making wine, wine does contain small amounts of iron in a form that is readily absorbed by the body. Wine also contains a fair amount of potassium, and most wines are low in sodium, which would make wine an acceptable drink for a person with high blood pressure. But all things considered, Dr. McDonald says, "except for calories, consumption of wine in moderate amounts contributes little to normal daily nutrient requirements. The same, of course, can be said for other alcoholic beverages."

Thus, if alcohol contributes a significant number of calories to your daily caloric intake, you should watch the nutritional value of the rest of your diet to be sure you don't develop nutritional deficiencies. Unfortunately, the more people drink, the less attention they are likely to pay to what they eat.

Although in small, well-diluted doses alcohol is an appetite stimulant that prompts a desire for food within five minutes of consumption, larger, more concentrated amounts suppress hunger. People who drink a lot tend to eat poorly. The toxic effects of alcohol are then compounded by the effects of chronic malnutrition, with liver and other diseases the likely result.

As if the emptiness of alcohol calories weren't enough, alcohol also deprives the body of nutrients from other foods you eat. When alcohol is metabolized by the liver, it uses up niacin and thiamin, which means that these B vitamins are not available for other essential purposes. Alcohol also interferes with the absorption and storage of other vitamins, especially folacin and B_{12}. And because alcohol is a diuretic that increases the output of urine, it can cause the loss of such water-soluble minerals as magnesium, potassium, and zinc.

The Hangover

You don't have to be a chronically heavy drinker to suffer the adverse effects of alcohol. One "night on the town" can do it, as millions have discovered the morning after. Hangovers have no respect for race, nationality, or socioeconomic status. Anyone who overdoes it can get one. To a hungover German, it's "Katzenjammer"—the wailing of cats. Italians call it "stonato"—out of tune. To the French it's "la gueule de bois"—woody mouth; in Spain "resaca"—surf of sea; in Norway "jeg har tømmermenn"—workmen in my head; and in Sweden it's "hont i haret"—pain in the roots of the hair. But by whatever name, the splitting headache, searing thirst, churning stomach, furry tongue, and shaky jitters of a hangover are an exacting price to pay for an evening's indulgence.

In many cases, the evening was not even that enjoyable. According to Dr. Morris Chafetz, former director of the National Institute on Alcohol Abuse and Alcoholism, those who drink under tense circumstances or who feel guilty about drinking are likely to have the worst hangovers. Fatigue also has a lot to do with it. Because alcohol anesthetizes the brain's early warning system that tells you when you're tired and ready to go to bed, you tend to stay up a lot later than you should. In fact, Dr. Chafetz says, you can get hangover symptoms without touching a drop of alcohol—just from pushing yourself too hard.

Alcohol also makes a direct contribution to the next morning's miseries. It draws water from body cells and increases the loss of water through the kidneys, causing the extreme thirst common to hangovers. Hangover headache may result from the swelling of cranial arteries, since alcohol causes blood vessels to expand. The nausea, vomiting, and heartburn of a hangover stem from alcohol's irritation of the lining of the gastrointestinal tract. Alcohol also delays the passage of food to the small intestine, interfering with proper digestion.

Then there are the *congeners*. These are chemical "contaminants" in distilled spirits that contribute to the characteristic flavors of the spirits. Congeners result from the fermentation and maturation of the liquor. Although alcohol is rapidly eliminated from the body, congeners are not, and they hang around to cause toxic effects the next day. In fact, researchers were able to produce hangovers in volunteers just by giving them water solutions of congeners devoid of alcohol.

Sensitivity to the type and amount of congeners in various drinks may be the reason why some people are adversely affected by some types of alcoholic beverages but not by others. Vodka and gin have the least congeners; blended Scotch has 4 times more than gin; and brandy, rum, and pure malt Scotch have 6 times the congener level of gin. Bourbon leads the pack, with 8 times as many congeners as gin and 30 times as many as vodka. Red wine contains substances similar to congeners to which some people are sensitive. In one study, hangovers were produced most often by brandy, followed by red wine, rum, whiskey, white wine, gin, and vodka, in that order.

The hangover has inspired a plenitude of remedies through the ages. Coffee, raw eggs, oysters, chili peppers, steak sauce, vitamins, antacids, aspirin, and sleeping pills are some modern American ones. The Norwegians swear by a glass of heavy cream, the Russians recommend salted cucumber juice, and the Swiss use brandy with peppermint —akin to the Bloody Mary of Americans who believe in the "hair of the dog" philosophy. But none of these is likely to bring much relief, and the "hair of the dog"—more alcohol—may actually make things worse. While the anesthetic effect of the alcohol may temporarily relieve the pangs of hangover, it only delays the moment of reckoning and interferes with *the only sure remedy: time and rest.* Coffee, a stimulant, and exercise are also counterproductive for that reason.

How to Drink for Pleasure Safely

What you drink, how you drink, and where you drink all influence the effect alcohol has on you. As with other aspects of nutrition, you can have your cake and eat it too if you understand some basic facts about how your body handles alcohol and you put these facts to work for you.

• Eat something before you drink, preferably something that is not sweet and that is high in fat or protein. Then wait fifteen minutes before drinking. Twenty percent of the alcohol you consume is absorbed immediately and directly into your blood through your stomach wall. The rest is subsequently absorbed through the small intestine. If you have food in your stomach before you drink, it will sponge up the alcohol, slow its absorption through the stomach, and delay its passage into your intestines. Fatty foods like cheese, meat, peanut butter, or whole milk are best for coating your stomach.

If you're drinking at someone else's house, dive into the hors d'oeuvres before you start drinking. At a restaurant you can order an appetizer or cocktail nibbles. But stay away from salty snack foods like chips, pretzels, and salted nuts. These make you thirsty and increase the likelihood that you'll drink too much.

• Lower the concentration of alcohol in your drink by diluting it with lots of ice and a mixer. But avoid carbonated mixers since these speed the absorption of alcohol. Water is by far the best mixer (it doesn't even add calories); juices are okay. The alcohol from distilled spirits is absorbed more rapidly than that in wine and beer, which contain nonalcoholic substances that slow absorption.

• Try some of the alcohol-free drinks such as nonalcoholic wine, beer, and champagne. They have the flavor of the real thing but at most only trace amounts of alcohol, and can be consumed as freely as your caloric requirements permit.

• Sip your drinks slowly. *It takes the average person's liver one hour to break down the alcohol from one drink.* If you consume alcohol faster than the rate at which the liver can clear it from your blood, you'll feel some of the effects of alcohol on your brain. The more you overwhelm the liver's capacity, the drunker you'll get. If you space your drinks an hour apart, you may be able to drink all night without getting tipsy, though I certainly wouldn't advise it. A quickly consumed drink not only produces a more potent immediate effect, but its effects last longer than that of a drink that's sipped.

The liver is sluggish about metabolizing alcohol in people who are unaccustomed to drinking, so these individuals have to be especially careful about how quickly the drink goes down the hatch. Also, some people seem especially sensitive to the effects of even small amounts of alcohol in their blood ("cheap drunks," in common parlance); for them, sipping slowly and stopping at one or two drinks is especially important. People who "hold their liquor well" are usually those who regularly consume several drinks a day, and their liver has become "primed" to more rapid breakdown of alcohol.

• Know your capacity and stick to it. Don't let companions cajole you into drinking more than you know you can handle comfortably. If your host or hostess keeps pushing drinks, ask for plain soda when you know you've had enough. If you start with a tall drink well diluted with ice and water and you sip it slowly, your glass will be ready for a refill less often.

• Remember, the smaller you are, the harder you're likely to be hit by a given amount of alcohol. Also, according to researchers at the University of Oklahoma, women are generally more sensitive to alcohol's effects than men. The same amount of alcohol produces a higher level of alcohol in the blood of women, and they act drunker than men do. This is true even among men and women matched for weight, drinking history, and previous food intake. The explanation may be that men have a higher percentage of water in their bodies, so a given amount of alcohol becomes more diluted in the body when consumed by a man. The menstrual cycle also has an effect: alcohol reaches its highest level in the blood just before a woman's menstrual period, and the lowest level occurs on the first day of menstrual bleeding.

• Drink only in a relaxed, pleasant atmosphere. To some that's like saying "go to bed only when you're not tired." Many people are inclined to drink—and most likely to drink too much—when they're tense and uncomfortable. The alcohol helps them "unwind" and masks their discomfort. But, according to Dr. Chafetz, a given amount of alcohol has a bigger wallop if consumed when you're emotionally upset, under stress, or fatigued. "If I had to come up with an unhealthy drinking situation, it would be the American cocktail party," he remarked. "Standing around uncomfortably in a crush of people, most of whom we don't know, makes us want to gulp that first drink"—and follow it quickly by a second and maybe a third.

• Don't mix drugs with drinks. *Alcohol enhances the effect of many drugs, and inactivates others.* Narcotics, tranquilizers, antidepressants, antihistamines, and sleeping pills become more potent when mixed with alcohol. In fact, some people have accidentally killed themselves by taking barbiturates and alcohol together, each in doses that separately would not come near to having a fatal effect.

Alcohol may also interact with certain antidiabetic medications, diuretics, and other drugs used to treat high blood pressure. And it can interfere with the action of anticoagulants, anticonvulsants, and the antibiotic tetracycline. Beer and wine can result in headaches, palpitations, nausea, and vomiting in persons taking antidepressant drugs called MAO inhibitors. If you are taking any medication, the wisest course of action is to check with your doctor or pharmacist before drinking. Don't assume it's safe to drink, even if you've tried it before without mishap when taking the same drug.

• Keep in mind that the alcohol content of different drinks varies widely—from 3.2 percent for some beers all the way to 80 percent for Polish spirits. But because you're likely to consume more beer or wine than distilled spirits, you can take in just as much total alcohol from the less concentrated drinks. It's the total amount of alcohol consumed over a given period of time that determines how drunk you're likely to get. See Table 14.2 on page 262 for some guidelines to how your consumption affects the concentration of alcohol in your blood and its effects on you.

• If you have overindulged in alcohol, *only time will help you to sober up.* In general, *it takes as many hours to recover as the number of drinks you've consumed.* There's no way to goad the liver into metabolizing alcohol any faster than it can. Walking around the block won't help because your muscles can't burn up the alcohol. You can turn sleepy drunks into wide-awake ones by giving them black coffee or putting them under a cold shower, but you won't sober them up. And, quite frankly, it's a lot safer to be sleepy if you're drunk!

If It's Your Party

There are a number of things you can do to help your guests have a good time without their having to pay for it afterward.

• Be sure to serve snacks with drinks and place them within easy reach of all your guests. Cheese and crackers (unsalted), vegetables with a dip made from mayonnaise and yogurt, cream cheese, or sour cream, and cocktail meats or fish are best from the standpoint of slowing alcohol absorption. My own favorites are two Middle Eastern appetizers—hummus and baba ghanoush—served with pita (Middle Eastern pocket bread), either fresh or toasted.

Hummus (Chickpea Spread)

1 large onion, minced
1 to 2 cloves garlic, minced
2 tablespoons vegetable oil
2 cups chickpeas (garbanzos), cooked (if canned, drain and rinse)
½ cup fresh lemon juice

1 tablespoon soy sauce
½ teaspoon salt (optional)
¼ cup sesame paste (tahini; see note)
½ cup sesame seeds, toasted and ground

Sauté the onion and garlic in the oil until they are soft, and set aside. In a food processor or blender, purée the chickpeas with the onion and garlic and the remaining ingredients. Yield: 3 cups. *Note:* If tahini is unavailable, it can be made in a blender from 1 teaspoon lemon juice, ½ teaspoon oil, 2 tablespoons water, and ¼ cup finely ground sesame seeds.

Baba Ghanoush (Eggplant Spread)

2 medium or 1 large eggplant (about 2 pounds), whole and unpeeled
¼ cup sesame paste (tahini; see note, above)
¼ cup fresh lemon juice
1 large clove garlic, crushed
¼ cup finely minced onion

1–2 teaspoons salt (or to taste)
Freshly ground black pepper (optional, to taste)
1 tablespoon olive oil or vegetable oil
2 tablespoons finely chopped fresh parsley

Prick the eggplant in several places with a fork, place on a baking sheet, and broil in a preheated broiler for about 20 minutes, turning several times so that the skin chars on all sides. When cool enough to handle, cut in half, scrape off the flesh into a bowl, discard skin, and mash the eggplant with the sesame paste, lemon juice, garlic, onion, salt, and pepper. Cover and refrigerate. Before serving, sprinkle with oil and chopped parsley.

• Always have nonalcoholic beverages readily available, and offer them when you take orders for drinks. Be sure to keep a tub of ice handy so that guests can help themselves.

• Serve your guests their drinks and measure the amount of alcohol you put in with a jigger or measuring cup. It's a favor to no one to be overly generous in pouring drinks. Remember, it's a drug that you're doling out, and it should be consumed in doses the body can handle. And don't race to refill every glass the moment it dips below the halfway mark. If they're not pushed to drink quickly, most people pace themselves and consume alcohol at a reasonable rate. Dr. Chafetz recommends keeping the bar in a room separate from the party to discourage self-service and too fast refills.

• Never serve "one for the road." Stop serving alcohol at least an hour before you expect the party to break up and substitute food or coffee. Although these won't help your guests to sober up, they also won't make them drunker and will give them time to metabolize the alcohol they've consumed before they leave.

• If guests appear to be intoxicated when it's time to go home, do everything you can to prevent them from driving. Call a cab, have another guest give them a lift, or have them spend the night with you. Take away their car keys if necessary. Although this may seem embarrassing, it might avoid an accident.

FOR FURTHER READING

Morris Chafetz, M.D., *How Drinking Can Be Good for You* (New York: Stein & Day, 1978).

PART FOUR

What to Do about Your Weight

15 ✍ OBESITY: MALNUTRITION, U.S.A.

WHILE the world worries about where to get enough fuel to heat homes and run machines in the coming decades, millions of Americans suffer from an energy crisis in reverse: an over-abundance of fuel for the body's needs. The result is obesity, by far the nation's most serious nutritional problem.

Paradoxically in a nation beset by dietmania, instead of shrinking, the caloric excess—and the resulting size of Americans—is growing year by year. A survey by the National Center for Health Statistics of 12,500 Americans aged 18 to 74 showed that in 1980, the average man weighed 6 pounds more and the average woman 4 pounds more than they had 20 years earlier. This increase in weight has outstripped a much smaller increase in height. The typical adult American male is now 20 to 30 pounds overweight and the typical female weighs 15 to 30 pounds too much. Worse yet, this calculation is based on an estimate of desirable weight that scientists now believe is 10 percent higher than it should be for optimal health. Even youngsters weigh too much—10 percent of elementary-school children and 20 to 30 percent of high-schoolers are overweight and already on the road to a lifetime of obesity.

How did such a rich nation reach this deplorable state? Precisely because of our riches—our rich food, our comfort, our labor-saving devices, our effortless means of transportation. The human body is, in simple terms, a biochemical machine. It requires energy to do work, and that energy comes from the calories derived from food. Through an extensive series of chemical conversions, the body can use food calories to run thousands of essential operations—the contraction of muscles, transmission of nerve signals, digestion of foods, respiration, vision, hearing, elimination of wastes, building of new tissues, production of vital chemicals, and many more.

And, like any well-designed machine, the body can store energy for future use. The primary means of storage is fat, or adipose tissue, which lies under the skin and surrounds the internal organs. You can

Table 15.1 • WE ARE GETTING FATTER

Ages	Weight gain in pounds (1962–1974)
Males	
18–24	7
25–34	7
35–44	8
45–54	5
55–64	7
Females	
18–24	5
25–34	6
35–44	6
45–54	4
55–64	−1

Note: The data represent national averages as determined by the National Center for Health Statistics.

think of fat and its potential calories as the "gas tank" of your body. But unlike a gas tank, the body has an almost limitless capacity to accumulate an energy reserve. The more you store, the fatter you are. Any energy—that is, calories—you consume in excess of your body's immediate needs is stashed away in the body's fat depots. This layaway plan undoubtedly contributed to the survival of the human species when periods of abundant food supply alternated with scarcity, and few, if any, means were available for preserving and storing foods.

Fat is a very efficient means of energy storage. Each gram of fat you store supplies your body with 9 calories of fuel, or 245 calories per ounce of stored fat. Each pound of *fatty tissue* can yield 3,500 calories, somewhat less than 245 multiplied by 16, because fatty tissue contains some water and protein as well as pure fat. If the body were to store carbohydrates or proteins for energy, you'd get only 4 calories per gram. Thus, your body gets better mileage out of a pound of stored fat than it would from a pound of stored starch.

When you expend more energy (calories) than is provided by the foods you consume, your body draws on its fat reserves to meet the extra demand. When the energy deficit—the amount of calories used minus the amount consumed—reaches 3,500 calories, you will have lost a pound of stored fat. Since the average person uses between 1,500 and 2,700 calories per day, even a twenty-four-hour fast would not result in the loss of a pound of fat. (Your scale might show a drop of several pounds, but this represents lost water, not fat, and is immediately regained when you eat again.)

Even though millions of Americans are "on diets" to produce an energy deficit, in the long run the vast majority are in *positive energy balance*—they consume more energy than they expend. It doesn't take much to produce creeping obesity. As little as 25 extra calories consumed a day—the amount in a tablespoon of ice cream or one plain graham cracker—adds up to 175 calories a week, or a total of 9,100 calories a year. That's enough to put on 2.6 extra pounds a year, or 26 pounds in a decade.

Dr. Richard Spark of Harvard Medical School notes, "We have demanded, and constructed, a society that has made it hard to stay thin." On the one hand, we're surrounded by a surfeit of calorie-rich foodstuffs that beckon us to overconsume at every turn. And on the other hand, our lives are increasingly sedentary, so mechanized that we have less and less opportunity to expend the extra calories we consume unless we really "work" at it through special exercise programs. It takes 40 minutes of driving a car to use up 100 calories—the same amount you'd use by walking briskly for 19 minutes or riding a bicycle for 12 minutes. Throwing the clothes in the dryer takes less personal energy than hanging them on the line. The same with using a dishwasher, writing on an electric typewriter, or riding a power mower. Even the 2 million Americans who produce our food don't have to work as hard as farmers did half a century ago.

"But," you say, "it's not worth it." Why should you spend all that time mowing lawns, hanging laundry, or washing dishes by hand? Why indeed! After all, you've worked hard to be able to afford the things that relieve you from drudgery at home and at work. But, if you're not going to use all that energy to do chores, either you must eat less or spend more leisure time in physical activities that consume the calories you don't otherwise expend. Preferably, you should do both.

How Many Calories Do You Really Need?

Just as your car's fuel requirements are determined by how it is constructed, how much it weighs, and how fast you drive it, the caloric needs of your body reflect its underlying basic chemistry, its size, and how hard you drive it.

Everyone starts from a ground floor called the resting, or basal, metabolic rate (BMR)—your idling speed, as it were. It's a measure of how many calories your body needs to maintain its vital functions when you're doing "nothing." Though you may be lying motionless, your body is always working: your heart beats, your lungs expand and contract with each breath, your kidneys cleanse your blood, your liver makes enzymes, your digestive tract breaks down and absorbs food, your cells manufacture essential chemicals, and so forth. These millions of individual actions require energy, measured in the calories you use per hour just to stay alive.

The following are among the factors that affect your BMR:

Your sex. The rate for men is slightly higher than for women.

Your weight. The heavier you are, the higher your BMR.

How much of your body is fat. Lean muscle tissue uses more calories than fat tissue. Therefore, at a given weight, the more fat and less muscle you have, the lower your BMR.

Your age. The older you are, the lower your BMR is likely to be, probably because for most people the amount of lean muscle tissue decreases with age and the amount of fat increases.

How much you sleep. Your BMR is about 10 percent lower when you're asleep than when you're awake.

The temperature. The colder the air surrounding your body, the higher your BMR needs to be to keep you at 98.6 degrees.

The Food and Nutrition Board has calculated that the average American adult male of 154 pounds uses up between 1,440 and 1,728 calories a day to sustain his BMR, and the average female of 128 pounds uses up between 1,296 and 1,584 calories a day for basic metabolism. You can roughly calculate your own rate. For women, add a zero to your weight in pounds and then add on your weight to the result; for men, add a zero to your weight in pounds and then add twice your weight to the result. For each decade over 20, reduce your calculated BMR by 2 percent.

For example, if you are a woman who weighs 120 pounds: *Add 1,200 plus 120 = 1,320, the approximate BMR for a 20-year-old.*

If you are a man who weighs 160 pounds: *Add 1,600 plus 2 × 160 (or 320) = 1,920, the approximate BMR for a 20-year-old.*

Now, if you are a man of 30 who weighs 160: *Subtract 2 percent of 1,920, or 38, from 1,920 = 1,882, your BMR.*

And if you are a man of 60 who weighs 160: *Subtract 8 percent (for the four decades past 20) of 1,920, or 153, from 1,920 = 1,767, your BMR.*

But none of us lives by BMR alone. We do things during the course of our waking hours that burn calories beyond our BMR. *The more active you are, the more calories you need to sustain your weight—that is, the more calories you can consume and still lose or maintain your weight.* Thus, if our typical adult male walked at an average pace of 3 miles an hour, he would use 200 calories in one hour instead of his BMR of 66. Our typical female would use 150 calories in that hour instead of 55. More strenuous activity, such as playing tennis, walking at 4 miles an hour, or scrubbing floors, would raise caloric expenditure to 300 calories an hour for the man and 240 for the woman. Heavy activity increases caloric expenditure even more. An hour of walking with a load up a hill, playing football or basketball, or swimming hard would cost our man between 450 and 720 calories and our woman between 360 and 600 calories. (Note that the caloric cost of activity includes your BMR. That is, if playing an hour of tennis is said to burn 400 calories, you don't add that on to your day's resting BMR; rather, you substitute the higher rate for one hour of the BMR.)

The bigger you are, the more work your body must do to carry itself around, so the more calories you'll burn at any activity. How hard and fast you work also affects caloric expenditure. Casual splashing about the pool with occasional bursts of stroking uses far less energy than the speedy, continuous swimming of laps. Cycling uphill in high gear uses far more calories per minute than a leisurely bike ride on a level surface. How hard you have to breathe to sustain your activity is a good indication of how many calories you're using to do it.

Table 15.2 shows the approximate caloric cost of various activities when each is done for one hour. But remember, the calculations are rough—you can't use them to construct a precise inventory of caloric expenditure for yourself. However, they will give you an idea of which activities are greater energy guzzlers than others. Remember, too, that you're not likely to perform each of these activities for one solid hour.

Table 15.2 • PERSONAL ENERGY COST OF VARIOUS ACTIVITIES

Calories used per hour	Activities	
120–150	Strolling 1 mph Light housework	Walking 2 mph
150–240	Typing, manual Riding lawn mower	Golf, using power cart
240–300	Cleaning windows Mopping floors Vacuuming Pushing light power mower Bowling	Walking 3 mph Cycling 6 mph Golf, pulling cart Horseback (sitting to trot)
300–360	Scrubbing floors Walking 3.5 mph Cycling 8 mph Table tennis Badminton Volleyball	Golf, carrying clubs Tennis, doubles Calisthenics (many) Ballet exercises Dancing (foxtrot)
360–420	Walking 4 mph Cycling 10 mph Ice skating	Roller skating Horseback ("posting" to trot)
420–480	Hand lawn-mowing Walking 5 mph Cycling 11 mph	Tennis, singles Water skiing Folk (square) dancing
480–600	Sawing hardwood Jogging 5 mph Cycling 12 mph Downhill skiing	Paddleball Horseback (gallop) Basketball Mountain climbing
600–660	Running 5.5 mph	Cycling 13 mph
Above 660	Running 6 or more mph Handball	Squash Ski touring (5+ mph)

Source: "Physical Activity and Cardiovascular Health," *Modern Concepts of Cardiovascular Disease* 41 (1972):25–30.

Rather, you may play golf for two hours, tennis for one, squash for half an hour, and swim for fifteen minutes. Adjust your caloric expenditure accordingly. (See Table 23.1, page 429, for a more detailed calorie-activity chart.)

A rough idea of how many calories (including your BMR) you need each day may be derived as follows: if you're extremely inactive, you'll need only about 12 calories per pound to sustain your body weight; if your day is characterized by light activity, your caloric requirements per pound increase to about 15; if you're moderately active, you may need up to 20 calories per pound; and if you're extremely active, you could require as many as 25 calories per pound if you want to maintain your weight. If you're a woman, two other factors can affect your caloric requirements—pregnancy and lactation. See Chapters 18 and 19 for more complete discussions.

Are You Overweight?

Some people who weigh too much don't recognize that fact. Their spouses may value extra padding or the "zaftig" look. Or they may feel discouraged about ever shedding the extra weight and so subconsciously deny their weight problem. Other people have the opposite problem. They always think they're too fat even though they're fine the way they are. Forever trying to get rid of pounds unnecessarily, they often drive themselves, and their families, crazy.

The fashion and film industries have made millions of Americans, especially women, nearly hysterical about their weight, to the point where it jeopardizes their emotional and physical health. For example, growing numbers of slender young women who want to be even thinner than they are are caught in a vicious cycle of starvation, binge-eating, and punishing purges. If they eat a "big" (i.e., normal) meal or splurge on a high-calorie dessert, they may induce themselves to vomit or run 10 miles to work it off. This eating disorder has a name, bulimia, and researchers say it is becoming increasingly common and may already afflict as many as 25 percent of college-age women.

Besides your height, your body build helps determine your ideal weight. A large-boned person should weigh more than one who is delicately boned but of the same height. The best height-weight charts take your "frame"—large, medium, or small—into account, or indicate a range of weight for different types of build. Another important consid-

Table 15.3 • ENERGY NEEDS THROUGH LIFE*

Ages	Daily caloric need	Range
Infants		
To 6 months	Weight in pounds × 53	43–66
6 months–1 year	Weight in pounds × 48	36–61
Children		
1–3 years	1,300	900–1,800
4–6	1,700	1,300–2,300
7–10	2,400	1,650–3,300
Males		
11–14	2,700	2,000–3,700
15–18	2,800	2,100–3,900
19–22	2,900	2,500–3,300
23–50	2,700	2,300–3,100
51–75	2,400	2,000–2,800
Over 75	2,050	1,650–2,450
Females		
11–14	2,200	1,500–3,000
15–18	2,100	1,200–3,000
19–22	2,100	1,700–2,500
23–50	2,000	1,600–2,400
51–75	1,800	1,400–2,200
Over 75	1,600	1,200–2,000
Pregnant	+300	
Nursing	+500	

*These daily caloric intakes are recommended by the Food and Nutrition Board of the National Academy of Sciences–National Research Council to meet the energy needs of average healthy persons. However, precise requirements may vary over a wide range, depending on height, weight, and level of activity.

eration is how much of your weight is lean muscle and how much is fat. A professional football player would be overweight by most charts, but compared to a sedentary person of normal weight who is the same height, a smaller percentage of the athlete's body is likely to be fat. It's fat, not pounds, that makes you overweight. A lean man carries about 5 to 10 percent of his body as fat, whereas a man who is moderately obese has 20 percent of his weight as fat. For a woman, for whom it is normal to carry a greater percentage of fat at any weight, leanness means about 10 to 20 percent fat, and moderate obesity, 30 percent fat. In extreme obesity, of course, the percentage of body fat can go much higher.

You can get a rough idea of how much fat you carry by having someone pinch your flesh between two fingers on the back of your upper arm midway between your shoulder and elbow. With your arm hanging relaxed at your side, have your assistant grasp the loose flesh between thumb and forefinger. As a general rule, if when squeezing slightly the distance between fingertips is more than an inch, you're probably carrying too much fat. Keep in mind that at any age, females have more fat than males, so the pinch test on a woman should produce a somewhat larger skinfold thickness than a man of the same age. Thus, for a teenaged boy, a skinfold thickness of only $^6/_{10}$ inch is defined as over-weight, whereas for an overweight teenaged girl, the skinfold thickness is nearly twice that.

But few people need measurements to tell them they're over-weight. Instead, remove all your clothes and take a long, hard look at yourself in a full-length mirror. Turn slowly, appraising your body from various angles. Look for flabby protrusions. If you're carrying too much "baggage," you'll know it right away.

Is Overweight Harmful?

The vast majority of dieters are motivated by "cosmetic" concerns —a desire to conform to the societal ideal of rib-showing slimness. But far more important is the fact that maintaining a lean body is conducive to good health and a long life. Actuarial studies have shown that as little as a 5-percent excess above ideal weight is associated with a diminished life expectancy. A 50-year-old man who is 50 pounds overweight has half the remaining life expectancy of a normal-weight man of the same age. Excess weight can aggravate existing health problems, causing more severe symptoms or the appearance of a disorder earlier in life than might otherwise occur. On the positive side, losing weight in-creases the number of years you're likely to live and live healthfully.

However, contrary to what you might think, it is also not healthy to be too thin. A twenty-four-year study in Framingham, Massachu-setts, and the latest insurance-company studies showed that the thin-nest people—those more than 10 or 20 percent below ideal weight—

DISTRIBUTION OF BODY FAT

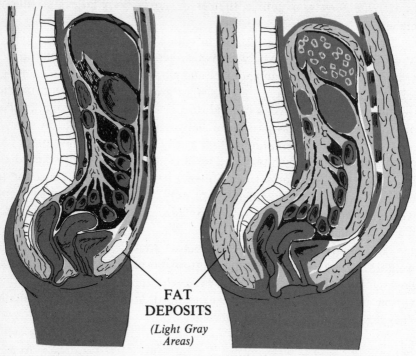

**FAT
DEPOSITS**
*(Light Gray
Areas)*

NORMAL   OVERWEIGHT

In the cutaway views of the human form above, the fat lies
under the skin and around the internal organs.

had a higher death rate than the heaviest people.

The following table (Table 15.4) shows "best weight" (in indoor
clothing) for men and women of different ages and heights. The figures,
from the Pacific Mutual Life Insurance Company, come from a new
study by the life-insurance industry of the effects of weight on mortality.
Though they do not take body frame into account, the weights listed
represent those associated with the longest life expectancy, according
to the study.

Experts in heart disease estimate that at least one-fourth of our
problems with cardiovascular diseases are attributable to obesity, which
forces your heart and lungs to work harder than they should. Obesity
is one of the leading causes of high blood pressure, which in turn can
cause death from heart and kidney disease and stroke. Hypertension is
twice as common among obese as among lean persons. Every extra

Table 15.4 • IDEAL WEIGHT IN POUNDS

Height	Age				
	20–29	30–39	40–49	50–59	60–69
Men					
5'3"	125	129	130	131	130
5'6"	135	140	142	143	142
5'9"	149	153	155	156	155
6'0"	161	166	167	168	167
6'3"	176	181	183	184	180
Women					
4'10"	97	102	106	109	111
5'1"	106	109	114	118	120
5'4"	114	118	122	127	129
5'7"	123	127	132	137	140
5'10"	134	138	142	146	147

pound of body fat requires an additional mile of blood vessels. Many people with high blood pressure are able to bring their pressure down to normal levels without drugs by losing weight and reducing their consumption of salt. Weight loss also can bring down blood-cholesterol levels and improve the body's ability to process sugars.

Obesity increases the risk of developing diabetes about fourfold. It also promotes heart attack, blood clots, varicose veins, gout, respiratory diseases, gastrointestinal disorders, gall bladder and liver disease, and arthritis of the weight-bearing joints. Fat women are more likely to suffer from toxemia during pregnancy and to develop cancer of the endometrium (lining of the womb) and the breast than women of normal weight. Recently, obesity has been linked to disorders of the menstrual cycle, including infertility.

Overweight people are clumsier, react to unexpected events more slowly, and are more likely to have accidents than normal-weight people. Compared to the general population, overweight people are more likely to die in automobile accidents. They are also more susceptible to complications from surgery, infections, and delayed healing of wounds. In short, being overweight is not good for your body.

Nor is it good for your mind. Contrary to the myth that fat people are happy people, some obese persons are caught in a devastatingly vicious cycle: miserably unhappy, they turn to food for solace, which in turn makes them fatter and even more unhappy. Fat people are often subject to ridicule and, because of the way society regards them, they tend to have a poor self-image, thinking of themselves as weak-willed, ugly, and shameful. They are also commonly victims of job discrimination. On the average, overweight executives earn $1,000 a year less than their normal-weight peers.

Why We Overeat

The reasons for packing in more calories than your body needs are legion, and most of us who watch our weight have invoked many of them at times when temptation overwhelmed restraint. Some you've undoubtedly heard or said so often you believe them to be written in stone. Actually, few, if any, are founded in immutable fact.

FAMILY FACTORS

Obesity does run in families. In families where both parents are of normal weight, only 7 percent of the children are overweight. But if one parent is fat, the chances of the children being fat as well leap to 40 percent. And if both parents are obese, 80 percent of the children are also obese. This suggests a strong hereditary tendency toward overweight, but it doesn't prove it. The family environment—especially the parents' eating and exercise habits—could also result in such statistics. The most recent comprehensive look at the question suggests that heredity does indeed strongly predict a person's adult weight. The study was conducted among hundreds of adopted people in Denmark by Dr. Albert Stunkard, obesity specialist at the University of Pennsylvania. Since Denmark keeps very careful and up-to-date records on adoptions, it was possible for Dr. Stunkard and his co-workers to obtain information about the adoptees' biological parents and natural siblings as well as their adoptive parents. No relationship was found between degree of overweight of the adoptees and their adoptive parents. However, adopted children—as adults—were much more likely to resemble the body weights of their biological parents.

While this study indicates that heredity is important, it does not mean you are doomed by your genes. Rather, it suggests that by controlling the "environment" to prevent obesity, especially early in life, people can prevent their "fat genes" from being expressed. This means taking care to avoid most empty calories and exercising vigorously on a regular basis. In other words, people with one or both parents who are significantly overweight may have to work harder than others to prevent obesity, but their genes do not necessarily doom them to a lifelong weight problem.

The fact remains that while genetics may set the stage for obesity, environmemt determines how the play turns out. At least two studies have shown that fat people are more likely than slender folks to have pets that are also overweight. In one study, 44 percent of overweight people had overweight dogs. Fattening snacks, double portions, and sedentary living can affect man and beast alike.

CHILDHOOD OBESITY

If a lifetime of obesity is not necessarily rooted in the genes, it must be influenced by events early in life. Indeed, early feeding patterns and attitudes toward food and eating can influence how much weight a child gains and how large his or her body's fat storage capacity gets to be. Fat is housed in special cells that can grow to be very large. Different people have different numbers of fat cells, which, once formed, remain in the body forever. As you lose or gain weight, the cells shrink or expand, but never diminish in number. The grossly obese adult who was obese as a child has on the average three times as many fat cells as his or her normal-weight counterpart, and the individual cells contain one and a half times as much fat. Fat cells multiply rapidly at several critical periods—particularly before birth, in infancy, and in early adolescence—and being overweight at these times may destine a person to a lifetime struggle with a tendency to gain weight. (On the other hand, if you become obese in adulthood, your existing fat cells enlarge but they don't increase in number unless the weight gain is extreme.)

Up to 80 percent of youngsters who are fat as 5-year-olds end up fat as adults. Their "thermostat" has been set at an early age. Even as early as 6 months of age, chubbiness may lead to adult obesity. Although most studies show a relationship after 2 years of age, one study in Rochester, New York, showed that 36 percent of infants who were obese during their first half year of life were also overweight between the ages of 20 and 36. But only 14 percent of those who were of average or below-average weight as infants grew up to be overweight adults.

In our grandparents' time, fat babies were considered the healthiest babies. Before antibiotics and other modern medical miracles, babies needed extra padding if they were going to weather those all-too-common attacks of diarrhea, pneumonia, and other life-threatening infections. Today, the tide is belatedly beginning to turn. Among the trend setters, baby fat is no longer chic. The desirable infant is lean and active, if not downright wiry. For a complete discussion of nutrition during infancy, see Chapter 19.

Adults often give babies food—such as a bottle or cookie—as a pacifier, regardless of what may be ailing the babies. As a child gets a little older, food, especially desserts or sweet snacks, may be offered or withheld as reward or punishment: "No pudding if you don't finish your vegetables"; "You've been such a good boy today I'm going to buy you a candy bar." Food becomes endowed with an emotional value that may carry over into adulthood. In times of psychic pain or pleasure, you reward yourself with ice cream, cake, or a steak dinner.

A study of 3,444 preschool children in twelve North Central states revealed that almost 25 percent of mothers used foods as rewards for good behavior; 10 percent used the deprivation of food as a punishment, and 29 percent used food as a pacifier. And the overwhelming majority of the foods so used were baked goods, desserts, sweets, and candy.

The mothers in the study were also preoccupied with the usually mistaken notion that their children didn't eat enough. They chronically overestimated the amount of food needed by preschoolers and encouraged overeating, using a variety of games and psychological inducements to get the children to eat more. In effect, the mothers were conditioning their children to overeat whether the children were hungry or not. See Chapter 20 on how to feed children.

THE WRONG SIGNALS

In the best of all possible worlds, you would eat only when you're hungry and only enough to meet your body's caloric needs. But we live in a real world that beckons many of us to eat at every turn. The whiff of a bakery starts visions of scrumptious treats dancing in your head. A dish of peanuts is set in front of you, and, hungry or not, you start nibbling at it, often not stopping until the last peanut is gone. The clock strikes noon, and even though you're still satisfied by a large, late breakfast, you eat lunch because "it's lunchtime." You've just learned that your junior colleague, and not you, is in line for a promotion and you're so furious you stop at an ice-cream parlor for a hot fudge sundae. Visiting your mother, who for years conveyed the unmistakable message "If you love me, you'll eat," you clean up a four-course dinner, plus seconds. You're exhausted after a hard day's work, and while watching television, you put away a bag of pretzels and three beers.

We are all beset each day with a thousand signals to "eat, eat" that come not from our bodies, but from the world we live in. Many people are able to tune out these signals, and some never notice them at all, saying quite simply, "No, thanks, I'm not hungry." The rest of us stand in awe of their "will power" and wonder where we were when this enviable character trait was passed out. How can they resist so painlessly when we so readily succumb to temptation? Don't they even notice that dish full of luscious chocolates? Don't they like them? No wonder they are so thin!

These seeming paragons of gustatory virtue are no more endowed with strength of character than you or I. There is no such trait as "will power" or "won't power." What does distinguish them from others is that they eat in response to their body's demands for food and not because someone urges them to eat, or because some delectable goody is waved before them, or because some emotional anguish needs assuaging, or because the clock says it's mealtime. Instead, they are said to be *"internally cued"* eaters. They eat when their brains signal physical hunger, they eat enough to satisfy that hunger, and they don't eat again until the signal of physical hunger reappears. And, as you might guess, they tend to be slender.

The rest of us march to a different drummer. We are *"externally cued"* eaters, eating in response to environmental stimuli. Some of us never even get hungry or, at least, notice that we are. And many of us are overweight, if not obese.

I know, because I used to be such an eater, and I used to be fat. I ate when I was depressed, and I ate when I was happy. I ate when I was trying to avoid an unpleasant task and when I was pleased with myself for accomplishing one. I ate when I was with others who were eating (even if I'd just eaten myself), and I ate when I was lonely. I ate when I was tired, nervous, uncomfortable, or cold. I ate when temptation beckoned in the form of an attractive aroma or display of food. I ate whenever there was food lying about and when I knew there was something I liked tucked away in the cupboard or refrigerator. In fact, I ate for every reason except the one reason that should have been my only stimulus to eat—because I was hungry. I actually had little trouble ignoring my body's hunger signals when I made up my mind not to eat anything. I could fast for a day without difficulty, and I often skipped breakfast and lunch if I knew a big dinner was in the offing. But despite this notable exercise of "will power," I was fat.

Recent studies indicate that sensitivity to external eating cues is probably the result of a superconsciousness about food and weight. But some cues may be programmed into certain people through early life experiences, and some may be inborn. Robert M. Milstein of Yale University, who tested 24 newborn infants for reactions to environmental cues, found that as early as one day of age, the children of obese parents are more responsive to visual cues and sweet tastes than those of normal-weight parents. Dr. Judith Rodin, also of Yale, showed that responsiveness to external stimuli could be used to predict which girls would gain weight at summer camp and which would not. She points out that not all overweight people eat in response to external cues, and not everyone who is externally cued becomes obese. But, she adds, "those who are externally responsive are highly vulnerable to putting on excess weight."

EXERCISE

You've heard the familiar lament—"I eat the same things you do, even less, yet I'm fat and you're thin as a rail. It's not fair!" Most of us tend to disbelieve such claims. Surely, our fat friends must sneak in those extra calories somewhere, maybe through bigger portions, second helpings, alcohol, snitched candy, cake, or cookies. And undoubtedly some do.

But study after study has shown that on the average, overweight people do not consume more calories than those who are not overweight. Since energy can neither be created nor destroyed, fat people obviously consume enough calories to maintain their overweight and too many calories to allow them to lose at their present level of caloric expenditure. But they do not necessarily eat more than other people.

At least two factors account for this apparent contradiction. One is that *body fat needs fewer calories to maintain itself than lean muscle tissue.* Studies of extremely obese individuals have shown that, pound for pound, they need a third to a half fewer calories to maintain their weight than people who are not overweight (though, of course, the obese need more total calories). Thus, if two people were exactly the same height and weight and got the same amount of exercise each day, but one was a between-seasons football player with 12 percent body fat and the other a sedentary office worker with 30 percent body fat, the football player could eat more calories without gaining an ounce than the office worker could. Of course, if the football player let himself get too badly out of shape, his muscle tissue would be replaced by fat and he'd start to gain unless he cut back on his eating. This, in fact, happens to a lot of retired athletes. Muhammed Ali's weight shot up 25 percent when he "retired" from boxing.

Which brings us to the second important fact—*exercise.* On the whole, overweight people are not as active as lean people, whose trim figures and laden plates they covet. Even when both lean and fat participate in the same sport, the lean move more and work harder at it, expending more calories than the overweight. I used to play tennis with a young woman who is my height but weighs 70 percent more than I do. She could really wallop the ball when it came directly to her. But if she had to move more than a few feet to hit it, it was my point.

Time and motion studies of girls at a summer camp showed that in a game of volleyball, the overweight girls hardly moved at all, hitting the ball only when it came right to them. But their lean playmates were in constant motion, using far more calories in the same game. This was also true of swimming. The fat girls merely paddled about in the water, but the lean ones swam hard and long in pursuit of one another and in vigorous races. A study in which pedometers were attached to housewives revealed that the lean women walked twice as far in a day than those who were obese—even though both did the same chores. So when you say of an overweight companion "He claims to eat less than I do but he must be doing something to make himself so fat," you may be wrong. He's not doing *something,* he's doing *nothing,* and that's why he's fatter than you are.

A study of runners in the San Francisco Bay area showed that on the average the men consumed 2,960 calories a day, but they weighed 20 percent less than inactive men their age who consumed 2,360 calories. Among women runners caloric intake was 570 calories more per day but weight was 30 percent less. Another recent study of 350 obese persons showed that in nearly 70 percent, the weight problem was related to inactivity, and in only 3.2 percent was it the result of increased food intake.

Not only does physical exercise force your body to use more calories while you're engaged in the activity, but it also revs up your engine (your BMR) for hours afterward. According to a study at the University of Southern California, four hours after completing strenuous physical activity, the participants' metabolic rate was 7.5 to 28 percent higher than if they had not exercised. Thus, exercise has a continuing benefit that could add up to a loss of several pounds a year beyond that produced by the exercise itself. Furthermore, a Cornell University study showed that when you exercise several hours—or even the next day—after a particularly large meal, your body uses more calories than usual to perform the same activity, helping you to compensate for some of the excess consumption.

Many people mistakenly think that exercise uses so few calories that it's of little value in weight control. Some even believe it's counter-productive because it stimulates the appetite and makes you hungrier than if you'd just sat around doing nothing. It's true that low-level exercise, such as a mile-long walk before eating or a short paddle about the pool, can be an invigorating boost to your appetite and result in your eating more than you would otherwise (which is why such activity is recommended for the elderly before mealtime). But more strenuous exercise has the opposite effect. Joggers, for example, commonly report that running takes the edge off their appetite.

Studies show that *the body is best able to match energy intake—* food calories—*with energy expenditure at moderate levels of physical activity.* When you're inactive or only slightly active, your body tends to overshoot in its estimate of caloric needs and you're likely to eat more than you burn up. At very high levels of activity, such as marathon running and long-distance cycling, the opposite problem occurs: you're likely to eat fewer calories than you use. Wisdom lies between these two extremes. It's as if the body has an innate "appestat" to balance food intake to activity, but it only functions accurately in the intermediate range of activity. This would account in part for the growing problem of overweight in an increasingly affluent society such as ours where our fingers, rather than our feet, do the walking.

NONCAUSES OF OBESITY

With rare exceptions, *obesity is not the result of any simple hor-monal abnormality* that physicians can correct. "Ninety-eight percent of the housewives who say they can't lose because they have low metab-olism are wrong," Dr. Rodin says. Rather, the studies indicate that most fat people probably start out metabolically normal, but as they gain weight they develop derangements in how their body handles nutrients. These derangements can result in more food being stored as fat and may explain the common lament of the obese that "everything I eat turns to fat." Even after they lose weight, they tend to store more calories as fat than persons without a weight problem.

Metabolic "abnormalities" seen in obese people can be provoked in persons of normal weight simply by overfeeding them. In a Vermont study of normal-weight prisoners, those who gained weight because they were fed two to three times as many calories as they normally consumed also experienced metabolic changes to those abnormalities seen in the obese. When the prisoners were no longer force-fed, they spontaneously lost weight and the metabolic abnormalities disap-peared.

Of course, there are individual differences in body metabolism—and, as we've already seen, people with a high percentage of body fat have a lower metabolic rate per pound than those with few fat stores—but there is nothing fundamentally abnormal about the metabolism of most overweight people. If they consumed fewer calories than they used up each day, their internal chemistry would become more normal and they'd lose weight.

Nor is a "low thyroid" or any other hormonal irregularity a common cause of excessive weight gain. Obese persons are no more likely to have below-normal thyroid function than persons of normal weight. Rather than the thyroid gland being sluggish, it's usually the person who's sluggish—who encourages his or her body to turn food to stored fat by getting little or no exercise. *The best way to stoke your metabolic furnace is not by taking hormone pills or shots, but by stepping up your activity.* Giving extra hormones to a person who already has a normal supply of his or her own only results in a shutdown of internal hormone production. Nothing is gained, and time, money, and hope are often lost as a result.

There is also no support for the notion that psychological disturbances are what cause some people to become fat. Rather, as studies by Dr. Albert Stunkard of the University of Pennsylvania suggest, psychological disorders are probably a consequence of being fat in a society that worships slimness. Self-disdain and rejection by others can produce severe emotional disturbances, which in turn may make it harder to cope with a weight problem. Although women in the lower social classes are far more likely to be obese, upper-class women who are overweight are more likely to be emotionally disturbed as a result of their weight problem. This strongly suggests that psychological disturbances among the obese are the result of value systems rather than causes of obesity. Overall, Dr. Stunkard found little difference in the amount and degree of mental illness between obese persons and those of normal weight.

Calories Always Count—or Do They?

The notion that calories from one type of food make you fatter than those from another is largely a product of wishful thinking and clever marketeering by diet mongers trying to make a fast buck—and often succeeding. Millions of Americans who struggle in vain against weight gain spurn potatoes, bread, pasta, and rice because they think carbohydrate calories make you fat. But they down generous servings of meat, cheese, tuna, chicken, and other high-protein foods in the illusory belief that protein builds lean muscle tissue, not fat, and that protein calories somehow "don't count."

Well, they're wrong. *All calories count,* be they from steak, bread, or butter. The calories from protein—4 per gram—count as much or more to your body's furnace as the calories from carbohydrates—also 4 per gram. And the calories from fat—which are more concentrated, at 9 per gram—provide equally acceptable fuel for your body to run on. *If you consume more calories than you use—whether from protein, carbohydrate, or fat—you'll gain weight.* And if you consume fewer calories than you use, you'll lose body fat. A high-carbohydrate diet is not necessarily a fattening one (see Chapter 5, pages 95–118). Witness the fact that obesity is rare among peoples in other parts of the world who live primarily on complex carbohydrates (starches) and only about a quarter of the protein eaten by the typical American. In fact, a study in laboratory rats published in 1981 showed that even when two groups of animals were fed the same number of calories, those consuming a high-carbohydrate, low-protein diet ended up leaner than those on a high-protein diet. Subsequent research in people by Dr. Michael Levitt at the Minneapolis Veterans Administration Hospital showed that up to a third of the calories in starchy foods are not absorbed by the human body. Rather, bacteria in the gut "digest" them and eliminate them as gas. So, a significant portion of the calories in complex carbohydrates actually don't count.

In addition to their low-fat content, diets rich in complex carbohydrates contain a lot of fiber, which helps to satisfy hunger and may also have a small calorie-sparing effect. Because undigestible fiber speeds the passage of digestible foodstuffs through the gastrointestinal tract, some foods that would otherwise add calories to your body may not be fully absorbed. Vigorous exercise, which increases the motility of your intestinal tract, has a similar effect.

16 &WHY "DIETS" DON'T WORK

AMERICANS, it seems, will swallow anything—dozens of eggs, hundreds of grapefruits, gallons of water, even wood pulp, vinegar, and seaweed—if it will keep them away, however temporarily, from the calorie-rich foods that have made them fat. We have been told we can lose weight by drinking alcohol (more fattening, gram for gram, than sugar), by consuming large amounts of vegetable oil (even more fattening than alcohol), by eating vast quantities of undigestible fiber (which may be socially less desirable than 200 extra pounds), by substituting sex for food (fine, if you can manage to work it into your schedule whenever your stomach cries "eat"—and you have an enthusiastic partner), and by eating anything you want (which is what made you fat in the first place). When it comes to diets as well as food, Americans are extraordinarily gullible.

Obviously, if any of these methods worked on a permanent basis for a significant number of people, there would be little or no market for the others. The fact that so many diet books have made their authors rich and famous is testimony to the failure of all of them to succeed.

At any given time, an estimated 20 million American adults are "on a diet" to lose weight. Another 20 million think they should be, and most of them expect to go on one sooner or later. In a year's time, these dieters will shed, collectively, hundreds of millions of pounds. And when they reach their goal, or get fed up trying, they will quit and the needle on the scale will begin its familiar upward climb.

Four out of five people who lose weight eventually regain it, often exceeding their previous high-weight mark. When determination to lose once again outweighs the desire to overeat, the "going on a diet" cycle will start anew. Dr. Jean Mayer, the obesity and nutrition specialist who is now president of Tufts University, calls it "the rhythm method of girth control." Others refer to it as the "yo-yo" syndrome.

But by whatever name, it's not healthy physically or psychologically. Studies indicate that the repeated gaining, losing, and regaining of extra pounds is more damaging to your physical health than just remaining overweight. That's why it's so important to forget all the gimmicks—the crash programs and diets you could not possibly follow for long—and find instead a permanent solution to your weight problem.

Some people, including me, are testimony to the fact that there is —at least so far—a lasting solution. It requires, first of all, that you *abandon the wishful thought that permanent weight loss can be achieved overnight.* The extra pounds you carry were not acquired in a few weeks or months. Chances are, they've accumulated gradually over a period of years and are maintained by decades of deeply ingrained habits. While you usually can get rid of them faster than they were acquired, you do have to give yourself a chance to learn a new way to manage food—a way to adjust caloric intake to output that you can maintain indefinitely. Since you don't expect to live the rest of your life on grapefruit and hard-boiled eggs or rice and water, that is not the best path to weight reduction.

The second requirement for permanent weight control is *an appropriate motive.* Your reasons for losing weight should be your own, based —for example—on your determination to protect your health or to look better for your own sake. Not to please your spouse or to acquire one, not to get the doctor off your back, not to fit into that dress you have to wear to a wedding in a few weeks, not to get that long-awaited promotion, not to impress your former classmates at the next reunion. You are losing weight because *you* want to, because you've had it with being fat, because you're determined once and for all to conquer your problem no matter how long it may take. *Successful, permanent weight loss is a lifetime decision.*

A final requirement is that you *give up the notion of a "diet."* A diet is something you go on and off. Permanent weight control means that the diet you go on today is the same as the diet you'll be on a year from now is the same as the diet you'll be on for the rest of your life. This is not really a diet, but an *eating management plan.* It allows you to lose weight while eating the same variety of foods and balance of nutrients that will enable you to maintain that loss—and good nutritional health—indefinitely. It will keep you from building up cravings for long-denied passions. It will teach you to deal with food—at home, in a restaurant, at a party, on vacation—in a normal, nonobsessed way. It will allow you to "cheat" on occasion without precipitating an uncontrollable binge. Your weight may fluctuate a few pounds here and there, but the extremes of the yo-yo syndrome will be gone forever. You will have learned once and for all how to eat thin in a world that beckons you to gorge on calorie-rich "goodies." You will not only learn how to resist temptation, but how not to be tempted in the first place.

I learned this lesson the hard way. I've spent much of my life watching my weight. From my early teens to my mid-twenties, it was mostly watching it go up. And nearly all that time, I was on a diet. Believe me, I tried them all—all the commercial versions of the day plus a few I devised on my own: cantaloupe and cottage cheese, liver and grapefruit, boiled chicken and carrots, Wheat Chex and apples, even graham crackers and skim milk. (I craved graham crackers and figured that I couldn't possibly eat more than my allotted 1,000 calories' worth of graham crackers a day. I figured wrong.) I also tried skipping breakfast and lunch, and, when that didn't work, I tried fasting every other day. I did manage to lose weight on many of those diets—5, maybe 10, pounds—only to gain it back again when I knuckled under to boredom and temptation. Then, fourteen years ago, desperate, disgusted, and fat, I made a decision: I stopped dieting and started to eat like a "normal" person. I ate every meal, and I ate all the foods I loved. But instead of becoming even more like the Goodyear blimp, I started to lose. Slowly, to be sure (7 pounds the first month, then only a pound or two a month thereafter), but painlessly and always in the same direction—down. *After two years of not dieting, I weighed 35 pounds less than when I had lived from one best-selling weight-loss scheme to the next.* And I never regained the lost pounds. Many people who knew me "when" ask for my weight-loss secret, their envy ill concealed. And most find my answer hard to believe—I simply stopped dieting. But the fact remains that they are still riding up and down the diet yo-yo string while I cut the cord years ago.

Why Fad Diets Fail

The Atkins diet, the Stillman diet, the Scarsdale diet, the drinking man's diet, the Air Force diet, the "Mayo" diet, the water diet, the rice diet, the macrobiotic diet, the grapefruit diet, the calories-don't-count diet, the eat-all-you-want diet, the sex diet, the liquid-protein diet, the Southampton diet, the Beverly Hills diet, the I-Love-New-York diet, the Eat-to-Win diet, the starch-blocker diet, the food-combining diet, the fiber diet . . . There are as many different ways to lose weight as there are people who need to lose it. And almost every one of them can work in the short run. Many work because they take choice out of your hands. By telling you exactly what and often how much you can eat, the diet usually limits the number of calories you can consume and bans the no-nos that contribute to overweight. Even the so-called all-you-can-eat diets help you cut back on calories because they're so boring you can't possibly consume more calories than you expend.

Let's say you go on a grapefruit-and-egg diet. To consume 1,000 calories a day—which would represent a 2-pound-a-week weight loss for an adult who burns 2,000 calories a day—you would have to eat ten hard-boiled eggs at 70 calories apiece and six grapefruits at 45 calories each. You'd soon get so sick of eggs and grapefruit that you'd probably eat even less than that amount after a few days and you'd lose weight. Far less extreme diets can quickly become tedious and result in a significant reduction in the number of calories you consumed when your choices were unlimited.

The all-you-can-eat high-protein diets are based on the myth that the body burns all the protein calories you consume when it digests and metabolizes protein. At best, if you ate only protein (virtually impossible), 30 percent of its calories would be used up by internal "processing." You can still get very fat on the remaining 70 percent of calories if you really do "eat all you want."

When you think of what's permitted in most fad diets, it's a good thing that few people can stick to them for long. *Every fad diet is nutritionally unbalanced in one way or another, and some are downright dangerous, even if followed by healthy people for a relatively short time.* Nutritionist Elizabeth B. Spannhake of Loyola University has made a nutritional analysis of nine popular diets. She reports, for example, that the Atkins low-carbohydrate diet is tainted by deficiencies in calcium, vitamins A and C, thiamin, riboflavin, and niacin because it excludes bread and cereal products and drastically limits servings of fruits, vegetables, and milk products (except fat-laden cheese). At the same time, it's loaded with protein, saturated animal fats, and cholesterol: bacon, eggs, sausages, cheese, roast beef, steak, fried chicken—a heart attack's delight. One woman I know who had a tendency to high blood cholesterol leaped from an already high level of 300 milligrams of cholesterol per 100 milliliters of blood serum to a whopping 740 milligrams—four times higher than normal—in just four weeks on the Atkins diet. Her horrified physician warned her to get off it immediately before she precipitated a heart attack!

Another popular low-carbohydrate diet—the "quick weight loss" or "water" diet—shortchanges you on calcium, vitamins A and C, and thiamin. It contains practically nothing besides eggs, cheese, meat, and water (plain or flavored but sugarless). No fruit, no vegetables, no grains, and, as a result, no roughage. Another name for it might be the "constipation diet" since it does nothing to stimulate the proper functioning of the bowels. And, like the Atkins diet, it's also high in choles-terol, although not especially rich in saturated fats.

The Scarsdale diet is the most recent twist on the low-carbohy-drate theme. It is a slight improvement over the aforementioned schemes because it limits fats and includes some fruits and vegetables and because the dieter is advised to follow it for no more than two weeks at a time. But it remains an unbalanced diet, too low in carbohydrates and too high in protein.

Moreover, *diets that promise quick weight loss are illusory.* The first 5 pounds or so that you lose on low-carbohydrate diets is water, not fat. It's the water your body is forced to excrete when it relies on protein and fats (from the diet and your body) for energy. The kidneys use water from your tissues and body fluids to wash out the toxic waste products from incompletely burned fats and unused nitrogen from protein. But as soon as you stop losing weight and resume eating carbohydrates, the body's normal main source of fuel, you regain the lost water and the lost pounds.

When you think about it, it's impossible to lose—as many of these diets suggest—10 pounds of *fat* in ten days, even on a total fast. A pound of body fat represents 3,500 calories. To lose 1 pound of fat, you must expend 3,500 more calories than you consume. Let's say you weigh 170 pounds and, as a moderately active person, you burn 2,500 calories a day. If your diet contains only 1,500 calories, you'd have an energy deficit of 1,000 calories a day. In a week's time that would add up to a 7,000-calorie deficit, or 2 pounds of real fat. In ten days, the accumulated deficit would represent nearly 3 pounds of lost body fat. Even if you ate nothing at all for ten days and maintained your usual level of activity, your caloric deficit would add up to 25,000 calories (2,500 calories a day times 10). At 3,500 calories per pound of fat, that's still only 7 pounds of lost fat. So if you want to lose fat, which is all you should want to lose, *the loss must be gradual—at most a pound or two a week.*

Fad Diets Are Health Hazards

A further problem of fad diets is the health risks associated with many of them. These are not hypothetical risks, but actual complica-tions that have occurred to people who've followed the bizarre diet schemes. Many of the victims were seemingly healthy to begin with and had no reason to suspect that they would fall prey to the disorders induced by their unbalanced diets. Here's a rundown on the problems peculiar to the various diet schemes.

The high-fat, high-protein diets, also known as low-carbohydrate diets. These are popular because fat in the diet makes dieting easier. It helps to stave off hunger because fat is digested more slowly than carbohydrates. Also, when the body burns fat for energy in the absence of carbohydrates, toxic substances called ketone bodies are produced that are claimed to suppress appetite (they really don't).

But—and this is an important but—a high-fat diet is fundamentally unhealthy. It can produce an increase in the blood levels of *uric acid,* which already tend to be high in overweight people, and precipitate an attack of gouty arthritis. And, since most such diets are high in *saturated animal fats* and *cholesterol* (from meat, eggs, and cheese), they can raise the blood levels of cholesterol and speed the development of atherosclerosis, the leading cause of premature death in this country. These diets can also cause abnormalities in heart rhythm.

A further risk stems from the *excessive protein,* which forces your kidneys to get rid of large amounts of nitrogen wastes. While a person with normal, healthy kidneys can usually handle this without difficulty, many people have marginal kidney disease and don't know it until the kidneys are overly stressed. The added stress of a high-protein diet could precipitate uremic poisoning, damage to the brain and nervous system, and, ultimately, death. Diets too high in protein also cause your body to lose calcium and bone. And, without fruits and vegetables, followers of low-carbohydrate schemes can developed symptoms of scurvy from a deficiency of vitamin C.

An accumulation of ketone bodies in the blood—ketosis—can cause nausea, vomiting, apathy, fatigue, dizziness, and low blood pressure. Ketosis is especially hazardous for pregnant women; it can, among other ill effects, result in impaired brain development of the baby. A woman I know in her early thirties asked me to recommend a physician who might find the cause of her extraordinary fatigue and lack of ambition and energy. She said she was so "collapsed" that she had stayed home from work for two days and did practically nothing but sleep. But she didn't feel any better afterward. She said she thought she might be anemic, so I asked her about her diet. She'd been eating plenty of meat, so anemia was an unlikely explanation. In fact, she was eating mostly meat and not much of anything else. As it turned out, she had been on the Atkins diet for a month and had been feeling rotten for the last three weeks. I suggested that she might save herself a doctor's fee if she resumed a more normal diet that included carbohydrates and especially fruits and vegetables. Three days later she came to me again, all smiles. "You must be right, because I did what you said and I feel fine now. No diet is worth feeling as lousy as I did."

Low-protein diets. In contrast to the above diets, which contain little or no carbohydrates, these have almost nothing but—cereal, pasta, fruit, and vegetables but no meats, cheese, or poultry. The diet is extremely unbalanced nutritionally, and, in addition to shortchanging you on such essential minerals as calcium and iron, it forces your body to break down its own muscle tissue to meet its needs for new protein. You lose not only fat, but also a lot of lean body mass and strength. The complications of low-protein diets are shared by those that rely on single foods, such as bananas or rice, which, in addition to being too low in protein, add the problem of vitamin and mineral deficiencies.

Protein-sparing diets. These spartan regimens are simply one step away from starvation. They involve a caloric intake of 200 to 400 calories a day in the form of an unpalatable liquid-protein preparation. The protein is added to what is otherwise a complete fast to keep the body from using its own organs and muscles to meet its protein needs. The dieter never has to face "real" food, which makes it easy to resist temptation, and the near-starvation results in the build-up of ketone bodies as the body relies entirely on its own fat for energy. The diets were designed to help extremely obese persons—those needing to lose 100 pounds or so—shed large amounts of weight relatively quickly before they get discouraged and give up trying. Protein-sparing diets were intended to be carried out only under strict medical supervision, often while the dieter was hospitalized. Their sudden burst of popularity among persons with little or no medical supervision—including those with relatively few pounds to lose—led to tragedy in some cases. For reasons that are still not clear, a number of dieters developed irreversible abnormalities of the heart rhythm that caused rapid death. There is no way to predict who will develop this fatal abnormality on a protein-sparing fast.

Fasting. This, of course, has even more complications than the protein-sparing regimen. It can precipitate gout and severe depression, as well as the loss of lean body tissue and sudden death due to heart-rhythm abnormalities.

Other Weight-Loss Gimmicks

Impatient with the slow results of dieting or unable to stick to a diet because of "breakthrough" hunger, many resort to pills, potions, and injections that promise painless weight loss. Again, the promise is often illusory and the health effects disastrous.

Water pills, or **diuretics,** merely dehydrate your body. Depending on how much water you were holding (which, in turn, depends on how much salt you've been consuming), you may lose 3 to 10 pounds of water taking diuretics, many brands of which are sold without prescription. But only water, not fat. As soon as you stop taking the pills, the water and the pounds come back. The dehydration associated with the unsupervised use of diuretics could interfere with proper muscle function and disrupt the balance of body salts, causing heart-rhythm abnormalities.

When you reach a plateau on a diet and suddenly seem to be getting nowhere despite a reasonable caloric deficit, retained water is likely to be the problem. It's a result of normal shifts in water balance as the body readjusts to its thinner, calorically undernourished self. The best way to prevent this kind of discouraging plateau is to cut back on the amount of salt you eat. It also helps to remember that as long as you're consuming fewer calories than you're using, you will continue to lose fat. It just may take a few extra days to show up on the scale. But water pills have no place in your weight-reducing scheme. They should never be taken unless prescribed by a physician for the treatment of specific health problems, such as high blood pressure or congestive heart failure.

Laxatives, like water pills, are also bad news as diet aids. Again, the weight you may lose is essentially water weight, not fat, since the way most laxatives work is to increase the water content of your stool. Sometimes passage of food wastes through your gut may be fast enough to reduce the number of calories your body absorbs from your diet, but not by enough to justify the risks. Hazards of laxatives include interference with the absorption of essential vitamins and minerals and loss of other essential elements, such as potassium. Laxatives can also cause permanent crippling of bowel muscle function, leading to chronic problems with constipation.

Fiber pills, taken five at a time, three times a day, with a glass of water, are intended to help fill your belly before meals, thus reducing the amount you consume at each meal. Actually, the amount of fiber in a day's worth of the tablets can be obtained from just one-third of a cup of an all-bran cereal. Manufacturers rightly emphasize that the pills won't work unless you also eat fewer calories than normal. In studies of the pills' effectiveness, both the pill takers and those who simply ate less lost weight. In fact, drinking water before meals may be more helpful than the fiber pills themselves. Whether or not they are effective, at least the fiber pills are probably harmless.

Appetite suppressants, like phenylpropanolamine (PPA) and amphetamines, may, or may not, help you to lose by reducing hunger pangs. But the price you're likely to pay is hardly worth it. These drugs are addictive, and you may become dependent on their antidepressive effects. As stimulants of the nervous system, they make you feel jittery and "hyper." As a further deterrent, bear in mind that once you stop taking the drug, you're more than likely to regain what you've lost. Advertising claims to the contrary, there is inadequate scientific proof that over-the-counter diet pills containing the nasal decongestant phenylpropanolamine or the anesthetic benzocaine are truly helpful in weight reduction. In 1980, the Food and Drug Administration withdrew from sale nine nonprescription diet pills that contained twice the allowable dose of phenylpropanolamine. Studies showed the drug could cause sudden, dangerous rises in blood pressure even in young, healthy people who were not overweight.

Thyroid, HCG, and other **hormones** are ineffective as diet aids. If your thyroid gland is functioning normally to begin with—as is true for the vast majority of overweight persons—taking additional hormone will have no effect. It will merely cause your own gland to cut back its hormone production. Those people who do lose weight while taking thyroid hormone lose primarily lean muscle tissue, not fat. And they gain back the lost weight when the hormone treatment is stopped. Thyroid hormone may also disrupt the function of the heart.

HCG, which stands for human chorionic gonadotrophin (a hormone produced by the placenta and derived from the urine of pregnant women), has been shown in careful studies to have no effect on weight loss. The unorthodox "fat" clinics that prescribe HCG accompany it with a very low-calorie diet. Those who attend these clinics lose money as well as pounds since it's the diet, not the hormone, that causes weight loss.

Surgery, in which a major portion of the small intestine is "bypassed" to reduce the amount of food your body absorbs, is a desperation measure used only for extremely obese people who have tried and failed at every other means of losing weight. Unfortunately, the operation is dangerous and can produce a number of serious, often life-threatening, complications, including liver failure and severe diarrhea. Although weight loss following the surgery has often been dramatic and painless, many of the operations have had to be reversed.

Psychotherapy is sometimes an effective aid in weight loss, especially for "binge" eaters. These are people who eat large amounts of food in a compulsive way. Once they start, they can't stop. They may gorge themselves to the point of abdominal pain and culminate the binge with self-induced vomiting. Psychotherapy, hypnosis, and self-help groups like Overeaters Anonymous have helped binge eaters to overcome their problem. But for the usual overweight person, psychological disturbances are rarely a cause of their weight problem; therefore, treating these disturbances is rarely a cure. However, psychotherapy or counseling may help some overweight people to overcome the emotional obstacles and self-loathing that stand in the way of successful weight loss.

Reducing salons and **health clubs** are okay if you can afford them. But they aren't essential to establishing a reasonable exercise and diet program that can help you trim down. Their main benefit is the moral support they offer and the fact that since you've paid good money to belong, you're more likely to follow the program. Beware of reducing organizations that promote strange diet plans or food supplements or exercise gadgets that you might not otherwise include in your weight-loss scheme. Gadgets that are claimed to help you trim off excess fat but that require little or no work on your part are worthless. It's a good idea to have a complete physical examination by your physician before joining a reducing club.

Weight-loss organizations like *Weight Watchers International* and *TOPS* (Take Off Pounds Sensibly) that promote well-balanced meal plans are excellent for those who can benefit from leadership, group support, and weekly monitoring of their progress in shedding unwanted pounds. Members share recipes and tips on reducing calorie intake and increasing caloric expenditure. However, the quality of the leadership varies from group to group. It is not necessary to purchase commercially prepared low-calorie meals unless you're already living on high-calorie TV dinners and have no time or interest in learning how to cook good-tasting food the low-calorie way. Overall, these reducing organizations are no more or less successful at producing lasting weight loss than any other sound weight-reduction program. However, they may be the best approach for some people.

17 ✤ WEIGHT CONTROL: SECRETS OF SUCCESS

LEST THE previous chapter discourage you from ever again trying to shed those extra pounds, let's say at the outset that there *is* a way to lose weight once and for all and still live in a world with normal people and normal meals. It's neither quick nor especially easy. But, take it from one who's tried it, it can work. It can work in the short run, albeit slowly, and, far more important, it can work in the long run. Though it's no guarantee you'll lose weight and never regain it, it will give you the tools for lifelong weight control because it involves a permanent change in the role food plays in your life and in how you consume and use calories. Once you learn to live normally with food, you won't have to exercise the constant restraint and eternal vigilance that undo so many dieters. You will also learn to tune out many of the external cues that now trigger your overeating.

The method, called *behavior modification*, can be applied in a group or on your own. Books to help you "go it alone" include *Act Thin Stay Thin* by Richard B. Stuart, Ph.D. (New York: Norton, 1977), *Eating Is Okay!*, by Henry A. Jordan, M.D., Leonard S. Levitz, Ph.D., and Gordon M. Kimbrell, Ph.D. (New York: Signet, 1976), and *Permanent Weight Control*, by Michael J. Mahoney, Ph.D., and Kathryn Mahoney (New York: Norton, 1976).

If the support of a group whose members are struggling with similar problems is helpful to you, join one. Some of these groups have been organized by individual therapists. Weight Watchers International and TOPS (Take Off Pounds Sensibly), both nutritionally sound weight-reducing organizations, have recently incorporated behavior-modification techniques into their programs. However, not every such group uses the behavior-modification approach, so check before you join if that's what you're after.

Behavior modification is not a diet—you really *can* eat anything you want, once you learn how to put food into its proper perspective. And it doesn't involve calorie counting, although it most certainly accepts the fact that calories count in weight gain and loss—both calories consumed and calories spent. Behavior modification does not promise a shortcut to a new slender you, but rather emphasizes gradual weight loss to give you time to unlearn your fattening eating habits and substitute slenderizing ones that will help you to maintain the loss indefinitely.

Know Your Fattening Eating Habits

Behavior modification rests on the hard-to-refute premise that overeating is a habit, or, rather, a collection of many habits, all of which lead to consumption of more calories than you need. The first step in changing any habit is to become aware of it. Do you "taste" practically a whole dinner while preparing it and then sit down to eat again with the family? Do you nibble half-consciously while watching TV or reading a book? Do you get carried away when something "irresistible" is set before you? Do you stuff your mouth whenever you're depressed, anxious, tense, angry, disappointed? Do you use food to calm your nerves or to reward yourself when you've completed a trying task? Do you eat whenever something is offered to you whether you're hungry or not? Do you overeat at restaurants because you're "paying for it anyway"?

The best way to inventory your fattening eating habits is to keep a diary in which you record every morsel of food or drink (except water or other noncaloric beverages) that passes your lips. Write down not only what you eat and how much but also the circumstances under which you eat it—time of day, place, who you were with, what you were doing, how you were feeling, and any precipitating events (for example, "fight with spouse" or "got raise"). (See Table 17.1 for prototype diary.) The diary should be kept daily for at least a week, preferably two. It will seem a terrible bother at first. But, according to Dr. Albert Stunkard, University of Pennsylvania psychiatrist who developed many of the behavior-modification techniques now used for weight control, you'll enjoy your eating diary once you realize how revealing it is. He's found that just having to keep track helps people cut down on how much they eat. When you know you're going to have to record that half-pint of ice cream you sneak in at midnight, you're less likely to eat it.

Substitute Slenderizing Strategies

My food diary revealed that I ate for a million and one reasons, all of which contributed to my weight problem. Every kind of negative

Table 17.1 • HOW TO CONSTRUCT A DAILY EATING INVENTORY

Time	Place	With whom	Eating cues	Mood	Degree of hunger (0–5)	Simultaneous activity	Food eaten	Amount
8:00 A.M.	Kitchen table	Children	Breakfast time	Harried—late for work	3	Read newspaper	Juice Toast Butter Jelly Coffee	4 ounces 2 slices 2 pats 1 tablespoon 2 cups
10:00 A.M.	Office desk	Alone	Fellow worker offered food	Nervous—problems with work	2	Working on calculations	Doughnut Coffee	1 1 cup
....	....	....	....	....	...	....	....	....
....	....	....	....	....	...	....	....	....
10:00 P.M.	Living room	Husband	Commercial break	Angry—fight with children	0	Watching TV	Peanuts	2 ounces

emotion sent me scurrying to the cupboard or refrigerator to assuage the psychic pain. Whenever I had to write something (which was nearly every day, since I was a newspaper reporter), I first made a stop at the candy machine. I ate whenever I was offered food or saw or smelled something I liked (which was almost everything). When I went grocery shopping, I couldn't even wait to get home—as I left the market I would rummage through the sacks and start nibbling on the way. I ate when I was cold (often, since I lived in Minnesota) or tired (also often, since I worked the late shift). *I ate for every reason except the right one —because I was hungry.* Hunger was rarely the cause of my overconsumption. In fact, once I made up my mind to do it, I had little trouble getting through a 24-hour fast. Therefore, for me, the single most important strategy was to learn to listen to my body and feed it whenever it was hungry, not because my mind "wanted something." I started by "training" my body to be hungry when it should be—at mealtimes. For the first time since my early teens, I ate three real meals a day, never skipping breakfast, lunch, or supper. If I was not especially hungry for one of them, I ate less, but I always ate something reasonably nourishing. This greatly reduced my tendency to nibble high-calorie snacks between meals. It also kept me from building up a voracious appetite for the next meal and hurriedly devouring everything in sight.

The strategy worked so well that I've become almost compulsive about mealtimes, especially breakfast and lunch, the meals that fuel my day's work. If I know in advance or even suspect that work or play will get in the way of a regular meal, I take something nourishing along with me—a container of yogurt, cheese and fruit, a sandwich—that I can eat "on the go." This keeps me from grabbing a candy bar, peanuts, sweet roll, or soda to stave off my hunger, and it reinforces the habit I have tried so hard to substitute for my old eating habits—that of eating only when I am physically hungry. At first I was a little embarrassed about pulling out my "emergency ration" on a train, at a meeting, or in the middle of a press conference. But I soon got over it by telling myself it was even more embarrassing to be fat.

A second highly successful strategy for me was to rethink the importance I placed on the different meals of the day and to realize that the typical American pattern of skimpy breakfast and lunch and huge dinner was contrary to my body's needs and to my ability to match my consumption to those needs. I'm a "morning person" and I use a lot of energy early in the day. So it seemed reasonable to fuel my body most when it needed it most—at breakfast and lunch. This has an added advantage because the body is less likely to store calories as fat when you're active than when you sit around or go to sleep soon after eating. Second, my eating diary showed that I have better self-control early in the day and that I'm inclined to overeat—as are many other people—when I'm tired in the evening. So I stopped thinking of the evening meal as my main repast for the day. Instead, for dinner, I usually eat a large salad, a piece of bread, coffee, and sometimes a miniportion of the family meal. More often than not, however, my share of dinner gets saved and becomes breakfast or lunch the next day. By eating less for supper, I find that I have more energy to do chores and projects or get some exercise in the evening. Now, if I'm going to skip any meal during the day (a rare event), it's supper rather than breakfast or lunch.

On days I'm planning to go out for dinner I cut back on the amount I eat for breakfast and lunch or I get some extra exercise (or both) to make room for the added calories I'll most certainly consume that night. But I don't skip those early-in-the-day meals. That would only leave me famished for the dinner out and less able to limit myself to reasonable portions and food selections.

To cut down on fattening snacks, I make sure that the cookies infrequently bought or made for my children are ones I can resist. The same for ice cream—we mostly buy ice milk in flavors I don't care for. We almost never have potato chips, pretzels, snack crackers, or nuts in the house. (Unsalted nuts for baking and cooking are kept in the freezer.) If overwhelmed by the urge to nibble, I make myself some popcorn without butter. For years, the strategy I used to prevent cravings for sweets was to allow myself one sweet "no-no" a day—such as two cookies, a sliver of cake, or a few bites of ice cream. Knowing that I could have these things—that they weren't forbidden—kept me from eating them by the box or pint when I could no longer resist. In truth, my "will power" is no stronger now than it was when I was 35 pounds heavier. I have just removed the temptations! And with the passing years, as my consumption of sweets and other once-favored snacks has diminished, I've noticed that I crave them less and less—if at all—and am satisfied by far less than formerly.

Leftovers were another of my problems. Having heard all through childhood that it's immoral to waste food because "the children in Poland are starving," I grew up cleaning my plate, the serving dish, even the pot, at every meal. During my freshman year at college, which was my first exposure to meals served family style, I gained 15 pounds eating the "leftovers" in the serving dishes.

My husband, who was raised in the same tradition (only for him it was the children in India who were starving), devised a superb solution. Every leftover beyond 1 or 2 tablespoons gets saved in a labeled margarine tub and after a few days, there are usually enough miscellaneous ingredients to make a wonderful soup, supplemented by additions of fresh celery and onions and herbs or whatever else appealing happens to be in the house. You'd be surprised at what can taste good together—even rice, pasta, and potatoes can be mixed in the same pot. With salad and bread, these soups serve as a complete evening meal for us once or twice a week. That is, unless I steal the leftovers for my own concoctions of stir-fried leftover rice, bulgur, kasha, noodles, or potatoes with miscellaneous leftover meat and vegetables and/or chopped fresh vegetables (onions, scallions, celery, bean sprouts, spinach, green pepper, whatever). If no meat or chicken is available, I sometimes scramble in an egg white for added protein. This dish, which is never the same twice, is a favorite breakfast or lunch for me, especially on cold winter days (see the recipe on page 112).

These are only a few of the tricks for restructuring fattening eating habits. Other possibilities devised by Dr. Henry Jordan and other specialists include the following:

• Eat more slowly. Put less food on your fork or spoon, chew it deliberately for far longer than you ordinarily would, and put your eating utensil down between bites. For a while, you might even count the number of bites, and after every four bites, wait two minutes before taking another—a taxing exercise, but instructive about speed. If you have companions at mealtimes, talk to them—but never talk with food in your mouth. The more slowly you eat, the less likely you'll be to gobble down a second serving before your body's had a chance to tell you it was filled up by the first. By eating slowly you'll also spend less time sitting at the table staring at an empty plate that cries out for refilling while your dining companions are still eating.

• Serve yourself on a smaller plate. Smaller portions will fill it up and you're less likely to feel deprived by "skimpy" servings.

• If you're still hungry after you've finished your first serving, wait at least twenty minutes before you reach for seconds. It takes that long for the satiety signal to register in your brain.

• Restrict all your eating to one or two places in your home—the kitchen and dining-room tables—and for everything you eat, whether it's a four-course dinner or just tea and toast, set yourself a place with a napkin and utensils and sit down to eat it. This helps to diminish the number of locations you associate with food and the chances you'll sneak in extra calories "on the run."

• If you nibble while you watch television, take up a hobby like knitting, woodworking, needlepoint, basketweaving, rug hooking—anything that will keep your hands busy and out of the cookie jar or bag of chips.

• By the same token, don't watch television or read while you're eating. Instead, concentrate on your meal: take in the sight, smell, texture, and taste of your food. This makes your meal more satisfying and thus helps you to eat less.

• If certain activities or times of day are associated with between-meal eating, change your routine. Walk the dog after dinner instead of plunking down in front of the TV set with a can of peanuts.

• Let your family and friends know that you're trying to cut down, and ask them not to offer you seconds or urge you to eat when you say "no, thanks." Many people offer food as a sign of affection. Tell them the most caring thing they can do is *not* to offer you something to eat.

• Go grocery shopping *after* you've eaten a satisfying meal. If you shop when you're hungry, you're likely to select more fattening foods than you otherwise would. And shop from a list that you prepare when you're not hungry.

• Rearrange your cupboard and your refrigerator so that when you open them, your eyes don't land instantly on something tempting. Store tempting items in opaque containers.

• Don't leave food out where you repeatedly see it and can easily reach for it many times a day. If you have a cookie jar, it should be behind closed doors. Even a bowl of fruit can tempt you to eat more calories than you intend to.

• Try to spend less time in the kitchen, where you're surrounded by food. The kitchen should be a place for preparing and eating meals, not for socializing.

• Don't set serving dishes on the table. Serve from the stove or refrigerator and put away the leftovers as soon as you've taken what you consider a reasonable portion. Never eat from the serving platter.

• Forget about "clean-plate clubs" and starving children in other countries. There are several possibilities for leftovers. If my remedy of soup and stir-fried leftovers doesn't appeal to you, you could feed them to the dog or—if you don't have a dog—save them for a neighbor's dog.

If all else fails, the garbage pail will do. It is no more immoral to "throw away good food" than it is to demean your humanity by treating yourself like a human garbage pail.

• Get someone else in the family to clear the plates and put away the leftovers. That way, you'll be less tempted to nibble after you've finished your meal.

• At meals eat your favorite things first. You'll be more likely to stop eating when you've had enough rather than after you've cleaned your plate.

The Importance of Exercise

In modifying your behavior to achieve lasting control over your weight, you can't afford to neglect the energy-expenditure side of the caloric equation. As you know, *energy in* must equal *energy out,* or the remainder gets stored as fat. The larger the right-hand side of the equation, the more leeway you have on the left. You can make the same kind of inventory for activity that you can for eating patterns. Construct a diary and record every significant move you make—or fail to make—in the course of a day over a period of a week or two.

Your exercise diary should state what you did, how much of it, or for how long. It can include such items as "(walked, drove, bicycled, jogged) to store and back, 1.5 miles," "(took elevator, climbed upstairs) three flights," "(carried groceries, pulled cart) four blocks," "(hung up, put in dryer) two loads of laundry," "(walked, jogged, cycled) around park, 3 miles," "swam laps, 15 minutes," etc. *You don't have to become an "exercise nut" to put activity back into your life. Little things add up,* like leaving your car at the far end of the lot instead of parking right in front of the store. Or getting off the bus a stop or two before your destination and walking the rest of the way. Or walking up—and down —one, two, or more flights of stairs instead of taking the elevator or escalator. Or using footpower instead of horsepower to go ten or twenty blocks (which uses the energy you have in surfeit and saves the energy the world is short of). When I dine in the company cafeteria seven floors above my office, I walk up four flights, ride up the other three, and walk down all seven. Lately, I haven't been using the elevator at all.

Even though my life is crammed with work, activities, and family chores, I have found that extending my use of personal energy by hanging up the laundry, walking instead of riding, climbing stairs, chopping by hand, etc., really doesn't cut significantly into the time I have available to carry on with the rest of my life. If anything, it has made me more energetic and efficient and thus has provided me with more time for fun. And by reducing tension, defusing anger, and relieving depression, it has, I think, made me easier to live with. In fact, the more I do with my body, the better I feel about it. And the less sleep I seem to need. Instead of eight hours of restless sleep, I'm "out cold" for five and a half or six hours and wake up fully rested and rarin' to go. While others are sleeping in, I jog or ride a bicycle.

Some Slimming Tips

When you're trying to lose weight, you need all the help you can get. The following tips are worth bearing in mind.

• Weight control is your personal responsibility. Don't assign anyone else to keep an eye on you. If someone else is your watchdog, you're likely to find yourself cheating when that person isn't looking.

• Don't let an occasional indulgence be an excuse for going completely overboard. If you've "blown" your diet by eating a brownie, that's no reason to blow it even further by eating ten brownies. When you're trying to lose weight, every brownie counts. Eating ten brownies in one day counts as much as eating one brownie a day for ten days. Your diet should not be so rigid that you cannot "write off" an occasional indulgence and make up for it by cutting back a little the next day or by getting some extra exercise.

• Don't start your weight-loss program just before vacation or the Christmas holidays, when you know it will be especially difficult to lose weight. By the same token, don't use such "prediet" periods as an excuse to pack in as much food as you can or you'll have more to shed later.

• Don't weigh yourself more than once in two weeks while you're trying to lose. Losing fat takes time, and you may get discouraged if you don't see daily progress on the scale. Once you've reached your desired weight, a weekly "checkup" on the scale will help you to maintain the loss. As soon as you see a few pounds creeping back, get rid of them before they add up to a noticeable gain.

• Cut back on salt, which holds water in your body and may mask a loss of body fat, depriving you of all-important encouragement on the scale.

• Keep your consumption of caffeinated beverages—that includes tea and colas as well as coffee—to a minimum since caffeine can stimulate your appetite.

• Drink a glass of water before meals and sip water or some other noncaloric beverage between bites of your meal. That will help fill you up without overloading you with calories.

• "Diet" food doesn't have to be tasteless and uninteresting. In place of high-calorie fats, oils, and dressings, season your foods generously with herbs and spices. Experiment a little until you find combinations you especially like.

• Try hot soup before your meals or *for* your meals. Because it must be eaten slowly and is filling, hot soup is likely to reduce the number of calories you might otherwise consume at the meal.

• Study a comprehensive calorie chart to familiarize yourself with foods that are unexpectedly rich in calories. Be sure to take note of portion sizes. A good, low-calorie food can easily become a fattening one if you eat too much of it. Conversely, by consuming very small portions of high-calorie foods you especially adore, you may be able to lose without changing the items in your diet, just the amounts.

• Beware of hidden fat, a concentrated source of calories. Some foods we ordinarily think of as highly nourishing and good diet foods are actually loaded with fat. These include hard cheeses, nuts and seeds, granola cereals, and most meats. Peanut butter, avocados, and tuna fish (especially if packed in oil) are also rich in fat. The caloric difference between a whole-milk product and one made from skim or low-fat milk can be as much as 100 calories per serving. Over the course of a day, substituting low-fat milk, cottage cheese, and yogurt for the high-fat varieties can mean a savings of several hundred calories. So can choosing only lean cuts of meat, trimming away all visible fat and preparing the meat (for example, by broiling) so that hidden fats drain off.

• In most recipes, far more fat is called for than is really needed to cook the food properly. Try using half the amount, and if that works out okay, try even less the next time. The new nonstick pans (for example, those coated with Silverstone) permit cooking without any fat if you wish. The new edible spray-on coatings made from vegetable oils also help reduce the amount of fat you consume. See Chapter 4 on low-fat living for further tips.

• Don't be fooled by frozen yogurt. With sugar as the main source of calories, it's as calorically rich as ice cream. The main difference is that frozen yogurt lacks much of the saturated fat that's in regular ice cream and ice milk. And instead of buying regular yogurt with preserves, get the plain kind, add fresh fruit or one or two teaspoons of jam and save 50 to 70 calories.

• Except under medical supervision, it's unwise for anyone to eat less than 1,200 calories a day. Below that, it's hard to meet basic nutritional needs. If you're cutting your caloric intake to 1,200 calories a day or less, or if—against all advice—you restrict yourself to just a few kinds of foods, take a daily multivitamin and mineral supplement to be sure you're meeting your micronutrient needs. Such supplements contain inadequate amounts of calcium and, for women, insufficient iron, so it's important to include in your diet foods that are good sources of these minerals (see Chapter 9).

HOW TO CONSTRUCT A WEIGHT-LOSS MENU PLAN

The following lists can help you construct a varied nutritious, calorie-controlled eating plan that does not lock you into a limited number of foods or restrict you to foods you don't especially like. If you stick to the portion guide for the calorie level you need to lose weight or maintain your loss, you don't have to count calories—they've already been counted for you, by the Institute of Human Nutrition at Columbia University. All you have to do is select the appropriate number and size of portions in the seven food-exchange lists.

FOOD EXCHANGES

List 1—Free foods
(no specific amounts)

Bouillon
Chicory
Chinese cabbage
Clear broth
Coffee
Endive
Escarole
Gelatin, unsweetened
Lemon
Lettuce (all kinds)

Lime
Mustard
Parsley
Pickle, sour or unsweetened dill
Radishes
Tea
Soy sauce
Vinegar
Watercress

Lists continue on next page

List 2—Vegetables
(½ cup cooked or 1 cup raw, except as indicated)

All leafy greens, except those in List 1
Asparagus
Bean sprouts
Beans, green or wax
Beets
Broccoli
Brussels sprouts
Cabbage (all kinds)
Carrots
Catsup (2 tablespoons)
Cauliflower
Celery

Cucumbers
Eggplant
Mushrooms
Okra
Onions
Peppers, red or green
Rutabaga
Sauerkraut
Summer Squash
Tomato or vegetable juice (6 ounces)
Tomatoes

List 3—Fruits

Apple, ½ medium
Applesauce, ½ cup
Apricots, dried, 4 halves
Apricots, fresh, 2 medium
Bananas, ½ small
Blueberries, ½ cup
Cantaloupe, ¼ medium
Cherries, 10 large
Dates, 2
Figs, dried, 1 small
Fruit cocktail, canned, ½ cup
Grapefruit, ½ small
Grapes, 12
Honeydew, ⅓ medium
Mango, ½ small

Nectarine, 1 small
Orange, 1 small
Papaya, ⅓ medium
Peach, 1 medium
Pear, 1 small
Pineapple, ½ cup
Prunes, dried, 2
Raisins, 2 tbs.
Strawberries, ¾ cup
Tangerine, 1 large
Watermelon, 1 cup cubed
Juices:
  Grapefruit, Orange, ½ cup
  Apple, Pineapple, ⅓ cup
  Grape, Prune, ¼ cup

List 4—Starches

Breads
  Any loaf, 1 slice
  Bagel, ½
  Dinner roll, 1, 2-inch diameter
  English muffin, ½
  Bun (hamburger or hot dog), ½ inch
  Cornbread, 1½-inch cube
  Tortilla, 1, 6-inch diameter

Cereals
  Hot cereal, ½ cup
  Dry flakes, ⅔ cup
  Dry puffed, 1½ cups
  Bran, 5 tablespoons

Vegetables
  Beans or peas (dried), ½ cup cooked
  Corn, ⅓ cup (½ ear)
  Parsnips, ⅔ cup
  Potato, white, 1 small or ½ cup
  Pumpkin, ¾ cup
  Winter squash, ½ cup

Crackers
  Graham, 2, 2½-inch
  Matzoh, 4 inches × 6 inches, ½
  Melba toast, 4
  Oyster, 20
  Pretzels, 8 rings

Wheatgerm, 2 tablespoons
Pasta, ½ cup
Rice, ½ cup

Desserts
Fat-free sherbet, ½ cup
Angel food cake, 1½-inch square

RyKrisps, 3
Saltines, 5

Alcohol
Beer, 5 ounces
Whiskey 1 ounce
Wine, dry, 2½ ounces
Wine, sweet, 1½ ounces

List 5—Proteins

Beef, dried, chipped, 1 ounce
Beef, lamb, pork, veal, lean
  only, 1 ounce
Cottage cheese, uncreamed,
  ¼ cup
Poultry, no skin, 1 ounce
Fish, 1 ounce

Lobster, 1 small tail
Oysters, clams, shrimp, 5 medium
Tuna (in water), ¼ cup
Salmon, pink, canned, ¼ cup
Egg, 1 medium
Hard cheese, ½ ounce
Peanut butter, 2 teaspoons

List 6—Milk

Buttermilk, fat free, 1 cup
Yogurt, plain, made with nonfat
  milk, ¾ cup

Skim milk, 1 cup
1%-fat milk, 7 ounces

List 7—Fats

Avocado, ⅛ of 4-inch diameter
Bacon, crisp, 1 slice
Butter, margarine, 1 teaspoon
French dressing, 1 tablespoon
Mayonnaise, 1 teaspoon
Oil, 1 teaspoon

Olives, 5 small
Peanuts, 10
Roquefort dressing, 2 teaspoons
Thousand Island dressing, 2 teaspoons
Walnuts, 6 small

Table 17.2 • DAILY PORTION GUIDE:
NUMBER OF PORTIONS FOR VARIOUS CALORIE LEVELS

	Calories			
List	*1,000*	*1,200*	*1,500*	*1,800*
1—Free foods	Unlimited	Unlimited	Unlimited	Unlimited
2—Vegetables	2	2	2	2
3—Fruits	3	3	3	3
4—Starches	3	5	7	9
5—Proteins	6	6	7	7
6—Milk	2	2	2	3
7—Fats	2	2	6	7

SAMPLE MENU FOR 1,500 CALORIE PLAN

List	Number of Portions	Possible Food Choices
		Morning
3	1	½ grapefruit
4	2	1 slice whole-wheat bread, and 1½ cups puffed cereal
7	1	1 teaspoon margarine
6	1	1 cup skim milk
1	—	Coffee
		Noon
5	2	½ cup tuna
4	2	2 slices bread
7	3	2 teaspoons mayonnaise, and 1 teaspoon oil
2	1	3 slices tomato
3	1	½ cup diced pineapple
1	—	Lettuce, pickles, lemon juice, vinegar
		Evening
2	1	½ cup string beans
5	4	4 ounces chicken (no skin)
4	2	½ cup mashed potatoes, and ½ cup sherbet
7	2	2 teaspoons margarine
3	1	2 dates
1	—	Lettuce, radishes, soy sauce, parsley
		Snack
6	1	1 cup skim milk
4	1	1½-inch square angel food cake
1	—	Coffee

Source: Nutrition and Health 1, 2 (1979), Columbia University Institute of Human Nutrition.

Pitfalls in Your Path

All of us who've tried to take off extra pounds know the trail to a trimmer figure is set with booby traps that spring on the unsuspecting, often spoiling the best-laid plans to lose weight. But if you're aware of these traps ahead of time and prepare strategies for coping with them, you can avoid most of the pitfalls most of the time.

SNACKING

Few of us are immune to the urge to nibble. Here are some slenderizing suggestions for coping with snacks, including ones recommended by Weight Watchers International.

• Don't buy high-calorie snacks to have in the house "just in case" unexpected guests drop in.

• To minimize your contact with food between meals, ask your children to take their own snacks, or prepare them yourself at mealtime and set them aside "prepackaged" for later consumption.

• Plan your own snacks for a certain time of day and prepare them ahead. Cut up a bag full of fresh vegetables or a bowl of fresh fruit and set it aside for consumption at assigned times during the day. If you work away from home, take "safe" coffee-break snacks with you from home to avoid being tempted by the high-calorie choices on the coffee cart or cafeteria line.

• Do nothing but eat at snack time. Don't read, watch TV, or talk on the phone. The object is to dissociate eating with other activities so that you won't think of food when you're doing other things.

• Know your most vulnerable times for nibbling (check your eating diary), and plan activities for those times that would make eating difficult or help you forget about it.

• One way to get in several snacks during the day without adding extra calories to your diet is to save parts of your meals to eat as snacks later on. Appetizer, dessert, and salad are ideal for this purpose.

• Don't skip or skimp on meals. That just lowers your resistance to snacking between times, and you may end up consuming more calories than if you had eaten a real meal.

• At a party, plant yourself far from the hors d'oeuvres. Find someone interesting to talk to—it'll help take your mind off the dips and chips, and it's hard to talk with food in your mouth.

• If you know you have a hard time ignoring cocktail snacks, ask the host or hostess if you may bring some hors d'oeuvres and prepare an attractive platter of cut-up raw vegetables with a low-cal dip seasoned with herbs. Many party-givers are already planning to serve such platters, in which case you might ask if you could bring your own "special" dip as an accompaniment.

DINING OUT

In a restaurant, you've got the "paying-for-it-anyway-so-why-not-eat-it" booby trap to sidestep plus the fact that it's hard to know from

the menu how many high-calorie ingredients—like cream and butter—
the chef may have used in preparing an otherwise innocent-sounding
meal. When eating at a friend's house, you don't usually have a choice
as to what to eat and you don't want to insult the cook by passing up
courses or merely picking at your food. Nor do you want to ruin an
evening out by counting calories and worrying about the consequences
of every bite. Many of the following tips for enjoyable but weight-
conscious dining out are derived from *Nutrition and Health,* the newsletter edited by Dr. Myron Winick, director of Columbia University's
Institute of Human Nutrition.

• No matter where you're eating, practice portion control. Most
restaurants give servings that are far larger than you would dish up for
yourself at home. You don't have to finish it all. Offer some to a
tablemate or take home a "doggie bag."

• If the regular dinner comes with four or more courses and you
know it's going to add up to more food than you want or need, order
à la carte even if it costs more. If you end up overeating, the dinner's
no bargain. Order two appetizers (less food than a main course) and
salad, or share a dinner with someone and get an extra salad or appetizer, if needed.

• Skip the parts of the meal you like less, or that the restaurant
doesn't prepare especially well, or that you can get at home "any old
time."

• For your first course, avoid pâtés (very high in fat and usually
eaten with lots of bread), cream soups, and quiches. A good choice
would be fresh fruit, vegetable relishes, juice, seafood cocktail, or clear
soup. Select your entrée from among lean meat (such as a roast), broiled
or roasted chicken or turkey, or broiled, baked, or poached fish. Ask
the waiter to tell the chef to hold the butter when broiling your portion.
Trim off all visible fat and skin. Avoid entrées that are prepared in
gravy, glazed, breaded, fried, in cream sauce, or au gratin.

• In ordering vegetables, ask for your potato baked or boiled and
season it with pepper and the barest amount of fat, if any. Avoid
vegetables that have been fried or are served with a cream or cheese
sauce.

• Ask for your meal without gravy and your salad dressing on the
side and use it sparingly. Or order oil and vinegar, which you put on
the salad yourself.

• For dessert, order fruit. (Check the appetizer list if no fruit is
listed under "Desserts.") Or skip the dessert and ask your tablemates
for a (tiny) taste of theirs. Or, get your own dessert, taste it, and divide

the rest among your fellow diners.

• In someone else's house, your best bet is to take—or ask for—small portions. If dessert is a high-calorie wonder, ask for a tiny serving and say something like "it looks scrumptious, but I'm really stuffed."

• If you're invited to cocktails to be followed by dinner, ask the host or hostess approximately when dinner will be served and arrive halfway through the cocktail hour to reduce your exposure to the hors d'oeuvres and alcohol.

• For business lunches, keep a list of places where you know you can order a relatively low-calorie meal.

• From time to time there'll be special evenings, events, and places where you'll want to ignore all the above suggestions. *There's nothing wrong with an all-out splurge now and again.* You shouldn't have to worry about your diet at your fortieth birthday party or your daughter's wedding. *Just get back to normal the next day.*

DRINKING

In figuring how much they eat, many people neglect to include the caloric contribution of alcoholic beverages. For the average American adult who drinks, 10 to 20 percent of the daily calories comes from alcohol. Ounce for ounce, alcohol has more calories than either carbohydrates or protein and nearly as much as fat. The caloric contribution from one cocktail a day can add up to 15 extra pounds a year, all other things being equal. Besides, alcohol, noted for its ability to "loosen" people up, also loosens the rein on your resistance to temptation (see Chapter 14).

If you're serious about weight control, limit yourself to one drink a day and stay away from high-calorie mixers and sweet liqueurs. For a relatively low-calorie drink, try a wine spritzer—2 to 4 ounces of dry wine mixed with club soda or mineral water. The alcohol content is low and you can nurse one drink for a long time. When you're ready for a refill, try plain soda or mineral water with a wedge of lemon or lime. And don't forget the calories you add to your meal if you cook with wine or beer. The alcohol evaporates during cooking, but the sugars and starches stay and add calories to the food.

If You Want to Gain Weight

There are some people (most of us consider them lucky, but, oddly enough, they don't think of themselves that way) who have the opposite energy problem. They weigh 10 or more pounds *less* than they should, and, try as they might, they can't seem to put on weight. If, during a time of extreme stress or illness, they happen to lose a few pounds, it often takes them many months to regain those pounds.

Persons who are too thin have been neglected by researchers and therapists because they are rare compared to the numbers of too-fat people and because the problem was long thought to be not particularly hazardous to health. However, it was shown in 1980 that being too thin may diminish life expectancy even more than being too fat. A very thin person may get chilled or fatigued more easily than someone of normal weight and may have an increased susceptibility to infection. Further, a "skinny" person often feels unattractive, has trouble getting clothes that fit properly, and may even look considerably older than his or her years.

Studies indicate that one cause of the problem is an inadequate number of fat cells. There are simply not enough places for the body to store extra energy. This is most commonly an inherited characteristic rather than a result of deprivation in early childhood. If you come from a line of too-thin people, don't expect miraculous results from your attempts to gain weight.

The first step in a weight-gaining program is to make sure that a medical disorder is not the cause of your problem. A thorough checkup is particularly important if you have previously been of normal weight and have recently lost a significant amount of weight without really trying. Emotional stress is a common cause of involuntary weight loss, but weight loss may also result from a serious underlying illness or hormone imbalance. Chances are, though, if you've been too thin all your life and one or both of your parents was also very thin, there's no illness at the root of your problem.

Some of the aids to gaining weight are the reverse of the advice commonly given to those who are trying to shed excess pounds. But other tips may surprise you. Here are some suggestions, including several from Barbara E. Echols and Dr. Jay M. Arena of Duke University Medical Center, authors of *The Common-Sense Guide to Good Eating* (New York: Barron, 1978).

• Try to increase your caloric intake by about 500 calories a day —that will put on a pound a week—by adding high-calorie foods to your meals or consuming them as between-meal snacks.

• Fat is the most concentrated source of calories, so you might use more vegetable oils and polyunsaturated margarines. But beware of saturated animal fats in meat and dairy products, as well as saturated coconut and palm oils commonly found in commercial baked goods and other processed foods. (And don't get carried away, because excessive amounts of polyunsaturated fats may also be hazardous.)

• Study a calorie chart to identify high-calorie foods that are low in bulk (for example, peanut butter and avocados), and increase your consumption of those that appeal to you.

• Avoid bulky, low-calorie foods with your meals lest they fill you up before you've consumed an adequate number of calories. Such foods would include clear soups, vegetables like cabbage and summer squash, and salad entrées. Eat your salad as a side dish after your main course and use lots of rich dressing.

• Concentrate on high-calorie vegetables, such as winter squash, dried beans, and potatoes, and don't skimp on rice, pasta, and bread.

• Don't drink water, tea, coffee, or other low-calorie drinks before eating or with your meal. However, a cocktail before dinner or wine with dinner can help you relax and may stimulate your appetite.

• Consume snacks two or three hours before meals so that the snacks won't ruin your appetite. An excellent time for a high-calorie snack is just before bed. A sandwich, puddings, fruit-flavored yogurt, creamed soups, cookies and milk, nuts, and crackers and cheese are good to snack on if you're trying to gain weight.

• If you find you can eat only small amounts of food at a time, plan substantial meals and divide them into five or six "doses" over the course of your day rather than trying to eat a large, complete meal at one sitting.

• Get some exercise on a regular basis. This will tone up your body, help you to relax, and improve your overall sense of well-being. Exercise will also help you to put on those extra pounds as muscle rather than flabby fat. But don't go overboard on exercise or you'll end up burning more calories than you can consume, and losing weight instead of gaining it.

• If you're a picky eater or if you've been eating poorly in terms of amounts and types of foods, you might benefit from a one-a-day vitamin-mineral supplement. If you're a menstruating woman, a supplement that contains iron may also help to improve your vitality and your appetite. But avoid megadoses and monolithic vitamins and minerals, which just further distort your nutrient balance.

• Be sure to get lots of rest. Many too-thin people are "nervous" types who are constantly on the move, rarely relax, and sleep poorly. Taking daily exercise, avoiding caffeine-containing beverages, and perhaps drinking a glass of warm milk (you can make this a calorie-rich drink by adding some honey or molasses) at bedtime will help to improve your ability to relax and sleep well.

• If you're a smoker, quit, and try food when you want to put something to your lips.

• While you're concentrating on how you eat, pay attention too to how you look. By choosing your clothes, your colors, and your hair style carefully, you can make your slimness an asset rather than a liability.

PART FIVE

Food for Special Lives

18 ❧ PREGNANCY: EATING FOR TWO, BUT HOW?

How MANY of these statements have you heard before?

A pregnant woman is eating for two, so she should eat twice as much as usual.

It's bad to gain more than 10 or 15 pounds during pregnancy.

If you're overweight and do not gain during pregnancy, you can easily lose 20 pounds when the baby is born.

Salt is bad for a pregnant woman. It makes her body swell and her blood pressure rise.

If you take high-potency prenatal vitamins, you don't have to worry about what you eat during pregnancy.

Those cravings a pregnant woman gets for strange foods are a sign her body is lacking certain nutrients.

An unborn child is like a parasite: it can get everything it needs from its mother even if she is poorly nourished.

You can make up for a haphazard diet before pregnancy by eating well for the next nine months.

All of the above notions are just that—*notions.* None of them is true. Yet many women believe them, and, as a result, these women may jeopardize their health and that of their unborn children. Sometimes, the doctors who care for pregnant women are as poorly informed as their patients about proper nutrition. A great deal of new information about maternal nutrition has come to light during the past decade or so, and much of it runs counter to long-standing beliefs. It is now known that *what* as well as *how much* a woman eats during pregnancy can make an enormous difference to the physical and mental development of her child. It can also affect her own ability to weather the trials of pregnancy, delivery, and care of the new baby.

Realizing they are now responsible for the nutritional well-being of another, completely dependent human being, many women use pregnancy as a time for making permanent changes for the better in how they eat. While this is certainly a laudable step, many experts say it may be too late. Optimal maternal nutrition actually begins long before egg meets sperm. A fertilized egg may fail to become implanted in the uterus of a poorly nourished woman, and the healthiest babies are born to women who were well-nourished and of normal body weight *before* they conceived.

So if you're not yet pregnant but plan to be, now's the time to review the preceding chapters and get yourself into tip-top nutritional shape. If you are already pregnant, all is by no means lost. You can start today to feed yourself and your developing child in ways that will mean a happier and healthier future for both of you.

Don't Cheat Your Baby on Weight

I still remember the anxiety I felt each month on the day I went to the obstetrician for a prenatal checkup. I was so afraid of being chastised about the weight I'd gained that I didn't eat lunch until after my late-afternoon examinations. Actually, the doctor never said a word about my weight, but I "knew" I wasn't supposed to gain more than 1 or 2 pounds a month if I was to end up with at most 15 extra pounds by my due date. In the seventh month, though, I gained 9 pounds and, in expectation of a severe talking-to, I burst into the doctor's office and announced that fact before anyone could weigh me.

Much to my surprise, the doctor said, "Don't worry. You look fine. You're not too fat. From the back, you don't even look pregnant." Little did either of us know then that the reason for the precipitous increase in weight was that I was carrying twins! (I gained 18 additional pounds during the last two months, and still ended up after delivery weighing less than I had when I conceived.) But I was astonished at the doctor's casual acceptance of my "enormous" weight gain.

I hadn't realized that the entire concept of how much a woman should gain during pregnancy was undergoing a radical revision. The old dogma that weight gain should not exceed 18 pounds, and is best held at 10 to 15, was finally being laid to rest by new evidence that such weight restrictions produced too many babies born dangerously small. In the old days, there was some reason to hold down the mother's weight, since this would likely result in smaller babies that were easier to deliver. But with safe, modern obstetrical techniques, restricting the baby's growth was no longer medically defensible. It had also been finally shown that, counter to prevailing obstetrical wisdom, large weight gain during pregnancy was not the cause of toxemia, a serious complication near term that involves swelling of tissues, high blood pressure, and loss of protein in the urine.

Despite the dogma, numerous surveys taken through the years both here and in Britain showed that the average woman gained 24 to 27 pounds during the nine months of pregnancy. Then in the late 1960s a study of 12,000 pregnancies by an obstetrician from Johns Hopkins University, Dr. Nicholson J. Eastman, revealed that babies had a better chance of surviving if their mothers gained 20 or more pounds during pregnancy. He concluded that if a woman hasn't gained at least 10 pounds by mid-pregnancy (20 weeks along), she should be considered a "high risk" case and given nutritional supplements to increase her rate of gain.

Dr. Eastman pointed out that a woman who gains only 14 pounds during the nine months of pregnancy has a net loss because she will lose more than that when the baby is born. In fact, about 20 pounds can be accounted for by growth of the fetus and its supporting tissues and fluid and by changes in the mother that are essential to a healthy pregnancy. On top of that, an extra few pounds are recommended to provide nutritional leeway for mother and baby. (See Chart 13.)

In addition to providing nutritional insurance *during* pregnancy, those few extra pounds help to protect the mother's health should anything go wrong *after* delivery. For example, I developed a serious infection following the Caesarian delivery of my twins and was unable to eat much for ten days. Despite my 36-pound prenatal weight gain, I ended up scrawny—7 pounds underweight. Even if you're healthy after delivery, you'll need some extra stored energy to meet the exhausting schedule of caring for a newborn infant. And if you breastfeed, those extra pounds are needed to make milk for the baby.

Studies subsequent to Dr. Eastman's have confirmed and extended his findings. Most recently, Dr. Richard L. Naeye of Hershey Medical Center in Hershey, Pennsylvania, studied the relationship of weight gain to the survival of the baby in 53,518 pregnancies. He showed that not only is weight gain during pregnancy important, but how much the mother weighed *before* becoming pregnant is also important to the baby's welfare. Women who start out underweight are more likely to deliver babies who are dangerously small, even if the women gain normally during pregnancy. And women who are obese to start with are more likely to develop serious pregnancy complications and to encounter difficulties in delivery that could jeopardize both baby and mother.

Among women who were of normal weight at the start of preg-

Chart 13 • WHERE THE WEIGHT GAIN GOES IN PREGNANCY

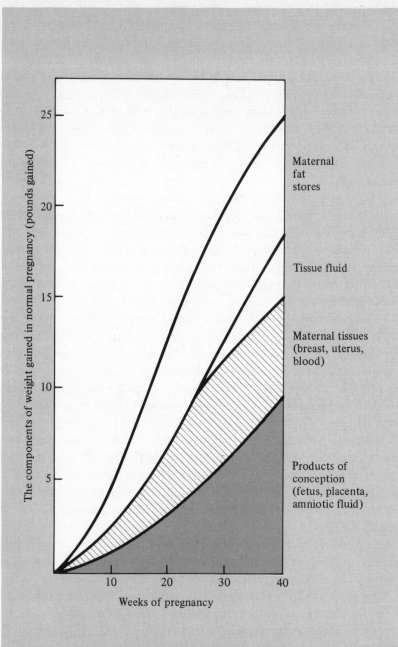

Maternal
fat
stores

Tissue fluid

Maternal tissues
(breast, uterus,
blood)

Products of
conception
(fetus, placenta,
amniotic fluid)

The components of weight gained in normal pregnancy (pounds gained)

Weeks of pregnancy

Source: Adapted from *Nutrition & Health*, 1979, Vol. 4.

nancy, Dr. Naeye's study showed, a prenatal weight gain of 20 pounds gave the best chances of having a healthy baby. If the mother was underweight to start with, she needed to gain 30 pounds. And if she was overweight before conceiving, a gain of 16 pounds produced the best results. And no matter what the mother's starting weight, gains of more than 32 pounds (for a single baby) were also associated with a greater risk to the baby.

Pregnancy is no time to try to get rid of prepregnancy fat. Chances are you'll omit from your diet some nutrients needed by your unborn baby for normal development. Also, when you lose body fat, it is broken down into substances called ketone bodies that are passed to the fetus, where they can cause irreparable damage to its developing brain and body.

The rate at which you gain weight during pregnancy is also important. During the first three months, you should gain only 1½ to 3 pounds. From the beginning of the fourth month on, weight gain should average about 1 pound every nine days (¾ pound a week), reaching a total of about 24 pounds by the end of pregnancy. *Be sure to watch your rate of gain all through pregnancy, so you won't be tempted to cut back toward the end* when you realize you've been gaining too quickly. The weight increase during the last three months represents mostly growth of the baby, so a cutback in calories then could compromise the baby's development.

How Much to Eat and What

Pregnancy can be viewed as an energy equation. It takes about 80,000 extra calories to produce a baby, and those calories should come from extra foods you eat. That averages out to about *300 calories a day more than you usually consume,* assuming you don't change your usual level of activity. If you do exercise less during pregnancy (and there's no reason why you should until perhaps the last three months, unless your doctor tells you otherwise), you will also have to eat proportionately less. The less you eat, the harder it is to pack in all the nutrients you and your unborn baby need. Bear in mind, too, that those extra 300 calories really don't amount to a lot of food. You can blow it all on one slice of pie or six chocolate chip cookies or three Cokes and miss getting the added nutrients you need.

Pregnancy is tissue-building time. You, mother, are constructing an entire new human being and all the tissues it needs to support its development. You can't make a proper cake without flour, liquid, salt, sugar, leavening, and eggs, and neither can you make a baby without the right ingredients. Those in greatest demand are protein, vitamins, and minerals. The baby's body is also made of fats and carbohydrates, but these are readily obtained from mother. Here's how pregnancy changes your nutrient requirements.

Protein. The amount of protein—the critical ingredient of new tissue—recommended for daily consumption *increases by two-thirds* during pregnancy, from 44 grams to 74 grams. To be sure the protein you eat is available to build tissues, you must also consume enough calories to meet the daily energy needs of you and your unborn child. Most Americans are already eating this amount of protein (half a chicken breast, a cup of cottage cheese, and one pork chop exceed that, without counting the protein from dairy products, eggs, vegetables, and grains). But women who are watching their weight or who eat only one square meal a day may be shortchanged on protein. If you don't consume enough protein, neither will your baby; growth retardation and/or mental deficiency can be the result. Adequate protein is also important to prevent the development of toxemia late in pregnancy.

In "As You Eat, So Your Baby Grows," an excellent booklet on good nutrition during pregnancy, nutrition writer Nikki Goldbeck lists the following foods as a guide to meeting your protein needs. Each item as listed contains approximately *15 grams of protein,* so you would need to eat five such items each day to get the recommended amount.

> 2 large or 3 medium eggs
> 2 to 2½ ounces meat, fish, or poultry
> 2 ounces natural cheese (Swiss, cheddar, muenster, etc.)
> ½ cup cottage cheese
> 2 cups milk (whole, skim, buttermilk) or yogurt
> 4 tablespoons peanut butter or ½ cup peanuts
> 1 cup cooked beans (kidney, lentils, chickpeas, etc.)
> ¾ cup cooked soybeans
> 2 cakes bean curd (tofu)
> ½ cup sunflower seeds

Remember, if you rely on vegetable protein to meet all or part of your protein needs, two or more vegetables should be combined to provide a proper balance of essential amino acids. You can obtain balanced vegetable protein by combining beans or nuts with grains or by combining any one of those with dairy products or eggs (see Chapters 2 and 24 for details).

Calcium. Calcium is needed in large quantities to build bones and in smaller amounts for a host of other vital body functions. The developing fetus will take much of the calcium it needs from its mother, even if she consumes inadequate amounts. But both mother and baby suffer if mother's prenatal diet is deficient in calcium. Calcium will be forced out of the mother's bones, weakening them, and bone growth in the baby will be inadequate.

A *50-percent increase* in calcium is recommended during pregnancy—to a total of 1,500 milligrams a day. Milk and other dairy products are your best sources of calcium. One cup of milk supplies nearly 300 milligrams of calcium, so drinking a quart of milk each day will nearly fulfill your need for calcium. It will also supply 40 percent of your daily protein. It doesn't matter if it's whole milk, skim milk, or buttermilk, but avoid adding chocolate because that reduces your body's ability to absorb calcium. You can obtain the calcium equivalent of a cup of milk from any one of the following: 1 cup of yogurt; 1½ ounces of cheddar cheese; 1 ounce of Swiss cheese; 2 cups of cottage cheese; or 1¾ cups of ice cream.

If you hate drinking milk, you can add it in liquid or powdered form to a wide range of prepared foods: soups, puddings, baked goods, casseroles, cooked cereals, meat loaf, among others. Some vegetables, including collard greens, kale, mustard greens, and broccoli, are also high in calcium. Oysters, sardines, and canned salmon (eaten with bones), and American-made tofu are also good calcium sources.

Some women may be unable to consume milk and other dairy products because they cannot digest the milk sugar lactose (see Chapter 13). However, very little lactose is found in natural cheeses, with the least in fermented cheeses. Cultured milk products like yogurt and buttermilk (brands without added milk solids) have reduced amounts of lactose, and some people with lactose intolerance can consume them without problem. Another alternative is acidophilus milk, available in some markets and health-food stores, or the addition of the enzyme lactase to ordinary milk. The enzyme, marketed as LactAid, can be purchased in pharmacies, health-food stores, or by mail (see pages 254–255 for the address).

With all these possibilities, it should not be necessary for any pregnant woman to take calcium tablets. It is far better to satisfy the calcium requirement with real foods, since these supply other essential nutrients at the same time.

Iron. Here the story is different. A woman's blood volume doubles during pregnancy, and iron is essential to the formation of healthy red blood cells. In addition, the developing fetus will take all the iron it needs from its mother, regardless of how meager her supply may be. An iron-deficient mother-to-be may end up anemic, exhausted, and susceptible to infection. Very few women start pregnancy with enough iron stored in their bodies to meet the greatly increased need for this trace mineral. And few eat enough iron-rich foods to keep up with the demand through nine months of pregnancy. Even if you do eat lots of iron-containing foods, only a small percentage of what you eat is actually absorbed, so it's hard to know if you're getting enough. Few doctors want to wait until their pregnant patients become anemic before deciding they're not getting enough iron. Therefore, *iron supplements of 30 to 60 milligrams a day are routinely recommended,* especially during the second half of pregnancy.

Good sources of iron include organ meats like liver and kidneys, dried fruits (raisins, prunes, apricots, etc.), prune juice, iron-fortified cereals, and dried beans. Even if you're taking an iron supplement, it's wise to include some of these foods in your regular diet. Iron pills tend to be constipating, so eating dried fruits or drinking prune juice may help counter that effect as well as give you added iron.

B vitamins. One of the least well known of the B vitamins, *folacin* (also called folic acid), turns out to be critically important to a successful pregnancy. *The need for folacin is doubled during pregnancy.* Folacin deficiencies are more common than most people realize, and during pregnancy they can result in spontaneous abortion or damage to the unborn child. This is particularly a problem for women who were taking the birth-control pill until shortly before conceiving. Folacin is found in leafy green vegetables, broccoli, asparagus, peanuts, mung bean sprouts, and liver. Many doctors advise taking a folacin supplement during pregnancy.

Recent studies suggest that some pregnant women need unusually large amounts of *vitamin B_6* to support the development of the baby's central nervous system. Researchers at Purdue University found that mothers of babies born in poor condition tended to have significantly lower amounts of B_6 in their diets and in their blood than mothers whose babies were born in A-one condition. Yet the mothers with endangered babies had consumed more than the recommended amounts of B_6, suggesting that for some women this level is not high enough. Vitamin B_6 is found in whole-grain (but not enriched) bread and cereal, liver, spinach, green beans, bananas, poultry, fish, meats, nuts, potatoes, and leafy green vegetables.

The need for other B vitamins—thiamin, niacin, riboflavin, and B_{12} —also increases during pregnancy, but for the most part these needs are met by the foods that supply the added calories during pregnancy. Good sources of B vitamins include liver, whole-grain bread and cereal, wheat germ, milk, and nuts. Supplements should not be necessary except in unusual cases.

Vitamin C. You need about *a third more* vitamin C during pregnancy than usual—80 milligrams a day altogether. This amount is readily supplied by commonly eaten foods—citrus fruits and juices, melon, strawberries, tomatoes, green pepper, and cabbage, especially if eaten raw. Vitamin C is particularly important during pregnancy because it enhances the body's use of iron, folacin, and vitamin A. But vitamin C tablets are unnecessary and may even be harmful to your child. Megadoses during pregnancy create a dependency on high doses of C in the unborn child. After birth, the baby may suffer from scurvy (vitamin-C deficiency disease) when consuming normal amounts of vitamin C.

Fat-soluble vitamins. *Vitamin A* is needed for the formation of healthy skin and the linings of internal organs, such as the lungs and gastrointestinal tract. A *25-percent increase* in consumption of vitamin A—to 1,000 retinol equivalents—is recommended during pregnancy. Two cups of fortified milk would supply this amount. Other sources of vitamin A include dark-green vegetables and deep-yellow or orange vegetables and fruits, organ meats like liver, and butter. *Vitamin A supplements should be avoided* because overdoses are poisonous. But it's practically impossible to consume too much vitamin A from foods, unless you go on a carrot-juice kick, which can cause you to turn yellow from too much carotene (provitamin A).

Without *vitamin D*, your body can't use calcium properly, so the need for this vitamin *doubles* during pregnancy—from 200 to 400 international units a day. A quart of fortified milk supplies this amount. To support their own *and* their baby's bone development, pregnant women between the ages of 19 and 22 need still more vitamin D—the amount in five glasses of milk. Other food sources of vitamin D include fortified margarine, butter, sardines, canned salmon, egg yolk, and liver. In addition, the vitamin is made on your skin when you're out in the sunlight. Like vitamin A, *overdoses of vitamin D are toxic* and can produce severe abnormalities in an unborn child; supplements should not be taken without a doctor's advice.

The recommended *25-percent increase* in *vitamin E* during pregnancy is readily obtained from vegetable oils, whole grains, and wheat germ. No supplement is needed.

Other minerals. Proper bone growth requires *phosphorus* and *magnesium* as well as calcium, and—like calcium—the recommended intake of these two minerals is 50 percent higher during pregnancy. However, these minerals are generally in plentiful supply in ordinary diets, so they rarely require special attention. Foods rich in phosphorus include meat, milk, cheese, soft drinks, and many processed foods containing phosphate additives. Magnesium is plentiful in salad greens, nuts, soy beans, seeds, and whole grains. Overconsumption of phosphorus in relation to calcium can lead to improper bone development. Dairy products are good sources of these minerals because they contain slightly more calcium than phosphorus.

Similarly, a *50-percent increase* in *zinc* consumption is advisable during pregnancy. A prenatal deficiency of this trace mineral may permanently damage the fetus. It is found most abundantly in animal protein foods (meat, eggs, seafood, and milk) and in whole-grain products.

To be certain of getting enough *iodine,* use only iodized salt or sea salt. And if your drinking water is not fluoridated, you might consult with your physician about the use of *fluoride* supplements to help protect the teeth that form before birth under the baby's gums. A study of 492 children by researchers at the University of Miami School of Medicine showed that fluoride supplements during pregnancy were both safe and effective in protecting the children's teeth against decay.

Salt. The need for salt (sodium) is *increased significantly* during pregnancy, and the notorious prenatal craving for pickles might reflect that need (although other maternal whims seem to bear no relation to nutritional deficiencies or excesses). It was long thought that too much salt during pregnancy caused toxemia. However, new evidence suggests that an inadequacy of protein is the more likely cause.

The Food and Nutrition Board of the National Academy of Sciences has concluded that "it is difficult to justify dietary sodium limitation in healthy women during pregnancy on the basis of either animal or clinical evidence."

Liquids. You need to drink plenty during pregnancy to keep your body operating like a well-oiled machine. *At least six to eight glasses of liquids a day* (in addition to milk) are recommended during pregnancy to help maintain the increased amount of body fluids and to prevent constipation.

Rely primarily on water, unsweetened fruit juices, and vegetable juices. Avoid soft drinks (nutritionally empty, calorically dense, and too high in phosphorus), and don't get carried away with coffee and tea. Excessive consumption of caffeine may cause fetal damage (see Chapter

12). Caffeine also acts like a diuretic, dehydrating you instead of adding water. And stay away from diuretics unless prescribed by your doctor for a specific medical problem. In addition to water loss, they cause your body to lose vital mineral salts.

Menu Planning

Now that you see how many extra nutrients must be packed into those 300 added calories you're entitled to during pregnancy, perhaps you'll better appreciate the importance of not wasting too many prenatal calories on junk foods. For your own and your baby's sake, it's best to make nearly every calorie count toward proper nourishment. Many different menus have been devised for pregnant women, but while the constituents vary, the pattern is always the same: three real meals a day (no skipping breakfast or lunch) plus two or three nutritious snacks. The precise ingredients you choose and the pattern in which you consume them can be highly flexible—a matter of personal taste, habit, and life style. You can eat dinner in the morning and breakfast before bed, if it suits you. The important thing is to get in the right amount of food in each food category each day without overloading on calories. You can divide up the foods in any way you like. Here's what you should aim for:

• One quart of fortified milk or its equivalent.
• Three to four servings of meat, fish, poultry, cheese, eggs, or vegetable-protein combinations each containing 15 grams of protein. For every two glasses of milk you miss, add one protein serving.
• One to two servings of fruits or vegetables rich in vitamin C.
• Two servings of a green leafy vegetable.
• One deep-yellow or orange fruit or vegetable at least five times a week.
• Four servings of grain products. One thick slice of bread or two thin ones or one cup of cereal counts as one serving. Whole-grain products are richer than refined ones in the required nutrients.
• One to two tablespoons of vegetable oil.
• Six to eight glasses of liquids, in addition to milk.

When it comes to snacks, think of foods that are nourishing as well as delicious: ice cream (if you can afford the calories), milk puddings, fresh or dried fruits, nuts and seeds, popcorn, whole-grain cereal, or cheese and crackers.

ONE DAY'S SAMPLE MENU DURING PREGNANCY

BREAKFAST	Orange juice, Bran flakes with peaches, Milk
MORNING SNACK	Peanut butter and jelly on whole-wheat toast, Milk, Pear
LUNCH	Vegetable juice, Egg salad on lettuce, Tomato slices, Pumpernickel bread (2 slices)
AFTERNOON SNACK	Yogurt, Carrot sticks, Water or other beverage
DINNER	Chicken, Carrot-raisin-apple salad, Baked potato, Green peas, Apple juice
EVENING SNACK	Cheese and crackers, Milk, Dried apricots

Source: Prepared by Columbia University Institute of Human Nutrition, as printed in *Nutrition and Health,* 1, 4 (1979).

To get yourself started down the right nutritional road, you might consider keeping an *eating diary* for a week to be sure you're consuming the proper foods in needed amounts. As your pregnancy continues, do a spot check now and again to be sure you're still eating properly. If you follow the dietary plan described above, you should not need supplements of any vitamins or minerals except iron and possibly folacin. Far better to spend your money on the foods you need than on pills.

As one expert, Dr. Roy M. Pitkin, obstetrician at the University of Iowa in Iowa City, wrote: "The traditional practice of prescribing vitamin-mineral supplements for the pregnant woman is . . . probably unnecessary. Among the disadvantages of routine supplementation are cost and the potential for a false sense of security regarding nutritional status." On the other hand, Dr. Pitkin adds, "the practice is not dangerous as long as toxic overdoses are avoided and it should therefore be viewed as an option."*

Alcohol Can Harm Your Baby

In the Old Testament, an angel admonishes Samson's mother: "Behold, thou shalt conceive, and bear a son; and now drink no wine or strong drink" (Judges 13:7). Did the ancients know something about the effects of alcohol on the fetus that we have only just rediscovered within the past decade? Although several reports at the beginning of the century suggested a link between consumption of alcohol by mothers and abnormalities in their babies, it wasn't until 1973 that doctors

*In *Nutritional Disorders of American Women,* edited by Myron Winick, M.D. (New York: Wiley-Interscience, 1977).

began to take such findings seriously.

That was when Drs. David W. Smith and Kenneth Jones at the University of Washington in Seattle published a description of eight children of alcoholic mothers. These children were suffering from what the researchers called *fetal alcohol syndrome.* The characteristics of the syndrome may include growth retardation before and after birth; mental deficiency; delayed development of both gross and fine motor activities; structural abnormalities of the face and skull; and abnormalities of the joints and heart.

Since the initial description of fetal alcohol syndrome by the Seattle researchers, several large studies have confirmed these researchers' suspicion that excessive alcohol consumed during pregnancy can cause irreparable damage to the unborn child. Although many pregnant women who drink a lot also smoke cigarettes, eat poorly, and may use other drugs as well, the damage observed in their offspring appears to be caused primarily by alcohol. Even nonsmoking, well-nourished alcoholics have babies with fetal alcohol syndrome. Also, experiments done with rats and mice have shown similar fetal effects when otherwise well-nourished pregnant animals were fed alcohol.

As studies of alcohol's effects have broadened, they've suggested a further link to a pervasive behavioral and learning problem in children—hyperactivity, or minimal brain dysfunction. This observation in the children of alcoholic mothers is supported by studies in animals. The offspring of rats fed alcohol during pregnancy were abnormally active and didn't learn tasks like running a maze as quickly as the offspring of rats whose mothers were not fed alcohol.

Most of the research has focused on the children of heavy drinkers, but *there is some evidence that as little as two drinks a day can increase the risk* of having children with certain birth defects, including learning difficulties. Such children also are more likely to be born dangerously underweight.

A safe level of alcohol during pregnancy has not yet been defined. In the meantime, government experts and the American Medical Association recommend that a pregnant woman consume *no more than two drinks on any one day,* even if she only drinks once in a while.

Coping with Common Eating Problems

Pregnant women are often beset with a host of digestive upsets that may interfere with good nutrition. Nausea and vomiting, heartburn, constipation, and the ability to eat only small amounts of food at a time are certainly not conducive to a hearty appetite.

During pregnancy, your digestive processes slow down. Muscle movements in your gastrointestinal tract are slower and your stomach secretes less acid and digestive juices to process the foods you eat. As a result, food spends a longer time than usual in your stomach. At the same time, the muscle between the esophagus and stomach is more relaxed, and may allow some of the acid contents of the stomach to rise into the esophagus, causing heartburn. The slowed movements of the digestive tract also may produce constipation.

Fortunately, most of these problems are short-lived, and various tricks of the maternity trade can help you overcome the limitations of other problems.

"Morning sickness." Despite its name, cyclic nausea and vomiting may occur in the afternoon or evening as well as in the morning. It afflicts half of all pregnant women, usually between the second and fourth months of pregnancy. Sometimes it continues nearly to the end of pregnancy. Typically, the nausea occurs soon after getting up in the morning, and any breakfast that is eaten is likely to wind up down the drain. Although its precise cause is unknown, there is some indication that it's related to a drop in blood sugar.

Eating lots of small, protein-containing meals throughout the day helps many women. It's best not to let yourself get too hungry. The time-honored remedy of eating dry crackers immediately upon awakening—before you've even lifted your head off the pillow—also helps. *Put the crackers on your night table before you go to bed.* Save your morning juice or fruit for the end of breakfast. Or have it at some other meal. Also, give yourself extra time to get ready in the morning, since the stress of rushing contributes to the problem. If you go to work, carry something with you for a midmorning snack. If your "morning sickness" strikes in the evening, try the dry-crackers routine or a substantial snack half an hour before the expected onset.

Heartburn. Stay away from antacids and baking soda. They don't help, they may upset your body's acid-base balance, and they can destroy the B vitamin thiamin. To reduce the likelihood of heartburn, avoid fried foods, sweets, rich desserts, pickles, spices, and other foods that irritate the stomach or are hard to digest. Sometimes a mildly acidic food like yogurt or buttermilk is helpful. Learn to eat slowly, and eat small meals. Try to avoid emotional upsets during meals or shortly after eating, since they can stop your digestive processes cold.

Constipation. Don't use laxatives or resort to frequent enemas.

Instead, eat plenty of *foods high in fiber*—fresh fruits and vegetables, dried fruits, and whole-grain breads and cereals—and *drink lots of liquid.* In addition to what you drink during the day, have two glasses of water before you go to bed, and drink something hot right after getting up. Make sure you get a reasonable amount of exercise.

Limited capacity. As your baby grows, there's less and less room in your abdomen for your own digestive organs. You may be unable to eat much at any one time. That's okay; just eat more often. *Divide your meals up into six small ones,* or three small main meals and three substantial snacks. As long as you get in the required nutrients, it doesn't matter how you eat.

Special likes and dislikes. The nutritional significance of cravings for certain foods during pregnancy is not known. It may have something to do with hormonal influences on your sense of taste. It matters little whether you give in to these cravings or not as long as they don't interfere with your remaining nutritional requirements. Don't, for instance, indulge a desire for chocolate by eating half a pound. And don't succumb to cravings for nonfood items, like clay or dirt, that afflict some women during pregnancy; these can block the body's use of vital nutrients like iron.

Sometimes certain foods absolutely turn women off during pregnancy. I, for one, developed a nine-month-long distaste for red meat, which I formerly enjoyed. There's no reason for you to eat foods that don't appeal to you during pregnancy as long as you eat other foods that provide the nutrients they would otherwise supply.

Fatigue. Many women find, especially during the first and last months of pregnancy, that they're simply too tired to care about fixing meals. Here's where *the prospective father can make a real contribution* to the nutritional welfare of mother and baby by helping with menu planning, grocery shopping, and meal preparation. Many evenings during my pregnancy I would lie down to rest "for a few minutes" after work, and not open my eyes again until my husband rang the dinner bell. When I thanked him for preparing dinner, he reminded me that pregnancy is, after all, a shared responsibility.

Financial problems. Pregnancy can put a decided crimp in an already tight food budget. Knowing that it doesn't pay in the long run to compromise on maternal and fetal nutrition, *the federal government has set up a food supplementation program* for low-income pregnant women (and for nursing mothers and young children). Called the federal WIC Program (Special Supplemental Food Program for Women, Infants, and Children), it provides at no cost about $20 worth of high-protein, high-mineral, and high-vitamin foods each month for persons who are "nutritional risks" because of low income and inadequate nutrition. Dietary counseling goes along with the subsidy. Check with your local Department of Health for further information about the WIC program.

As a parting word, remember that what you eat and don't eat during pregnancy may make a big difference to your baby's chances for a healthy and happy life. A baby's diet before it's born may be more important than at any other time in life. And it's entirely up to you to see that the prenatal menu is a good one.

FOR FURTHER READING

Nikki Goldbeck, "As You Eat, So Your Baby Grows," a practical sixteen-page pamphlet. At some health-food stores and bookstores or by direct mail ($1.50) from Ceres Press, PO Box 87, Woodstock, New York 12498.

Phyllis S. Williams, R.N., *Nourishing Your Unborn Child* (Los Angeles: Nash, 1975). A guide and natural-foods cookbook for pregnant women.

Judith E. Brown, R.D., *Nutrition for Your Pregnancy* (Minneapolis: University of Minnesota Press, 1983). Accurate, up-to-date information about how nutrition affects pregnancy.

Diane Klein and Rosalyn T. Badalamenti, *Eating Right for Two* (New York: Ballantine, 1983). A complete nutrition guide and cookbook for a healthy pregnancy.

19 ❧ HOW TO FEED
YOUR BABY

H UMAN MILK *is for the human infant; cow's milk is for the calf.*"
This seemingly obvious point, made more than sixty years
ago by the late Dr. Paul Gyorgy, discoverer of riboflavin and
vitamin B_6, amused his medical colleagues, who were then enamored
of formula feeding. Formulas were a symbol of an affluent society, of
mothers no longer stuck with what nature had foisted on them, liber-
ated from the round-the-clock need to be feeding stations for their
infants. Physicians and advertising convinced mothers that cow's-milk
formulas were actually better for their babies than the thin fluid that
emerged from their breasts.

As the twentieth century wore on, breast feeding gradually became
passé among those who could afford formulas and were willing to
contend with the business of preparing and sterilizing baby's food. By
1930, most women who still nursed their babies were from the lower
social classes, a demographic pattern that continued for another two
decades. Finally even the poor turned to formulas, and by 1970, three-
fourths of all mothers were feeding their babies only with a bottle.

As we have seen, a diet born of affluence is not necessarily the best
one. In the past decade, the back-to-nature movement and widely publi-
cized discoveries about the unique virtues of breast milk for human
infants have brought breast feeding back in fashion. Today, more than
half of new mothers leave the hospital intending to nurse their babies;
as recently as 1971, less than a quarter had expressed this intention.
Now it's mostly the affluent, well-educated mothers who nurse, but
between 1971 and 1978 breast feeding also doubled among lower-
income mothers. By 1984, 62 percent of all mothers were breast feeding
their newborns, and 47 percent were still nursing when their babies
were two months old.

What's So Special about Mother's Milk?

Dr. Gyorgy was right. Each mammalian species produces milk
uniquely suited to support the growth of infants of that species. Since

no two species have precisely the same needs, no animal's milk is exactly like that of any other. A calf is certainly different from a human baby. It has to grow quickly, putting on lots of muscle and extending its bone structure to allow early independence from its mother. Brawn, not brains, is the focus of the calf's early development. The human infant, by contrast, has a very long period of parental dependence and doesn't reach its full physical size for more than a dozen years. But while the body grows slowly, the central nervous system—the brain—develops rapidly and extensively.

The constituents of cow's and human milk reflect these developmental differences. Cow's milk has four times as much protein as human milk, and different proteins as well. Dr. Gerald Gaull, pediatric researcher at Mount Sinai School of Medicine and the New York State Institute for Basic Research in Mental Retardation, reports that 70 percent of the protein in human milk is easily digestible *whey protein,* whereas cow's-milk protein is 80 percent casein, which forms a hard curd in the acid of the stomach and is harder for a human infant to digest.

Cow's-milk protein is very low in the *amino acid cystine,* which newborn humans require in their diet. But it is high in another amino acid, *phenylalanine,* which the human infant has a limited ability to metabolize, possibly causing a toxic build-up of the substance in the baby's blood. As you might expect, human milk is well endowed with cystine but has little phenylalanine. Also in short supply in cow's milk, but plentiful in human milk, is the *amino acid taurine,* which preliminary studies suggest may play an important role in brain development and in how efficiently the body handles cholesterol. The human infant can make only limited amounts of taurine, so if more of this amino acid is needed, it must be supplied by the baby's diet.

The *fats* in human milk are also different from the fats in cow's milk. In cow's milk, saturated fatty acids predominate, whereas human milk has mostly unsaturated fat. Human milk is rich in the enzyme *lipase,* which predigests the fats even before they reach the baby's intestines. Cow's milk doesn't have much lipase, and as a result some of the fat combines with calcium and is excreted by the human infant undigested, leading to a loss of both calories and calcium.

Although cow's milk contains more *calcium* and *phosphorus* than human milk (presumably needed by the calf's rapidly growing skeleton), calcium is better absorbed from human milk and breast-fed infants have higher levels of calcium in their blood than those who are bottle-fed. As for the *milk sugar lactose,* human milk is loaded with it. Dr.

Gaull suggests that the galactose that results from the digestion of lactose is needed to synthesize essential brain chemicals that contain galactose.

Another difference from cow's milk is the amount of *cholesterol,* which is higher in human milk. With all that's been said about the risks of a high-cholesterol diet, you might not regard this as an advantage. However, cholesterol is required for the synthesis of bile acids, needed to absorb fats that are important to the baby's development. It also may contribute to immunological defense against harmful organisms in the infant's intestinal tract.

Indeed, the most talked about difference between human and cow's milk—and possibly the most significant one—is the *immunological weapons* carried by mother's milk. Human milk has as many infection-fighting white blood cells as blood does, and those in milk are even more active in destroying bacteria than the ones in blood. Human milk also contains a kind of antibody that helps to defend the infant gut against invasion by foreign organisms and proteins. Furthermore, recent studies have shown that the nursing mother, who necessarily maintains close contact with her infant, produces antibodies to disease-causing organisms that threaten the baby and then passes these antibodies to the infant through her milk. The nursing mother, in other words, acts as an antibody factory for her infant, manufacturing the specific weapons the baby needs to stay healthy.

Dr. Michael Klagsbrun, a Harvard biochemist, recently discovered a powerful substance in human breast milk that stimulates the growth and division of human cells. This may be the factor responsible for the maturation of the gastrointestinal tract in breast-fed babies, helping to protect the babies from intestinal diseases and food allergies. Subsequent studies conducted at Vanderbilt University have identified "epidermal growth factor" as a growth stimulant in mother's milk.

Why Mother's Milk Is Best

In 1978, the American Academy of Pediatrics, long an advocate of breast feeding, and the Canadian Pediatric Society issued a sweeping endorsement of mother's milk. Calling it "the best food for every newborn infant," the two prestigious societies recommended that physicians encourage all mothers to breast-feed their infants. Ideally, they said, breast milk should be practically the only source of nutrients for the first four to six months in the lives of most infants.

Behind that statement lies a number of established and strongly suggested benefits of breast feeding.

BREAST-FED BABIES ARE HEALTHIER

Dr. Allan S. Cunningham, pediatrician from Cooperstown, New York, showed that during their first year of life, breast-fed babies had only about a third as many serious illnesses as bottle-fed babies. Among the latter, respiratory infections occurred fifteen times as often, vomiting and diarrhea nearly three times as often. What's more, bottle-fed babies were admitted to the hospital nine times as often as babies who were breast-fed.

At the Kaiser-Permanente Hospital in Hayward, California, doctors found that of 107 infants admitted over a recent two-year period with gastroenteritis (infection-caused diarrhea and vomiting), only one was being breast-fed. Similarly, among 339 infants hospitalized in Britain for diarrhea, 338 were bottle-fed.

In Iowa City, Dr. Randolph Paine compared 40 babies who were breast-fed for the first six months of life with 66 babies who were bottle-fed from birth. The breast-fed babies made an average of 1.6 visits to the doctor for illness during the first half year, compared to 2.8 visits for bottle-fed babies. During the time that breast-fed babies were receiving only mother's milk, 78 percent had no visits for illness, compared to only 3 percent of the bottle-fed babies. Dr. Paine found that even a short period of breast feeding helped to protect the infants from illnesses requiring medical attention.

Premature babies who are breast-fed are less likely to develop a severe and often fatal intestinal disorder called necrotizing enterocolitis. Tests indicate that some factor exists in fresh human milk that protects against the disorder. The factor is destroyed, however, if the milk is heated or frozen. This raises questions about the benefits of human milk banks for hospitalized premature babies who must be tube-fed, because the milk in such banks is usually stored frozen and must be sterilized.

Studies by Dr. Stephen S. Arnon at the California Department of Health Services in Berkeley have shown that breast-fed babies get milder forms of a potentially fatal infection called infant botulism. Earlier studies by Dr. Arnon linked severe cases of infant botulism with crib death (sudden infant death syndrome).

It was once thought that breast-fed babies had fewer infections because breast milk was cleaner than formula. There was no chance of it becoming contaminated with infectious organisms the way formula can. Now there's every reason to believe that the healthfulness of breast milk most likely results from the protective, immunological factors it contains—factors that are simply not present in cow's milk.

Here are some advantages of breast milk to the baby.

Breast milk may prevent allergies. A Finnish study published in 1979 showed that babies breast-fed for more than six months were less likely to develop severe or obvious allergies than those nursed for a shorter period and weaned to formula. Breast feeding seemed to be most helpful to babies from allergic families. The researchers recommend that such babies be given breast milk as their only source of milk for at least the first six months of life. Breast milk contains a type of antibody that can coat the infant's intestinal tract and prevent the absorption of allergy-provoking proteins. Breast feeding also prevents the development of cow's-milk allergy, one of the most common feeding problems in young infants.

Breast-fed babies are leaner. Once considered a disadvantage of breast feeding, this fact is now regarded as a plus since fat babies are more likely to grow up to be fat adults. Many pediatricians no longer use rapid weight gain as the main measure of good health in infancy. What matters is how much weight babies gain in relation to how much they grow in length. Breast-fed babies determine for themselves how much milk they drink. But when a bottle-fed baby slows down before the preordained amount of formula has been consumed, the adult holding the bottle is likely to nudge the baby into drinking more. The result is a kind of forced feeding that could become a lifelong habit and prevent the baby from developing control over his or her own appetite.

Breast feeding may lead to lower cholesterol. The reason is not yet known, but studies involving a total of 420 adults who have been followed by researchers since before birth have shown that those who were breast-fed exclusively for more than two months have less cholesterol in their blood as adults, even if their current diets are high in fat.

BREAST FEEDING HELPS MOTHER, TOO.

Women who nurse have an easier time *shedding excess fat* accumulated during pregnancy. Nature provides some 35,000 calories of stored fat—10 pounds worth—to support milk production, and the mother who doesn't nurse has to lose this fat on her own. At least one study showed that mothers who nursed lost more weight during the first three months after childbirth than those who fed their babies formula.

The hormones produced by the nursing mother *help the uterus to contract* and return quickly to its normal, nonpregnant state. And women who feed their babies breast milk and no other food have a longer period of infertility following childbirth. This *helps to space pregnancies,* but it cannot be relied on as a method of birth control. Nursing mothers can become pregnant, even if their menstrual periods have not yet returned.

. . . but Not Perfect

Thanks to a host of contaminants, both environmental and personal, a mother's milk can transfer a variety of potentially harmful substances to her baby. This is especially true for chemicals that are stored in fatty tissue, which the mother's body draws on to produce breast milk.

CONTAMINATION FROM WITHOUT

Although so far only one baby is known to have been harmed by the environmental pollutants transmitted through breast milk, the effects of such contaminants on nursing infants have not been systematically studied. Some doctors are concerned about possible long-term consequences and the fact that the chemicals are being passed on to yet another generation of Americans. The following are among the causes for concern.

PCBs. Analyses by the Environmental Protection Agency of breast-milk samples from women in ten states suggest that nine in ten nursing mothers across the country have measurable amounts of polychlorinated biphenyls, or PCBs, in their milk. These chemicals have been used in a wide range of industrial products and processes and have been polluting the environment for half a century. Although further production of PCBs has been banned, the chemicals are persistent substances that are stored in body fat. The EPA found that breast milk contained an average of 1.8 parts of PCBs per million parts of breast milk, with some samples having more than 10 parts per million. In many cases, the amounts of PCBs found in breast milk were higher than is allowed in commercial foods. Studies with monkeys have linked very high levels of PCBs in breast milk with hyperactivity and mild retardation in the offspring.

Even so, the American Academy of Pediatrics has stated that most women have little to worry about from PCBs. The academy encourages all women to breast-feed unless they know they've had an unusually high exposure to PCBs—through their jobs, for example, or through the consumption of large amounts of freshwater fish taken from PCB-contaminated waters, such as the Saint Lawrence Seaway.

Any woman who is concerned about PCB levels in her milk can have it laboratory tested. The test takes about three weeks. State health departments or regional offices of the EPA may be able to provide information on testing breast milk for chemical contaminants.

DDT and other pesticides. Like PCBs, DDT and its chemical cousins are stored in body fat. Although most of these pesticides, known collectively as chlorinated hydrocarbons, are now banned, they still show up in mother's milk. In addition to DDT, a recent study by the EPA uncovered dieldrin, oxychlordane, heptachlor, and heptachlor epoxide in the milk of most of the 1,400 women tested in forty-six states. The agency said that the small amounts of these pesticides in milk pose *"no immediate health hazard to either mothers or their newborn children"* but that the *"possible long-term consequences of these minute amounts are uncertain."* However, neither the agency nor others who have studied the problem believe that this possible pesticide contamination outweighs the known advantages of breast-feeding.

Occupational chemicals. A six-week-old Nova Scotia baby who was being breast-fed became jaundiced and developed an enlarged liver. The doctors who treated her traced the illness to a toxic dry-cleaning solvent used in her father's plant. It seems the baby's mother frequently visited her husband at lunchtime, and the chemical—perchloroethylene —accumulated in the woman's body fat. When she began nursing, "perc" was transferred to her milk and passed on to the baby. The chemical has been shown to cause liver cancers in mice, and is now being treated as a carcinogen in American industry. About 500,000 workers are exposed to perc in the dry-cleaning industry alone, and many of them are women.

But perc is only one possible industrial contaminant of breast milk. Hundreds of thousands of women in the work force are exposed through their jobs to chemicals that could contaminate their breast milk. Working women may inhale fumes of heavy metals, such as lead, mercury, or cadmium, or pesticides or plastics chemicals that could get into their milk.

If you work with toxic chemicals now or did in the past, or if you live in an area where the chances of exposure to toxic chemicals are high, the American Academy of Pediatrics advises you to *have your breast milk tested before you start nursing* lest you inadvertently pass on a poison to your baby.

POLLUTION FROM WITHIN

There are other breast-milk contaminants that the nursing mother herself is responsible for. The following are among them.

Smoking. Nicotine and probably other chemicals accumulate in the breast milk of women who smoke cigarettes. Moderate smokers (one-half to one and one-half packs a day) were found by Vanderbilt University researchers to have from 20 to 512 parts of nicotine per billion parts of breast milk. Although no hazard to the infants was uncovered from this amount of nicotine in the milk, infants exposed to nicotine in the womb are born smaller and are more likely to die shortly after birth than the babies of women who do not smoke. In another study at Johns Hopkins University, smoking mothers were more likely to produce inadequate amounts of breast milk than those who didn't smoke. In fact, studies in animals have shown that nicotine can inhibit breast-milk production. The Vanderbilt researchers said that while they would not recommend that smoking mothers refrain from breast feeding, they would *urge all nursing mothers to stop smoking.*

Drugs. Many drugs, both prescription and over-the-counter, taken by a nursing mother can be passed on to her baby through her milk. The infant's immature kidneys and liver may be unable to excrete or detoxify these drugs fast enough, allowing trace amounts in mother's milk to build up to high levels in the baby that can cause a wide range of toxic effects. Some babies may become allergic to the drugs their mothers take while nursing. Among the drugs that can reach potentially harmful levels in the suckling infant are the painkillers aspirin and Darvon; the antibiotics penicillin, ampicillin, chloramphenicol, nalidixic acid (NegGram), sulfonamides, and Flagyl; the psychoactive drugs Valium, lithium, Thorazine, chloral hydrate, methadone, and heroin; radioactive iodine and other thyroid drugs; the anticonvulsant Dilantin; amantadine; anticancer drugs; and ergot derivatives. For many other drugs, current information is not sufficient to say whether they are safe for nursing mothers. *Women who are nursing should not take drugs without first consulting their physicians.* Even something as seemingly innocent as aspirin, taken in sufficient quantities, can lead to dangerous hemorrhage in a new baby.

Alcohol. The concentration of alcohol in a woman's milk is about the same as that in her blood. Now that doctors appreciate the adverse effects of alcohol on the fetal brain, they are increasingly hesitant to give nursing women the go-ahead to drink. While an occasional drink is most likely harmless to the nursing infant, most experts suggest that until more information is known, nursing mothers refrain from regular alcohol consumption or consumption of more than one drink on any given day.

Caffeine. Like alcohol, caffeine reaches the same level in mother's milk as in her blood. A nursing woman who drinks a lot of coffee or other caffeine-containing beverages throughout the day can pass significant amounts of this stimulant to her baby. Since infants cannot break down caffeine, it can accumulate in their blood and they may become "jittery." However, an occasional cup of coffee can be drunk two to three hours before nursing.

Other dietary items. Certain foods a nursing mother eats may adversely affect her baby. Although the notion that women who are breast feeding should not eat chocolate is thought by some to be an old wives' tale, researchers at State University of New York at Buffalo found that a caffeinelike substance in chocolate, theobromine, can reach high concentrations in breast milk and may accumulate in the nursing infant.

Studies by Swedish pediatric researchers suggest that a common cause of colic in breast-fed infants may be allergy to cow's-milk proteins that reach the baby through mother's milk. Of 19 colicky babies, 13 got over their problem when their mothers stopped drinking cow's milk. In 12 the colic returned when the mothers resumed consumption of cow's milk, and disappeared once more when the mothers again stopped drinking milk. Ordinarily, however, breast-fed babies are less likely to become colicky than those who are fed cow's-milk proteins directly in their formulas.

The Nursing Mother

More than 95 percent of women are physically able to breast-feed successfully, and can produce enough milk to feed their babies so long as no one, including the women themselves, throws psychological obstacles in their paths. *Anxiety is the main cause of an inadequate milk supply.* It doesn't matter what size breasts you have—larger breasts merely have more fat, not more of the mammary glands that produce milk. Nor should the shape of your nipples make a difference. If your nipples are flat or inverted (sunken), they can usually be manipulated during pregnancy so that they stick out enough for the baby to grasp by the time it is born. You can also wear a breast shield in your bra between feedings. The Woolwich Breast Shield is available through the La Leche League International, 9616 Minneapolis Avenue, Franklin Park, Illinois 60131; The Nesty Milk Cup can be obtained from Marianne Alstrom, 34 Sunrise Avenue, Mill Valley, California 94941.

Mothers who had Caesarian sections can also nurse, although they may get off to a slower start. So can mothers with diabetes and Rh negative blood. Regardless of the state of your health, it's a good idea to discuss your interest in breast feeding with your doctor during pregnancy. Also, discuss the matter with your husband, since your nursing will affect his life, too.

Even women who have stopped nursing or who took hormone shots to dry up their milk can often re-establish breast feeding weeks or months later. In fact, women who have adopted children have been able to nurse, although the preparation takes months and a lot of determination. The La Leche League can provide information and instruction for adoptive mothers who want to nurse and natural mothers who want to resume nursing.

Although nursing your baby will save you time and money spent on formulas, bottles, and sterilizing, it's not a free lunch. As in pregnancy, mother must fuel her own furnace adequately to meet her baby's needs. Based on present-day prices, the additional food a nursing mother requires costs one-third to one-half the amount she would have to spend on formula.

The kinds of *nutritional requirements for lactation are similar to those of pregnancy, only greater*—well-balanced meals containing plenty of protein and dairy products, extra calories from nutritious foods, and probably a vitamin-mineral supplement. Although the precise requirements vary with the amount of milk a woman produces, on the average a new nursing mother should be eating *about 500 calories a day more* than she did before becoming pregnant (assuming her prepregnancy diet was normal). You'll be amazed at how much food you can eat and still lose your pregnancy fat. If you continue nursing beyond the first six months of your baby's life, you may need even more extra calories—up to 1,200—to keep up with your growing baby's demands for food.

But even if your diet is poorly balanced and calorically inadequate, your body won't shortchange your baby. Nutritious milk will continue to be produced—but at your expense. So to maintain your own good health and strength at this demanding time, it's wise to pay close attention to what you eat. If you find that certain foods seem to upset the baby, avoid them. Excessive sweets or an overabundance of fruit may cause diarrhea in the nursing infant. (But don't mistake the frequent loose bowel movements of the typical breast-fed baby for diarrhea. It's normal for a baby to have a bowel movement during or just after nursing).

In addition to food, the nursing mother must pay careful attention to drink. *Without adequate liquids, your body will quickly become dehydrated and your milk supply will fall off.* A nursing mother should increase her liquid intake to at least *3 quarts of fluids a day,* including one quart of milk (whole or skim). That's a lot of drinking—much more than you're probably used to. You may find that the best approach is to paste up "Drink" notes and keep glasses around the house as a reminder. Or make it a habit to down an 8-ounce drink every hour on the hour all through the day.

Although a woman on a well-balanced diet should have an adequate supply of vitamins, most obstetricians recommend that nursing mothers continue to take the *multivitamin-mineral supplements* they used during pregnancy. A supplement of vitamin B_6 may be essential for mothers who prior to pregnancy were long-term users of the birth-control pill. And mothers who are vegans (strict vegetarians who consume no animal products) must take vitamin B_{12} supplements if they nurse. However, most pediatricians discourage nursing by vegans unless the mothers are willing to include dairy products and eggs in their diets while breast feeding.

When to Supplement the Breast

It takes several days after delivery for your milk to come in. Right after giving birth, the breast produces a watery looking substance called *colostrum,* which is loaded with antibodies that help protect the baby from illness. Colostrum is especially made for the newborn baby. It's low in fat and carbohydrates and easy to digest. It's also a laxative that helps the newborn baby to excrete the meconium (accumulated dark fecal matter) and prepare the digestive tract to receive the milk that gradually replaces colostrum. If your newborn baby is given bottles of milk, suckling on the breast is reduced and the establishment of your full milk supply delayed. However, after several weeks of nursing, it's okay to introduce an occasional bottle in place of the breast, allowing you to be separated from the baby for six to eight hours. You can hand-express your milk during the separation, should your breasts become uncomfortable or start to leak. Some mothers express the milk into a bottle, sterilize and refrigerate it to feed to the baby the next day.

To simplify matters, your "freedom bottle" can be a ready-made commercial formula that comes in sealed jars. When it's time to give it to the baby, the cover is removed and replaced by a nipple. No sterilizing is necessary. You may want to keep some bottles of prepared formula on hand for such occasions. They are also very handy for traveling, when it may be difficult or impossible to nurse.

Formulas

Although they differ from breast milk in some important ways, commercial infant formulas are not bad foods for babies. A mother who is unwilling or unable to nurse, or who must stop nursing before the baby is three or more months old, should not worry that she is somehow endangering her baby. Formulas are not replicas of breast milk, but the processing they go through makes them a vast improvement over what the cow produces to feed her calf.

The *casein* (cow's-milk protein) in formula is partially broken down to reduce its potential for causing allergies. The *amount of protein* in formula is much lower than that in cow's milk and more closely resembles the protein content of breast milk. *Lactose* (milk sugar) is added to formula, bringing it closer to the sugar content of breast milk, to help stimulate the growth of "friendly" bacteria in the infant's gut. And *polyunsaturated fats* are substituted for milk fat to increase the amount of fat the infant is able to digest and absorb.

The *salt content* of cow's milk is reduced in preparing formula, and *vitamins and iron* are added to prevent deficiencies of micronutrients. In fact, when it comes to vitamins and possibly iron, formula may represent an improvement over what nature offers the human infant. For example, formula contains more vitamin K than breast milk, and vitamin K deficiency is more common among breast-fed infants than among those who are bottle-fed. Breast-fed infants sometimes get rickets as a result of vitamin D deficiency, but formula is supplemented with this vitamin, which is so crucial to normal bone growth. As for iron, iron-supplemented formulas contain more, but the iron in breast milk is more easily absorbed. And breast milk has the upper hand when it comes to *zinc*. Although zinc concentrations are similar in formula and breast milk, the zinc from mother is better absorbed by the infant than the zinc in formula. Human milk is also ten to one hundred times richer in *copper* than cow's-milk formulas.

Formulas also contain *food additives*—emulsifiers, thickening agents, acid adjusters, and preservatives. Although none of the chemicals used is known to have adverse effects on health, Dr. Derrick B. Jelliffe and E. F. Patrice Jelliffe of the University of California School of Public Health in Los Angeles point out that the added chemicals "introduce further unknowns, certainly not found in the original product for human infants."

Nonetheless, Dr. Lewis A. Barness, head of pediatrics at the University of South Florida College of Medicine in Tampa, insists that formula can't be bad for babies. He points out that in the two decades during which breast feeding was a rarity in this country and babies were fed cow's-milk formulas, "most artificially fed infants lived and grew, and indeed may have grown bigger and faster than those who were breast-fed." He adds that mothers *"who cannot or will not nurse should not be made to feel guilty. Babies do grow and thrive on formulas, provided proper hygiene is used."*

Like breast milk, modern infant formulas can provide complete nutrition for the first four to six months of your baby's life. But if you're feeding by bottle, remember not to overfeed your baby. Weight Watchers International, an organization that tries to cope with the long-term consequences of overnutrition, cautions:

• Don't insist the baby finish every bottle. Breast-fed infants take varying amounts of milk at different feedings; bottle-fed babies should have the same privilege.

• Don't worry if the baby refuses to eat at the appointed hour or sleeps through most of a feeding. Babies naturally lengthen the time between feedings as they get older, and they should be allowed to learn to eat only when they are hungry.

• Don't shove a bottle in the baby's mouth at every cry. Babies cry for a lot of reasons—soiled diaper, need for suckling or cuddling, gas, thirst—not just for hunger. *Try other pacifiers first, including a bottle of water, before offering food if it's not a regular feeding time.* Most babies are not given enough water, especially in hot weather. They have a lot of surface area compared to their total body size, and they can lose lots of water through evaporation.

One last word of caution about cow's milk: *skim milk or formulas based on skim milk are generally considered inadequate and inadvisable for babies during the first two years of life.* Skim milk provides proportionally too few calories and too much protein, sodium and other minerals to be good for a rapidly growing infant. Skim milk is also lacking essential fatty acids and vitamins C and E, even if it's fortified with vitamins A and D. Although not necessarily a disadvantage, babies fed skim milk gain less weight than those on regular formula, even if the skim-milk diet is supplemented with the missing nutrients and the babies are also given as much solid food as they want. The high concentration of protein in skim milk may also be too much for the infant's kidneys to handle properly. Skim milk is a fine food, but it's best to wait until after your baby's first birthday to introduce it.

Soy-milk formulas are an acceptable alternative to breast milk for babies who are allergic to cow's milk, as well as for the few babies who may also be allergic to breast milk. A number of studies have shown that babies grow just as well on soy-milk formulas as they do on formulas based on cow's milk.

What to Do about Solid Foods

The age at which baby takes the first spoon of cereal or downs a jar of puréed fruit seems to have become a status symbol among American parents, who proudly report the fact as if it were a measure of superior developmental achievement. As a result, solid food is being foisted upon American babies at ever earlier ages. Some babies are getting cereal before they're one month old, and it's commonplace to start feeding cereals and fruits between two and three months.

Yet nearly every expert on infant nutrition says this is too early for the baby's well-being. These *experts recommend starting solids no sooner than four months of age, and preferably not until the baby is six months old.* There are at least two good reasons for this view. First, the young infant's digestive tract is immature. It cannot digest the starches in most baby foods, and it tends to let through relatively large, incompletely digested substances, including proteins, that could then trigger allergic responses. If you wait until the baby is six months old to begin feeding cereal, you will have given the baby's digestive tract a chance to mature and act as a better screen against foreign proteins. Dr. Lloyd J. Filer, Jr., professor of pediatrics at the University of Iowa College of Medicine, points out that solid foods given sooner than six months of age "contribute no special nutrients or energy not already provided by milk or formula, so why risk possible allergic reactions?"

The second reason for delaying solid foods has to do with calories and overnutrition. Cereal and fruit and other solid baby foods contain more calories than the same amount of milk—two to three times more in some cases. To fill baby's stomach, he or she must consume more calories of solids than of milk. The extra calories simply go to fat (which is not the same as growth), and the baby may be started down the road to lifelong overnutrition.

Pediatric researchers from the University of Iowa point out that not until 5 or 6 months of age is an infant "able to indicate desire for food by opening its mouth and leaning forward, and to indicate disinterest or satiety by leaning back and turning away. Until the infant can express these feelings, feeding solid foods will probably represent a type of forced feeding." They note that most infants are fed solid foods far too early as a result of social pressures, aggressive marketing by the infant-food industry, and the belief that solid food helps the infant to sleep through the night. If such food does help the baby sleep, they say, it's because it contains more calories than milk and "is therefore a type of overfeeding not conducive to establishing habits of eating in moderation."

Once your baby is ready for solids, start gradually, offering only one food such as a high-protein, iron-fortified cereal for the first month, and then others, introduced one at a time at weekly intervals. That way you'll be able to tell at once if a new food is causing an allergic reaction and you can readily eliminate it. Although strained fruits are frequently given as one of the first solid foods, most experts recommend concentrating on foods that have fewer of their calories from carbohydrates and more from protein, especially if the infant's only other source of nutrients is breast milk. Avoid those baby foods that have added starch. Since baby foods are now required to have nutritional labeling, it's easy to know what you're buying (see Chapter 27 for further information).

Baby-food manufacturers no longer add salt or sugar (except in puddings and in some strained fruits) to their products, and if you make your own puréed foods for your infant, you'd be wise to do the same. Your baby's taste buds are better off not getting used to the taste of salt and sweet. Baby food is not supposed to appeal to anyone except babies, and they won't know the difference. Similarly, avoid using vegetables and fruits that have been processed and canned for adults, since these have far too much salt and may contain excessive amounts of lead (from the can) that could be harmful to infants.

MAKE YOUR OWN BABY FOOD

Some excellent guidelines for making baby food "from scratch," mostly using fresh or frozen products can be found in *Feed Me, I'm Yours,* a 1974 book by Vicki Lansky, a nutrition-conscious mother from Wayzata, Minnesota, who collaborated in preparing the book with six other mothers, all members of the Childbirth Education Association of Minneapolis/St. Paul. If unavailable through your local bookstore, the spiral-bound book can be obtained from Meadowbrook Press, 18318 Minnetonka Boulevard, Deephaven, Minnesota 55391. It is also published in paperback by Bantam. Two of Mrs. Lansky's recipes follow.

Cottage Cheese Fruit

½ cup fresh, raw, or cooked fruit   4–6 tablespoons orange juice
½ cup cottage cheese

Combine ingredients in blender jar and blend at high speed until smooth. Serve cool.

Vegetable Soup

¼ cup cooked puréed vegetables   1 tablespoon margarine or butter
1 tablespoon whole-wheat or   ¼ cup liquid (water, broth, or
white flour   milk)

Combine ingredients in a sauce pan and warm.

Another good source of baby-food recipes made without added salt, artificial colors or flavors, and minimal sugar is *No-Nonsense Nutrition for Your Baby's First Year,* by Jo-Ann Heslin, Annette B. Natow, and Barbara C. Raven (Boston: CBI, 1978).

A final warning about solid foods. As with bottle feeding, there can be a tendency to push the baby into eating more than he or she wants. The University of Iowa pediatric researchers say that "infants should be permitted to stop eating at the earliest sign of willingness to stop— not to a point of maximum consumption. *No attempt should be made to get the infant to . . . finish the last spoonful in the dish.*"

Dr. Calvin W. Woodruff of the University of Missouri School of Medicine offers this rough guide to the feeding of solid foods, based on the developmental abilities of the average infant and nutritional recommendations derived by the American Academy of Pediatrics:

- Start with semisolid foods (thin baby cereals and other strained foods) at 6 months.
- Move into foods with lumps (including table foods that the baby can easily chew or mash) at around 9 months.
- By the end of the first year, the baby should be ready for most foods from the family table.

Vitamin Supplements

Most young infants are given vitamin supplements as routine nutritional "insurance." According to Dr. Woodruff and others, this is unnecessary and potentially dangerous except in a few rare instances, such as babies who cannot absorb fats or who must be on restricted diets because of allergies or metabolic disorders.

Babies are born with enough *iron* stored in their liver to last for three months. Although it was once thought that breast milk, like cow's milk, contained insufficient iron for an infant beyond three months of age, it's now known that the iron in breast milk is better absorbed, so nursing babies need less. However, if a baby is fed formula, one that is fortified with iron should be used. According to the National Academy of Sciences, mother's milk also supplies enough *vitamin C* for infants, so neither supplementation with vitamin C nor with fruit juices is necessary.

Some experts, including the National Academy of Sciences, recommend supplements of *vitamin D* for breast-fed infants (formulas are already supplemented with this vitamin as well as with vitamin A). If your baby is light-skinned and gets out into the daylight on a fairly regular basis, this should be unnecessary. Inadequate vitamin D could be a problem, however, for breast-fed "winter" babies or for dark-skinned infants living in relatively cold climates.

The need of infants for *fluoride* supplements is a matter of debate. Little fluoride gets into mother's milk, and cow's-milk formulas are also low in this mineral, which helps to prevent dental decay. If the baby drinks fluoridated water, a supplement is unnecessary, but if your water is not fluoridated, a supplement may be prescribed.

Feeding Your One Year Old

The young mother was perplexed. Seemingly overnight her one-year-old son, who until now had gobbled down every meal, reaching eagerly for her hand when she didn't shovel the food in fast enough, was refusing some foods and even refusing to eat more than a few bites of some meals. Was he sick? Was she doing something wrong? How could he survive, let alone grow, on the tiny amount he ate some days?

The mother needn't have worried. Her son was perfectly healthy and normal—in fact, typical of children his age. During a baby's first year of life, birth weight triples. Infants seem perpetually hungry, downing each meal as if it were their last. Then, at around the first birthday, feeding habits begin to change. Growth rate slows, a baby develops more of a mind of his or her own, and other activities—like walking, squishing the cereal between fingers, throwing the peas one by one to the floor, or pouring the milk into the spaghetti—seem infinitely more interesting than eating. This is commonly the time when eating problems begin. Mother, anxious to get balanced meals and enough food to support normal growth and activity into her child, tries with every means at her disposal—including an endless variety of games and tricks—to get her baby to eat more and to sneak in at least a few spoons of those green peas he or she now seems to hate. And, as Dr. Benjamin Spock points out in *Baby and Child Care* (New York: Pocket Books, 1968): "the more mother frets and urges, the less the child eats. And the less he takes, the more anxious the mother is. Meals become agonizing. The problem may last for years." On the other hand, the famous pediatrician adds, if you don't make a battle of it, your child will probably "eat a reasonably balanced diet from week to week, though it may be somewhat lopsided from meal to meal or day to day." Here are some tips to help you over the hurdles when your baby's appetite and tastes suddenly change:

Your baby won't starve. It's normal for a baby's appetite to fall off dramatically somewhere between 10 months and 3 years of age. If it didn't, you'd have a 200-pound monster by the age of 10. Let your toddler's appetite determine how much he or she eats, not some game like "Open Sesame." Since you really can't force-feed a baby or toddler who's determined not to eat, there's no point in trying. No child, given a reasonable selection of healthful foods, will deliberately go hungry and deprive his or her growing body of the foods it needs.

Tomfoolery at the table is out. A child who insists on playing at the table instead of eating, or who repeatedly tries to climb out of the chair, is probably not hungry. Casually take the food away. Dr. Spock says that if the child immediately whimpers for food, give one more chance—but only one more. Otherwise, take the food away, take the child away from the table, and end the meal.

But don't mistake natural curiosity for no interest in eating. Around the age of one, children like to experiment with their food as well as with everything else. They learn by touching and feeling, by squeezing the applesauce through their fingers, or mashing the peas, or finger painting with the cereal. Draw the line, however, at throwing food on the floor, turning over the bowl, or dumping the drink.

Cut out snacks if the child won't eat meals. A toddler who refuses lunch but knows that a hungry whimper an hour later will bring something yummy is likely to go on refusing lunch. If your child refuses to eat at mealtime, but gets hungry between meals, you have several choices: change the time of meals, making them further apart; offer water or juice to drink between meals, or serve the next meal earlier. As the toddler gets older, this last option becomes less attractive because it can disrupt the family meal. Better to say "I'm sorry, but I have nothing more to give you until supper" or "I can give you your supper salad (or appetizer) a little early, but that's all" and offer carrot and celery sticks or fruit or something similar that's not too filling to tide the child over.

Green vegetables are not essential to life. Most toddlers take a dislike to several or all the vegetables—especially the green ones— that they consumed with seeming relish as infants. Don't panic. If you play your cards right, the dislike will be temporary and your child won't become malnourished in the meantime. Give only the vegetables the child will eat, occasionally offering ones that had been refused earlier. Substitute fruits (unsweetened) since they contain most of the same vitamins and minerals found in vegetables. Sneak extra chopped or puréed vegetables into foods you know will be eaten, such as soups or spaghetti sauce (children will neither taste nor recognize grated zucchini in the sauce). While most parents want their children to eat everything and be adventurous about trying new foods, most children shudder at strangeness and want only the foods they know they like. Fear not. Few of us stay that way forever, refusing to eat mushrooms, onions, green peas, spinach, celery, squash, lettuce, broccoli, beans, and all the other favorite childhood "hates."

A balanced diet is not an everyday affair. Babies may want to live on practically nothing but mashed potatoes at one meal, beets the next, and applesauce the third. The following day, they may refuse all fruits and vegetables and instead go on a meat binge. Or they may refuse all solids and drink only their milk. But experiments with very young children have shown that when the child has access to a reasonable selection of good foods, over the course of a week the nutrients consumed tend to balance out. Don't worry unless the fixation on a very limited number of foods goes on for weeks. Assuming the child is otherwise healthy and normal, at that point your physician may recommend a vitamin supplement to fill in the temporary nutritional gaps.

Fat Babies Are Out of Fashion

In some families, the opposite kind of feeding problem prevails: the baby eats too well. Dr. Filer advises against putting overweight infants on a "diet" because this might deprive them of nutrients needed for real growth. But you can safely slow weight gain just enough so that as the baby gets taller, he or she will "grow into" a normal weight. Here's what you can do without compromising your baby's well-being:

• Don't start solid foods before your baby is four months old, and preferably not until six months of age.

• Avoid baby foods like puddings, meat soups, and creamed vegetables that are loaded with calories from starches and sugars.

• Don't give your baby cookies, candy, or ice cream. For teething babies with itchy gums, try a rubber teething ring. For desserts and toddler snacks, stick to unsweetened fruit or low-fat yogurt perhaps "sweetened" with a mashed banana.

• Between feedings, satisfy the baby's thirst and urge to suck with water, not milk or fruit juice. After the first year, you can gradually wean the baby to low-fat or skim milk.

• Serve the toddler what you consider a reasonable amount of food and, if more is requested, say that there is none or that you're saving it for another meal.

• Give your baby and toddler ample opportunity for exercise. Babies who spend the day in a crib, infant seat, or playpen don't expend enough energy to learn proper appetite control or to burn up the calories their stomachs demand.

If you're going to err on the matter of your baby's weight, it may be better to favor the lean and hungry look. Several studies in laboratory animals have shown that animals that are undernourished early in life live longer than those that receive what is considered a "normal" diet. In studies by Dr. Morris H. Ross at the Fox Chase Cancer Center in Philadelphia, the life expectancy of male rats was nearly doubled by underfeeding them after they were weaned from their mother's milk. He concluded that "dietary practices that promote rapidity of growth and early maturation are not conducive to long life."

FOR FURTHER READING

Vicki Lansky, *Feed Me, I'm Yours* (Deephaven, Minn.: Meadowbrook Press, 1974).

Margaret Elizabeth Kenda and Phyllis S. Williams, *The Natural Baby Food Cookbook* (New York: Avon, 1982).

Ellyn Satter, R.D., *Child of Mine: Feeding with Love and Good Sense* (Palo Alto, Ca.: Bull, 1983).

Sue Castle, *The Complete New Guide to Preparing Baby Foods* (New York: Doubleday, 1981).

Alice White, *The Total Nutrition Guide for Mother and Baby: From Pregnancy through the First Three Years* (New York: Ballantine, 1983).

Susan Tate Firkaly, *Into the Mouths of Babes: A Natural Foods Cookbook for Infants and Toddlers* (White Hall, Va.: Betterway, 1984).

20 ❧ CHILD FEEDING
IN THE JUNK-FOOD
GENERATION

M ARK, age 2½, won't let anything green pass his lips unless it's mint-flavored ice cream.

Joyce, who is 4, refuses to eat the carrots on her dinner plate because "some sauce got on them." Robert refuses to eat anything because the meat is "touching" the noodles and there are mushrooms in the gravy.

Jason, age 5, won't eat Chinese food because "everything's mixed together." Erik, of the same vintage, is willing to dine Oriental-style but only after he's carefully separated all the ingredients into individual piles that "don't touch."

Becky, a first grader, seems to live on thin air: a bowl of cereal and a glass of juice for breakfast, half a sandwich and milk for lunch, cookies and milk after school, and three bites of dinner. Yet she's not sickly and is growing normally.

Johanna cleans her plate all right, just as her parents insist. But she's still thin as a rail. The mystery is solved when Johanna's mother finds the remnants of countless suppers at the bottom of the sweater drawer. The clue to a similar puzzle at Jennifer's house comes when the vet remarks that the family dog is getting too fat.

Michael, age 8, eats his favorite foods first, one at a time—noodles, meat, and bread, in that order—then announces that he's "too full" to eat the broccoli and salad. Gary does him one better. He starts with his milk, moves on to the potatoes, then with a pained expression on his face and hands on his stomach, he asks to be excused because he's "got a stomach ache." Then he's fine again ten minutes later, when it's time for dessert.

Peggy grimaces as her mother sets her dinner down. "I hate that, you know I hate that, and I'm not eating it," she whines.

Matthew's parents can't understand why an active, growing child is not hungry for dinner night after night, until they discover that his weekly allowance is being spent after school at the candy store around the corner.

John's mother has to find a new hiding place for the cookies every few days. John, who always finishes his meals and usually asks for seconds, forages for sweets after school and in the evening. He has always been a chunky kid, but now at 12 he is getting fat.

If you don't recognize your child somewhere among these, then you probably don't have one! Or, by some miracle, you've managed to raise a nutritional saint. Actually, nutritional "freak" is a more apt description than "saint."

For it is truly the rare child who manages to go from toddlerhood through teens without some dietary quirks. In the "old days," I'm told, children sat respectfully at the table and ate whatever they were given —even if they had to choke it down. But I have a feeling that those times of idyllic dining with children are more myth than fact.

Whether they existed or not, there is no going back. We live in a world where children are encouraged to express themselves; where the best nutritional guidance at home is constantly undermined by television advertising, peer pressure, vending machines, and fast-food outlets; where so many interesting things (interesting to a child, anyway) compete for the child's attention that eating meals may be no more attractive than taking a bath. Still, it's the parents' responsibility to see that their children are well nourished.

Meeting Basic Needs

Children are always growing, from birth until the end of adolescence. Therefore, in addition to the nutrients needed to maintain their present selves, they need nutrients to form new tissue. In relation to body weight, a child's requirements for basic nutrients are greater than an adult's. A child of 5 weighing 44 pounds, for example, needs as much iron and calcium and even more vitamin D than a man of 25 who weighs 154. Although total quantities are smaller, pound for pound, 5 year olds need twice as much protein, thiamin, riboflavin, niacin, and vitamins A and C and three times as much B_6 and B_{12} as 25-year-old men. This means that the calories a child consumes need to be more densely packed with nutrients. There's less room for "empty calories" in a child's diet because more of what is consumed has to count toward meeting daily requirements (more later about how to achieve this).

But it doesn't mean a young child should be eating as much food as an adult. Parents commonly overestimate the total food needs of a preadolescent child. A child who eats with her family is usually served on a full-size plate with portions nearly as big as the portions her parents get. She may finish her favorite food, eat a few bites of the others, and be full. Parents become anxious about the fact that "she eats like a bird," not realizing that birds eat a lot for creatures their size and their daughter probably does, too.

A 1 year old consumes about 1,000 calories a day. The average 3 year old needs about 300 more calories than the 1 year old, and the 6 year old needs about 400 more calories than the 3 year old. That comes to 1,700 calories for a child of 6, 1,000 less than a 154-pound man and 400 less than a 120-pound woman.

Of course, children of all ages need the same kinds of nutrients as adults, and these nutrients generally come from the same food groups. For a preadolescent child, the recommended daily food plan is as follows (see Table 1.2, page 18, for details):

- Three servings of milk or milk products.
- Two servings of meat or meat substitutes.
- Four or more servings of fruits and vegetables.
- Four or more servings of breads and cereals.

The hitch lies in defining a serving. Family restaurants that provide a children's menu know, and so should you, that a child's serving is considerably smaller than an adult's serving. As nutritionists Eva May Hamilton and Eleanor N. Whitney of Florida State University suggest in their book *Nutrition: Concepts and Controversies* (St. Paul: West, 1979), a good rule of thumb for determining a child's-size serving of meats, fruits, and vegetables is to allow 1 tablespoon for each year of the child's life. Thus, a 2 year old would get 2 tablespoons of mashed potatoes and a 4 year old would get twice that amount. Remember, 4 tablespoons is not very much—only a quarter of a cup. That may not seem like enough to fill a cavity in your tooth, but it's enough for the average 4 year old.

Also remember that a rule of thumb is just a guide; it's not rigid. On some days your 4 year old may devour twice as much food as on others. While children are continually growing, they are not continually growing at the same rate. And their appetites will wax and wane with their rate of growth. I always know ahead of time when I'm going to have to let the cuffs down on my boys' trousers. Suddenly they're cleaning their plates, asking for seconds, and eating huge bedtime snacks—my clue that a growth spurt is in the offing.

Activity also has a lot to do with a child's appetite and nutritional status. Active children need more calories than inactive ones, and that means that active children have a better chance of getting in the required nutrients. They also have more room in their diet for "treats" that may be relatively deficient in essential nutrients. A child who spends six hours a day in school, comes home, has a snack, and then devotes the rest of the afternoon to trading baseball cards and doing homework is not likely to be "starved" at 6:00 P.M. The youngster who plays after school, whether he or she skates, sleds, swims, or plays touch football, is far more likely to work up a hearty appetite for dinner. Many parents have noticed that their children have a bigger appetite during the warm months when they play outside for hours every day than in the winter when they become after-school shut-ins.

Adequate physical exercise year round, preferably on a daily basis, is important to a child's development for many reasons other than as an appetite stimulant. As you will see, exercise also helps the overweight child to control his or her rate of gain. In fact, it is lack of exercise, not overeating, that is primarily responsible for obesity in youngsters.

Breakfast Is the Most Important Meal

No doubt you've heard this spiel so often that the next person who says it will get the eggs your child won't eat cracked over his or her head. But, like it or not, it's the truth. You can't expect a child to get through the morning, pay attention in class, and concentrate on his or her work on no fuel any more than you would expect to drive from New York to Washington on a gas tank reading "empty." A ten-year study by the University of Iowa Medical College showed that schoolboys became careless and inattentive in the late morning if they had skipped breakfast, but their schoolwork improved noticeably if breakfast was eaten. In addition, a child who skips breakfast is likely to be more susceptible to infection and fatigue than one who eats a morning meal.

Yet children omit breakfast more than any other meal of the day. And probably many more children would skip it if not for the prepared-breakfast-cereal industry. That industry is often—and justly—accused of subverting the dietary goals parents set for their children by creating a desire for overly sweetened "junk" cereals. But cereal manufacturers at least deserve credit for promoting a breakfast of fruit juice, toast, milk, and cereal and for providing an "instant" breakfast food that youngsters can serve to themselves or parents can dish up with only one eye open.

If you are convinced that a good breakfast is all-important, you can raise your children to think the same. All you have to do is make eating breakfast—a *real* breakfast, not overly sweetened instant junk food—an inviolable rule from the preschool years onward. Prepare a decent breakfast for your youngsters every day, and make sure they have enough unrushed time in which to eat it. *If you eat a decent breakfast yourself, your children will learn from the example you set.*

Many breakfasts can be made the night before with only a few minutes of cooking or heating up required the next morning. Here are some suggestions to make breakfast a relatively painless, but still nourishing, affair that's likely to be eaten with pleasure.

Broaden your repertoire. Whoever said breakfast has to be cereal or pancakes or bacon and eggs? If you don't feed your children that propaganda and instead give them leftover spaghetti, a hearty soup, rice pudding, a blender shake, homemake pizza on a muffin, a hamburger, a grilled-cheese sandwich, or peanut butter and jelly on whole wheat for breakfast, it may never occur to them that the rest of the world doesn't also eat that way. A breakfast of leftovers or a sandwich can be both nourishing and fast. You can even make the sandwich the night before, set it on a plate in the refrigerator, and have the child serve himself or herself while you're out jogging!

Your children can be the only ones on the block privileged to start the day with one of the following:

Rice Pudding Cereal

3 cups cooked rice (see note)
2 cups skim milk
1 whole egg plus 1 egg white, beaten

1–2 tablespoons sugar
¼ cup raisins
Cinnamon to taste

Combine all ingredients in a saucepan and mix well. Cook over medium heat, stirring often, until cereal thickens (about 5 minutes after the milk comes to a boil). Yield: 3 to 4 servings.

Note: Prepare the rice the night before to save morning time, or make extra for supper and use the leftovers.

Spaghetti Pancakes

1 whole egg plus 1 egg white, beaten
¼–⅓ cup grated Parmesan cheese
Pepper to taste

3–4 cups cooked spaghetti (see note)
Margarine for frying

Combine the egg, cheese, and pepper, and add to the spaghetti, mixing well. Melt the margarine in a heated 10-inch skillet, and add the spaghetti mixture. Pat down flat to make a pancake. Cook over medium heat until the bottom browns, about 10 minutes. Dot with more margarine, cut the pancake in half down the middle, and flip over with a spatula one-half at a time. Brown the pancake on the other side. Yield: 3 to 4 servings.

Note: Spaghetti can be prepared the night before; we make extra at supper and use the leftovers the next morning.

Pizza Patty

4 English muffins, sliced in half
¼ cup tomato sauce (see note)
8 slices tomato

8 slices muenster or other cheese
Grated Parmesan for sprinkling (optional)

Smear muffin halves with tomato sauce. Top each half with a slice of tomato and a slice of cheese and sprinkle with Parmesan. Toast under the broiler or in toaster oven until the cheese melts and starts to brown (about 3 to 5 minutes). Yield: 4 hearty servings.

Note: Leftover sauce comes in handy. Or skip the sauce and sprinkle the muffin with your favorite pizza spices (e.g., orégano, garlic, pepper).

Other delicious and nutritious breakfast recipes can be found on pages 92–93 in Chapter 4. Or try peanut butter and sliced banana on cranberry-nut bread (page 136) or oatmeal-raisin muffins (page 385) with a glass of milk.

If your children are old enough to prepare their own breakfast, they might consult one of the many cookbooks for children for easy-to-manage suggestions, such as the following one from *Love at First Bite*, by Jane Cooper (New York: Knopf, 1977):

Ape Shake

1 cup milk
½ cup plain yogurt

1 tablespoon honey or molasses
1 banana, broken into small chunks

Put all the ingredients into a blender jar and blend at high speed for about 10 seconds or until well mixed.

Don't buy sugared cereals. If they're not in the house, your children can't eat them. If your children refuse to eat any other kind of cereal, forget cereal altogether. After a while, though, they'll probably give in and try the ones you do buy. Many of the sugar-coated cereals contain a tablespoon or more of added sugar in a 1-ounce serving. And in breaking away from sugared cereals, don't add sugar to unsweetened cereals. Sprinkling sugar on cereal is a habit you can get out of just as you got into it. I, for one, never knew people did that until I was an adult because no one in my family put sugar on cereal. Instead, the bowl was garnished with raisins, sliced bananas or peaches, even strawberries or blueberries in season. If you want to compromise and can keep your children from dipping into the box when you're not looking, you can sprinkle a small amount of a sugary cereal on top of one that offers a better balance of nutrients. I sometimes use granola, which is too high in sugar and fat to be eaten alone, for a garnish on an unsweetened whole-wheat, oat, or bran cereal.

Rediscover hot cereal. There's nothing more warming and satisfying on a cold winter morning than a piping hot bowl of cooked cereal. In addition to the traditional fare of oatmeal, rice, and wheat cereals (farina or whole wheat), you might try some of the more exotic grains like bulgur or kasha (buckwheat groats). By cooking hot cereals with milk, you significantly increase their nutritional value and add to their ability to stick to the ribs. A little wheat germ will improve their protein and vitamin content as well.

One of our family favorites is a concoction I call hearty oatmeal (see the recipe on page 92). It can be completely set up in a saucepan the night before and held in the refrigerator until morning. It cooks in five to ten minutes, depending on the kind of oatmeal you start with.

Plan ahead. If you're nearly nonfunctional first thing in the morning or if you're short of time, you can do most of the preparation for breakfast the night before and make the last-minute part almost as simple as saying Apple Jacks.

For example, you can prepare separately the liquid and dry ingredients for nutritious pancakes (see the recipe on page 92) and refrigerate the liquid, to be combined with the dry ingredients in the morning. Or you can mix the egg batter for French toast, soak the bread in it, and keep it overnight in the refrigerator covered with plastic wrap. Better still, make extra French toast or waffles on a nonrushed morning and store it in the freezer, to be heated in the toaster on less leisurely days. See the recipes on pages 92–93 for nutritious, nonsyrupy serving suggestions.

Before going to bed, you can set the table or at least fill a tray with the requisite number of juice glasses, pieces of silverware, napkins, and cups. Make frozen juice the night before. You can even set up the coffee pot to be plugged in or turned on in the morning.

If your job or other circumstances—or your children's plain refusal to eat anything first thing in the morning—make it impossible to get a decent breakfast into them before school, many schools in every state offer a school breakfast program, with the federal government paying all or part for needy families. Similar breakfast programs are available at some day-care centers as well. For information on how to organize a school breakfast program, contact the regional office of the U.S. Department of Agriculture, Food and Nutrition Service, or write to: Margaret Lorber, The Children's Foundation, 1420 New York Avenue, NW, Suite 800, Washington, D.C. 20005.

Tips for Balancing Your Child's Diet

During the preadolescent years—and sometimes the adolescent years as well—many children are willing to eat only a limited selection of food. Sometimes whole food groups—for example, all vegetables or all meats—are refused. The more limited a child's selection, the greater the risk that he or she will be short on certain essential vitamins and minerals. But in nearly all cases, there's a nutritionally sound way around this problem without resorting to pills and tonics. Many of the following suggestions are derived from *Eating Your Way through Life* (New York: Raven Press, 1979), by Judith J. Wurtman, Ph.D., a mother and a biologist at the Massachusetts Institute of Technology. Dr. Wurtman's chapter on feeding children is especially perceptive and helpful.

KEEP A RECORD OF WHAT YOUR CHILD EATS

Many parents who worry about whether their children are eating enough, or enough of the right things, are astonished to discover just how much the children consume when a careful record is kept for several days or for a week. And for the child who truly is malnourished —either in total number of calories consumed (too much or too little) or absence of certain nutrients—such a record can show where improvement is most needed.

Dr. Wurtman suggests that you make a list of the different items your child is likely to eat, divide the day up into the various times during which food or drink is likely to be consumed, and then, whenever your child eats or drinks something, record the amount under the proper column (see Table 20.1 on page 377 for guidance on setting up an eating diary).

In just two days, you may have all the clues you need to tell why your child eats no supper (maybe he eats everything in sight between 3:00 and 5:00 P.M. when he's truly hungry), or why she's so chubby (maybe her between-meal hunger is often satisfied with cookies or her thirst quenched with sweetened fruit drinks, pop, or whole milk, or she's served portions twice too big for someone her age and height). If you discover a time of day when your child seems hungriest, perhaps you can feed him his main meal then and give him a nutritious snack in place of supper. At the least, make sure that what's consumed at hungry time is nourishing as well as filling (see the section on snacks in this chapter, pages 383–385). Or, you may find that your thin-as-a-rail child who gets full after a few bites may need to eat six small meals a day instead of three big ones, or that she really eats quite adequately and there's no reason for concern.

IF YOUR CHILD WON'T DRINK MILK

For a growing child, milk is an important source of crucial nutrients, especially calcium, vitamin D, and riboflavin. Yet many children give up drinking milk the moment they're weaned from bottle or breast. Often even adding chocolate or other flavors to the milk is inadequate enticement. Don't panic. First, a number of milk products can supply adequate amounts of the needed nutrients, including yogurt (with or without fruit or flavoring) and cheese (natural is better than processed as a source of bone-building minerals). Cottage cheese and ice cream are about half as good as milk, but much better than nothing.

A second approach is to sneak milk—in liquid or powdered form —into many of the foods your child does eat. Bread, soups, puddings, cakes, cookies, pancakes, casseroles, and hot cereal are just some of the possibilities.

IF YOUR CHILD <u>CAN'T</u> DRINK MILK

Some children develop a milk allergy soon after birth. Others gradually lose their ability to digest milk as they get older. This is a common condition, called lactose intolerance, that is especially prevalent among blacks and Orientals. It may start as early as age two, causing cramps and diarrhea when significant quantities of milk are consumed. Such children may be given fortified soy milk to replace the nutrients ordinarily supplied by milk. Other possibilities include the use of acidophilus milk (pretreated with bacteria that digest the lactose) or addition of the enzyme lactase to regular milk. See Chapter 13 for details and shopping hints.

Lactose intolerance is rarely an all-or-nothing phenomenon. Many children are able to handle small quantities of milk used in recipes or consumed at the end of a meal. But if your child cannot handle any amount of milk, you're going to have to start reading labels carefully to find products in which no milk or milk solids (nonfat or whole) have been used. You may also want to make some milk-free foods at home, especially things like cake and bread. In *The Taming of the C.A.N.D.Y. Monster,* Vicki Lansky, a writer and practical-minded mother of two, offers a number of nutritious recipes without milk.

Milk-Free Banana Bread

¾ cup vegetable shortening
½ cup brown sugar (see note)
½ cup white sugar (see note)
2 eggs
½ teaspoon vanilla or orange extract

1 cup very ripe bananas, mashed
1 cup whole-wheat flour
¾ cup white flour
4 teaspoons baking powder
Dash of salt

Cream the shortening and the sugars together. Beat in the eggs and extract. Add the mashed bananas. Sift in flours, baking powder, and salt. Mix thoroughly. Bake in a greased loaf pan at 350 degrees for 55 minutes. Yield: 1 loaf.

[*Note:* Use less if less sweetening is desired.]

Milk-Free French Toast

1 egg
½ teaspoon water or orange juice
Dash of cinnamon

Drop of vanilla
1 slice milk-free bread
1 tablespoon milk-free margarine

Beat the egg in a shallow bowl with water or juice, cinnamon, and vanilla. Soak the bread in the liquid until the liquid is absorbed. Melt the margarine in a pan. Brown the soaked toast on one side, flip, and brown on the other. Serve with syrup (no butter) or jam, or make a sandwich by using a slice of ham or bacon between two slices of French toast. (My own choice is sliced banana and a sprinkle of cinnamon-sugar on top of the toast.)

For further tips on milk-free cooking, Ross Laboratories (625 Cleveland Avenue, Columbus, Ohio 43216) offers a booklet, "Good Eating for the Milk-Sensitive Person," with recipes that use their soy-based infant formula.

WHEN VEGETABLES ARE REFUSED

It is normal for small children to refuse to eat all but a few vegetables. Carrots, potatoes, corn, and peas are the usual favorites, but I have heard of children who will eat nothing but avocados and sweet red peppers. The more limited a child's selection of vegetables, the harder it may be to get in the needed amounts of vitamins, especially if the child refuses all things green or all things yellow or orange or won't touch salad. Fear not, all is not lost. Here are some suggestions.

• Sneak the nutrient-laden vegetables into foods your child loves and in which they won't be recognized. My boys, who won't touch squash (winter or summer) in any recognizable form, adore zucchini and pumpkin breads, zucchini frittata (grated zucchini omelet), zucchini pancakes, and tomato sauce prepared with chopped or grated zucchini. Carrots are easily concealed in stews, puréed soups, meatloaf, breads, and cakes. You may think this is a terrible way to teach a child to eat vegetables. But remember, it's only temporary. Periodically, you can try reintroducing a despised vegetable in its more natural form. Chances are your child will eventually come to like it.

• Have your youngster help prepare the vegetables or dinner salad. Participation encourages consumption. A 3 year old can learn to snap beans or shell peas. By 5, he or she may be able to peel carrots and potatoes. A child of almost any age can tear lettuce or add cherry tomatoes, olives, or artichoke hearts to a salad.

• Learn some different ways of preparing and serving vegetables to enhance their taste and eye appeal. Too many of us grew up either

Table 20.1 • WHAT DOES YOUR CHILD EAT? HOW TO KEEP
A DAILY RECORD

	Morning	Midday	Afternoon	Evening
PROTEIN FOODS				
Chicken or turkey				
Beef				
Pork				
Lamb				
Tuna or salmon				
Fish				
Peanut butter				
Dried beans or peas				
Eggs				
Bean curd				
Yogurt				
Cheese				
Cottage cheese				
GRAIN PRODUCTS				
Bread				
Roll				
Muffin				
Cereal				
Pancakes or waffles				
Spaghetti or macaroni				
Rice				
Bulgur or kasha				
Hominy				
VEGETABLES				
Carrots				
Beans				
Peas				
Potatoes				
Broccoli				
Beets				
Salad				
Other				
FRUITS				
Orange or grapefruit				
Apple				
Banana				
Pear				
Other				
DRINKS				
Milk				
Water				
Juice				
Fruit drink				
Soda pop				
Shake or malted				

Table continues on next page

Table 20.1 continued

	Morning	Midday	Afternoon	Evening
SNACKS AND FATS				
Jam or jelly				
Margarine or butter				
Cream cheese				
Cookies or cake				
Ice cream or ice milk				
Frozen yogurt				
Ice pop				
Candy				
Crackers				
Dried fruits (raisins, etc.)				
Nuts or seeds				
Pudding (milk or gelatin)				

Source: Adapted from Judith J. Wurtman, Ph.D., *Eating Your Way through Life* (New York: Raven Press, 1979).

on mushy vegetables that were overcooked or that came out of a can. Children prefer vegetables that are brightly colored and on the crunchy side. Today, fresh and frozen vegetables (including a wide range of tasty combinations, with or without special sauces) are readily available. Try steaming or stir-frying fresh green beans, carrots, or broccoli instead of boiling them. Color, taste, texture, and vitamin content are greatly enhanced if you keep vegetables out of water. One of our boys' favorites is the following:

Stir-fried Green Beans

1 pound fresh green beans	1 large clove garlic, minced
1 tablespoon vegetable oil	⅓ cup broth (bouillon) or water
2 scallions, chopped	1 tablespoon imported soy sauce

Trim the ends of the beans and cut the beans in half or leave whole. Heat a wok or skillet, add the oil, and heat 30 seconds. Add the scallions and garlic, stirring for about 30 seconds. Then add the beans and stir to coat them with oil. Add the broth and soy sauce and stir-fry until the beans are tender-crisp.

• Broccoli cooked this way is also appealing. (When our boys were toddlers, we called broccoli "baby tree" and, although it was green, they loved it from the start!) Cut the tough stems crosswise into thin slices and add these to the oil first. Carrots can either be parboiled for three minutes before frying or fried raw using some additional sauce.

I recently tried stir-fried grated pumpkin which one of the boys loved and the other hated. (A batting average of .500 isn't bad.)

• Many children who won't eat cooked vegetables enjoy them raw. Try carrot and celery sticks, tomatoes, slices of green or red sweet peppers, even turnips, cauliflower, green beans, and peas. Serve them as snacks, appetizers, or in lieu of salad. Many children love dips with raw vegetables; the act of dipping makes eating vegetables more fun. Nutritious dips can be made from yogurt, low-fat cottage or ricotta cheese, buttermilk, or mayonnaise with herbs and spices. You might also try powdered dip mixes or dried soups (though these are very high in salt) mixed with yogurt or mayonnaise. Better yet, experiment and create a delicious dip on your own.

When time is short, we mix this one for the boys.

"Instant" Vegetable Dip

2 tablespoons mayonnaise   1–2 teaspoons ketchup
2 tablespoons low-fat yogurt

Mix all the ingredients together and serve with cut-up raw vegetables (for example, carrot and celery sticks, sliced red sweet pepper, sliced cucumbers).

Another favorite is made with

---

1 tablespoon crumbled blue   1 tablespoon mayonnaise
  cheese   2 tablespoons low-fat yogurt

Combine all the ingredients and serve with cut-up raw vegetables.

GETTING IN OTHER SOURCES OF ESSENTIAL NUTRIENTS

Fruits, many of which are liked by most children, can be good sources of the vitamins and minerals missed by children who won't eat vegetables. Peaches, cantaloupe, apricots, nectarines, watermelon, and prunes are good sources of vitamin A. Citrus fruits (oranges and grapefruits) and fruit juices, strawberries, watermelon, and tomatoes are excellent sources of vitamin C. Bananas provide ample amounts of potassium, important to proper muscle function. And dried fruits—

raisins, dates, prunes, and dried apricots—are good sources of iron.

Whole grains, in breads and cereals, supply large amounts of B vitamins. Your child may refuse "brown" bread, but you can make pancakes and muffins using part or all whole-wheat flour. Or you can make your own light-colored bread using part whole-grain flour and part enriched white flour. My husband is the family breadmaker. See page 109 for a recipe of his our children loved even when they refused commercial whole-grain breads.

Wheat germ, rich in B vitamins and vitamin E, can be added unbeknownst to children to a variety of foods, including meat loaf, pancakes, hot cereal, and baked goods. Or it can be mixed in with peanut butter or tuna salad. Try *oatmeal* in place of bread crumbs in meat loaf or use crumbs from whole-grain bread.

As for protein, you're not limited to meat, poultry, and fish. A *peanut butter* sandwich, that perennial childhood favorite, is an excellent protein source. So is grilled *cheese.* Many *high-protein pastas* are now available; served with grated cheese or meat sauce (a few children actually go wild for clam sauce), they provide adequate protein for children and parents alike. And some children who wouldn't otherwise touch tuna fish will eat it minced in a casserole with noodles and cheese.

We've never had any luck with *dried beans and peas,* both fine sources of protein, but many children who spurn them under ordinary circumstances will eat chili, baked beans, or puréed bean or pea soup. For youngsters who "hate" *nuts,* you can sneak an additional protein boost into breads and muffins by grinding nuts to a meal and mixing this with the dry ingredients.

DRINKS CAN BE A NUTRITIONAL DISASTER

Probably the most insidious undermining of good nutrition in the early years comes from the soft-drink industry. Catering to children's innate preference for a sweet taste, the industry has succeeded in drawing millions of youngsters away from milk and natural fruit juices and hooking them on pop and other artificially flavored drinks that offer nothing of nutritional significance besides calories. What's more, many soft drinks contain large amounts of phosphorus (as additives) that impair the body's ability to use calcium (already in short supply if the child isn't drinking much milk).

The best way to counter the soft-drink hard sell is not to bring these products into the house. If your refrigerator is stocked with fruit juice, milk, or water, a thirsty child will reach for these instead of Coke or Kool-Aid. Although some soft drinks are laced with vitamin C (artificially added), they are not a substitute for natural fruit juices, which, in addition to vitamin C, contain vitamin A, several B vitamins, magnesium, and potassium.

PILLS AND POTIONS: DON'T TAKE THE EASY WAY OUT

Many parents, concerned about their children's intake of vitamins and minerals, stuff their children with pills, fortified snacks, and meal substitutes like granola breakfast bars and chocolate (candy) food sticks. If you think these compensate for serious nutritional deficiencies in your child's diet, you're kidding yourself. Multivitamin-mineral tablets rarely contain adequate supplies of several important nutrients, especially iron and calcium. And fortified snacks provide a few, but by no means all, of the needed micronutrients. Neither is a substitute for real food, yet they create a false sense of security about the nutritional adequacy of a child's diet.

TEACH YOUR CHILD TO COOK

Start as early as you dare—age 3 is not too soon for certain tasks —to involve your child in food preparation. To keep his or her interest, you may want to start by baking cookies. If so, make nutrient-packed ones, using ingredients like oatmeal, raisins, or peanut butter, and explain what the various ingredients are and why they're used. Nutritious blender shakes with banana and egg are even simpler, and quickly enough prepared to hold a very young child's interest in "cooking." I've already mentioned involving children in the preparation of vegetables and salads as a way of stimulating an interest in eating vegetables.

But don't intimidate your kitchen-bound child with a long list of dos and don'ts. Make only enough rules for the sake of safety. If a child starts young, by the age of 7 he or she should be able to prepare many dishes alone. If you play your cards right, in fact, you may be able to retire from routine K.P. at an early age!

WHAT NOT TO DO AT MEALTIME

There's nothing that fills up a child's stomach faster than "knots" caused by tension, anxiety, coaxing, and criticism. Children who feel they are under constant scrutiny at the table are likely to lose their appetite in a hurry. Comments on table manners ("use your fork," "use your napkin," "don't talk with food in your mouth," "your hands are filthy," "get your elbows off the table," etc.) should be reserved for after the meal. Nor is the table the proper place for lectures on morality, behavior, school grades, or other such topics guaranteed to be unpleasant for the child. All you'll accomplish is to associate mealtime with misery, to aggravate existing eating problems, and probably to introduce some new ones. Try to keep the conversation light and pleasant. If you find you simply can't stand to watch the way your child eats without saying something critical or corrective, then eat at separate times or create a special "kids' table" and sit where you can't see what's going on.

Don't wheedle, cajole, or bribe your child into eating certain foods or cleaning his or her plate. And don't lay on the guilt with "I spent hours in the kitchen trying to make a good supper, and all you can say is 'Yuk.' " By threatening to withhold dessert if the peas and carrots are not eaten, or by presenting dessert as a reward for having eaten well, you further enhance the value to the child of the part of the meal that's nutritionally least important. Some experts have suggested reversing the bribe—"If you don't eat your cake, you can't have your carrots" —but I know of no one who's actually put this approach to a proper test.

If Your Child Eats Lunch at School

Even if your child takes a lunch to school that you carefully prepared to be nutritious as well as delicious, that's not necessarily what your child will eat. Children who eat together away from parents' watchful eyes routinely swap part or all of their lunch with one another. Or a nonhungry child may give away most of his or her lunch or toss it in the garbage can. Now and again ask your child what was eaten for lunch and see if it matches what you packed. If an apple or box of raisins was traded for a Devil Dog, you might want to know that. Sometimes a compromise can be reached by including some cookies and a piece of fruit. Or you may want to give the child something to trade away without giving up the fruit. Also, you might discover that tuna-salad sandwiches are always traded, perhaps for cream cheese and jelly, or that all sandwiches made on dark bread are traded for those on white.

The National School Lunch Act, administered by the Department of Agriculture, which pays for the lunches of needy children, requires every public school to make lunches available to its children. Lunches served in school must provide at least a third of a child's daily recommended allowances for certain nutrients. They must include milk, a protein-rich food, vegetables, fruit, bread or other grain food, and butter or margarine. Vast quantities of school lunches end up in the garbage instead of in the children's stomachs. To reduce waste and improve nutrition, some cities have capitulated to well-established childhood preferences and have begun serving balanced meals based on pizza, dressed-up burgers, and the like.

Still, some consumer groups are concerned about the fact that many school lunches contain too much fat and starch, are tasteless and unappealing, and encourage children to skip the part that's good for them to get to the cake, ice cream, and chocolate milk. Or children may skip the lunch entirely and eat candy, soda, and ice cream from school vending machines. Parent-Teacher Associations in many schools have taken an active role in monitoring and improving the types of foods served in school and in changing the items available in vending machines. Check with the PTA at your child's school to see if a study of the lunch program has been made and what you can do to help.

The Center for Science in the Public Interest (CSPI), 1501 16th Street NW, Washington, D.C. 20036, has a helpful guide for parent activists interested in the school lunch program. It's called "School Food Action Packet" and can be purchased by writing to the CSPI.

Snacks

It's the rare child who doesn't get hungry between meals and clamor for snacks. Small children, after all, have small stomachs relative to their caloric needs and can't hold enough food to sustain them for five or six hours. And few can consume enough calories in just three meals to meet their daily energy requirement. Besides, a child who's hungry is likely to be cranky, belligerent, accident-prone, and generally unpleasant to be with.

It's no surprise, then, that about a fifth of children's calories are consumed as snacks. But snacks don't have to be, as Vicki Lansky puts it, "C.A.N.D.Y.—Continuously Advertised Nutritionally Deficient Yummies." Snacks can be an important supplement to your child's diet, providing essential nutrients along with calories. To achieve this, parents have to take a firm stand on what is and what is not allowed and when. That doesn't necessarily mean "no sweets." Most children adore sweets (they come by it naturally; you don't have to blame yourself), and there's no good reason why they can't have them from time to time. But they'll be better off not thinking that every meal must end with cookies, cake, pudding, or ice cream or that every between-meal hunger pang must be subdued with a sweet.

Better choices include fruit (fresh or canned in water or light syrup) with or without cheese, cheese and crackers, yogurt, half a sandwich with milk or juice, a bowl of cold cereal and milk, nuts (preferably unsalted), popcorn (lightly salted and unbuttered), cut-up raw vegetables (many parents keep a bag of these in the refrigerator so that they're handy when hunger strikes) with or without dip. Dried fruits are a nutritious snack, too, but very hard on the teeth. They are best served when teeth can be brushed soon after eating.

To satisfy that sweet tooth once in a while, make your own cookies and cakes. That way you can control the amount of sweetener (most recipes could stand a 25- to 50-percent reduction in sugar) and the type of fat used (most commercial baked goods contain saturated fats to prolong shelf life). You can also pack them full of nutritious ingredients like oatmeal, nuts, raisins, wheat germ, bran, fruits, and vegetables. Even better choices are minimally sweet quick breads and muffins, also laden with nourishing ingredients. Recipes for some of my family's favorite breads can be found on pages 136–137. The following muffins are also winners:

Banana Bran Muffins

¾ cup unbleached white flour
½ cup whole-wheat flour
¼ cup sugar
1 tablespoon baking powder
1½ cups whole-bran cereal

¾ cup skim milk
1 cup mashed bananas
1 egg
¼ cup vegetable oil
½ cup chopped nuts (optional)

Preheat the oven to 400 degrees. In a small bowl, combine the flours, sugar, and baking powder and set aside. In a large bowl, mix together the cereal, milk, and banana, and let stand for 1 to 2 minutes until the cereal softens. Add the egg and the oil to the cereal mixture and beat well with a spoon. Stir in the flour mixture and nuts until just combined. Divide the batter among 12 greased muffin cups. Bake the muffins for about 25 minutes, or until golden brown. Yield: 1 dozen muffins.

Oatmeal-Raisin Muffins

1 cup rolled oats
1 cup buttermilk
1 cup whole-wheat flour (or half whole wheat and half white)
1½ teaspoons baking powder
½ teaspoon baking soda

½ teaspoon salt
¼ cup vegetable oil or melted margarine
¼ cup packed brown sugar
1 large egg, beaten
½ cup raisins

In a large bowl combine the oats and the buttermilk and let the mixture stand for at least 30 minutes. Preheat the oven to 350 degrees. In small bowl combine the flour, baking powder, baking soda, and salt and set the bowl aside. After the oats have soaked, stir the oil, sugar, and egg into the oat mixture and blend well. Stir in the flour mixture and raisins to moisten. Do not overmix. Divide the batter among 12 greased muffin cups (about ¾ full). Bake for about 25 minutes, or until a toothpick inserted in center of a muffin comes out clean. Yield: 1 dozen muffins.

The best way to keep your children from snacking on "C.A.N.D.Y." is not to have such things in the house. Many parents justify their regular purchases of soft drinks, cookies, candy, and ice cream by "buying them for the children." Then they watch with dismay as the children they bought them for devour them at a rapid clip! Remember, *if such foods are not around when a child gets hungry, he or she can't eat them.* Or, if you prefer to keep cookies in the house at all times, serve the child one or two and make it known that that's all he or she is going to get. *Never bring the whole box to the table.*

After-school snacks are a problem in some households because children often come home famished and for the next several hours devour everything in sight, only to spoil their appetite for supper. A better plan is for parents to determine the snack ahead of time and serve it right after school. Then, no more food until the evening meal. Close to suppertime, a thirsty child is best offered water rather than milk or fruit juice. If you're not at home after school and your children are old enough to take their own snacks, leave a note as to what is available for their snack that afternoon. Until adolescence, you can probably succeed in controlling the amount and kind of snack foods even in absentia.

TV and Other Nutritional Subversives

The average American child is said to spend more hours in front of the TV set than in school (not implausible when you count weekend and holiday viewing) and to witness more than 15,000 commercials a year for sugary foods. "Television advertising," says Dr. Wurtman, "is probably the most persistent force undermining good eating habits." Messages that promote well-balanced meals and nutritious foods "tend to be overwhelmed by the huge number of ads for junk foods that appear during prime TV time for children," she points out. Even though young children can't rush out to buy these nutritionally deficient items, the ads condition children to crave sweets and set the stage for continuing battles with nutrition-conscious parents.

Colman McCarthy, writer, runner, and concerned father of three, became so distressed by the "salesman in my living room telling lies to my children" that he got rid of the TV altogether. While this may be too drastic a solution for most, a number of less severe strategies can help you counter the sugar-coated messages beamed to youngsters over the boob tube.

Fight propaganda with facts. You can explain even to a three-year-old that you don't buy certain things because they don't help her grow up strong and healthy. No sermon is necessary, just matter-of-fact statements like "I want you to have healthy teeth; that's why I won't let you eat candy whenever you want it" or "I give you milk instead of Kool-Aid because I want you to have strong bones." As the child gets older, your explanations can become increasingly sophisticated so that the connection between good foods and good health is better understood. Chances are it won't be long before you hear your children repeating your pitch to their friends who overindulge in the forbidden foods.

Restrict viewing of commercial television. Public broadcasting, with its marvelous programs for young children, has given good nutrition a major, if indirect, boost by keeping youngsters away from seductive commercial messages. "Sesame Street" and "Mr. Rogers' Neighborhood" have spared millions of youngsters the constant barrage of ads for candy and sugar-coated cereals on early-morning cartoon and other commercial shows for children. The longer you can keep your children from watching such programs, the better chance you have of countering the multimillion-dollar effort to undermine nutritional health among the nation's youngsters.

Expose the hidden message. When your children do start watching commercial television, fortify them against undue influence by pointing out the gimmicks that advertisers use to get people to buy their products. This can quickly become a fun family game that extends to all sorts of commercials, not just those for food. "Tuned-in" children are quick to take up the sport of unmasking the sponsor's sales pitch—it's often more fun than the programs themselves! Among those my sons have picked out are the ads for a sweetened cereal with "eight essential vitamins and minerals" *("but they never tell you how much")* and one for a razor that's "the best we've ever made" *("but maybe all their razors are lousy").*

Blunt the commercial appeal. Dr. Wurtman suggests that parents should react with disgust at ads for foods that don't deserve to be eaten by any self-respecting child. She also suggests comparing these items to foods sold for pets, since ads for pet foods nearly always emphasize good nutrition. Ask: "If chocolate cupcakes with marshmallow centers are not good for our dog, why should they be good for you?"

Adopt smart supermarket strategy. Supermarkets often sabotage the efforts of parents trying to do right by their children's diets. Junk foods are strategically placed in markets to catch the eye of every sweets-loving youngster. Many well-intentioned parents have been worn down by children screaming from their perches in shopping carts for Cookie-Crisps, Oreos, or bags of candy. Here you have several alternatives. If possible, leave the children at home when you shop. Buy them an approved treat—fruit, raisins, nuts, sugar-free gum. Make out a shopping list before you go to the store and tell your children that you won't be buying anything that's not on the list. But whatever you do, don't give in to demands for foods you've decided not to buy. If your children discover that wheedling, whining, or screaming long enough will get them what they want, you're going to lose every such battle. Be firm, explain yourself, and stick to your guns. Eventually, most children stop asking.

If Your Child Is Overweight

The main environmental cause of childhood obesity is not overeating, but underactivity. Study after study has shown that the vast majority of fat children eat less than their more slender age mates, but they also expend far fewer calories. Therefore, the ideal solution to the problem is to program more movement into your child's life. If team sports are spurned (as they often are by fat children), try a swimming program, dance class, skating, cycling, walking, hiking, jogging, or some other noncompetitive activity.

Experts on child nutrition strongly advise against putting a child on a diet. Certainly you can *and should* restrict consumption of calorie-laden, nutritionally deficient foods. And a child who eats too much of good foods should be given smaller portions and encouraged to eat more slowly. But a child who is eating normal amounts of nourishing food cannot be placed on a calorie-restricted diet without compromising the intake of nutrients needed for proper growth and development. The goal for overweight children is not to get them to reduce, but to slow their weight gain enough so that they grow into a normal body weight as they increase in height.

But don't assume that you don't have to do anything about a child who's chubby because "he'll grow out of it." Fat cells acquired in childhood are permanent residents for the rest of one's life. If a child acquires too many in his early years, he'll have a lifelong battle trying to keep them from filling up (see Chapter 15).

FOR FURTHER READING

U.S. Department of Agriculture, *What's to Eat? And Other Questions Kids Ask about Food,* 1979 Yearbook of Agriculture (Washington, D.C.: U.S. Government Printing Office, 1980). For nine- to twelve-year-olds. (Free copies may be available through your U.S. senator or U.S. representative.)

Vicki Lansky, *The Taming of the C.A.N.D.Y. Monster* (Deephaven, Minn.: Meadowbrook Press, 1978).

Polly Greenberg, *How to Convert the Kids from What They Eat to What They Oughta* (New York: Ballantine, 1980).

21 ✒️ ADOLESCENCE: FEEDING THE FAST-FOOD FREAKS

Gordon was 14 and each day, it seemed, he said less and less and ate more and more. It was costing his family a fortune to keep him in food—not to mention clothes, which he seemed to outgrow every few months. There was no telling what might be left in the refrigerator when it was time to make dinner. And sometimes he ate the ingredients for the family's breakfast before he went to bed. He could polish off half a loaf of bread and a package of cold cuts, followed by a quart of milk and a box of cookies, all at one sitting. Nothing was sacred if Gordon was hungry and liked what he found.

Although chubby all through childhood, Gordon actually slimmed down as he shot up during adolescence. By 17, he was 6 feet, 2 inches tall and weighed 220 pounds of mostly muscle and big bones, perfect for playing high-school football.

Gordon's appetite, which continued essentially unabated for nearly four years, may seem extreme, but it is hardly unusual. During the teen years, caloric and nutrient requirements are greater and, except during infancy, growth is more rapid than at any other time of life. Adolescents, especially physically active boys, can eat you out of house and home. Some need as many as 4,000 calories a day just to maintain their weight, and even more if they're in training for a vigorous sport like football. Girls, too, have a growth spurt during adolescence that increases their need for calories and certain nutrients. In girls, the adolescent growth spurt begins about two years sooner—at 10 or 11—and is usually over by 15. Boys typically start their period of rapid growth at 12 or 13, and it doesn't end until about 19. Adolescent growth contributes about 15 percent to final adult height, yet accounts for fully half of adult weight.

Primarily because of differences in sex hormones, boys add mostly lean tissue (muscle and bone), ending up with about 8 percent body fat, whereas girls add proportionately more fat, reaching an average of 20 percent body fat. The higher percentage of body fat and the lower level of physical activity typical among adolescent girls mean that girls need fewer calories than boys do, even if they both weigh the same. Whereas boys between the ages of 11 and 18 need on the average 2,700 to 2,800 calories a day, girls require only 2,100 to 2,200. Many adolescent girls eat considerably less than this, hopping from one low-calorie diet to another in an effort to match the skin-and-bones models of American fashion. Yet adolescent girls have to pack into their fewer calories nearly as many nutrients as boys do. Adolescent girls need as much calcium, zinc, phosphorus, iodine, vitamins C, D, B$_6$, B$_{12}$, and folacin as adolescent boys, but they have to get them while consuming 20 percent fewer calories (see Table 21.1). That means there's less room in a teenaged girl's diet for junk food.

The Importance of Essential Nutrients

It should come as no surprise to anyone who has lived through adolescence that teenagers' diets often fall below recommended levels of certain nutrients vital to growth, especially the bone-building mineral calcium and the muscle- and blood-building mineral iron. Deficiencies in vitamins A and C and certain B vitamins (thiamin and folacin) are also not uncommon. Since 1965, intakes of iron, vitamin C, and thiamin have risen among teenaged boys and girls, but calcium levels have continued to fall (see Chart 14). In general, throughout the teen years, nutrient deficiencies are more common and more serious in girls, who consume fewer calories and are more likely to go on unbalanced fad diets to lose weight. Deficiencies affect youngsters in all socioeconomic groups, but are worse among the poor and minority groups.

Given the haphazard eating styles of adolescents—the skipped breakfasts, crash diets, catch-as-catch-can snacking on empty calories, irregular meals, frequent dining at fast-food joints—it's a wonder that adolescents are not more seriously malnourished than they are. As Dr. Jo Anne Brasel, nutrition specialist at Harbor-University of California, Los Angeles, Medical Center, says, "Most seem to muddle through reasonably well and somehow satisfy their nutritional needs in much the same erratic fashion they come to grips with the psychological changes necessary to move from the protected world of childhood to the independent world of the adult."

Nonetheless, nutrient shortages may compromise the growth and well-being of millions of American teenagers, possibly interfering with

Table 21.1 • A TYPICAL TEENAGER'S DAILY NUTRITIONAL NEEDS

Vitamins

Ages	Calories	Protein (g)	A (RE)*	D (µg)**	E (mg)	C (mg)	Thiamin (mg)	Riboflavin (mg)	Niacin (mg)	B_6 (mg)	Folacin (µg)**	B_{12} (µg)**	K (µg)**	Biotin (µg)**	Pantothenic acid (mg)
Girls															
11–14	2,200	46	800	10	8	50	1.1	1.3	15	1.8	400	3	50–100	100–200	4–7
15–18	2,100	46	800	10	8	60	1.1	1.3	14	2.0	400	3	50–100	100–200	4–7
Boys															
11–14	2,700	45	1,000	10	8	50	1.4	1.6	18	1.8	400	3	50–100	100–200	4–7
15–18	2,800	56	1,000	10	10	60	1.4	1.7	18	2.0	400	3	50–100	100–200	4–7

Minerals and trace elements

Ages	Calcium (mg)	Phosphorus (mg)	Magnesium (mg)	Iron (mg)	Zinc (mg)	Iodine (µg)**	Copper (mg)	Manganese (mg)	Fluoride (mg)	Chromium (mg)	Selenium (mg)	Molybdenum (mg)	Sodium (mg)	Potassium (mg)	Chloride (mg)
Girls															
11–14	1,200	1,200	300	18	15	150	2–3	2.5–5.0	1.5–2.5	.05–20	.05–20	.15–50	900–2,700	1,525–4,575	1,400–4,200
15–18	1,200	1,200	300	18	15	150	2–3	2.5–5.0	1.5–2.5	.05–20	.05–20	.15–50	900–2,700	1,525–4,575	1,400–4,200
Boys															
11–14	1,200	1,200	350	18	15	150	2–3	2.5–5.0	1.5–2.5	.05–20	.05–20	.15–50	900–2,700	1,525–4,575	1,400–4,200
15–18	1,200	1,200	400	18	15	150	2–3	2.5–5.0	1.5–2.5	.05–20	.05–20	.15–50	900–2,700	1,525–4,575	1,400–4,200

Source: Based on Recommended Daily Dietary Allowances (RDAs) established in 1980 by the Food and Nutrition Board of the National Academy of Sciences–National Research Council to meet the nutritional needs of healthy people. Those nutrients for which a range is given (for example, vitamin K: 50–100 micrograms) represent "estimated safe and adequate" daily intakes, since there were not sufficient data on which to base a definite RDA. Caloric values represent an average; precise caloric requirements depend on height, weight, and level of activity, and should be adjusted accordingly.
*RE = retinol equivalent.
**µg = microgram.

Chart 14 • WHAT TEENAGERS EAT

DAILY CONSUMPTION IN 1965 AND 1977

CALORIES

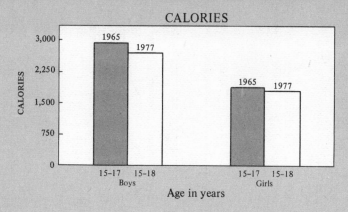

FAT

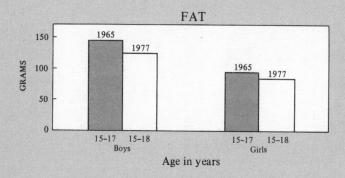

PROTEIN

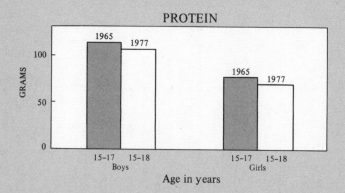

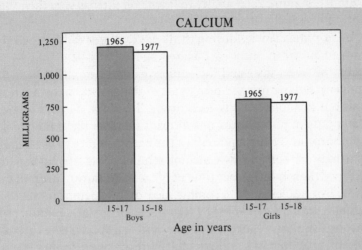

CALCIUM

MILLIGRAMS

1,250 1,000 750 500 250 0

1965 1977

15–17 15–18
Boys

1965 1977

15–17 15–18
Girls

Age in years

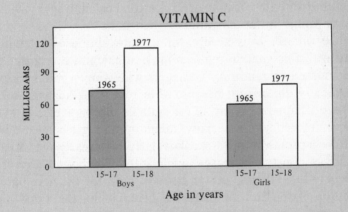

VITAMIN C

MILLIGRAMS

120 90 60 30 0

1965 1977

15–17 15–18
Boys

1965 1977

15–17 15–18
Girls

Age in years

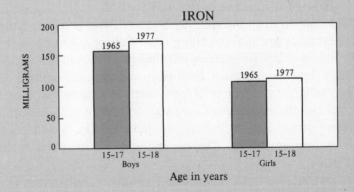

IRON

MILLIGRAMS

200 150 100 50 0

1965 1977

15–17 15–18
Boys

1965 1977

15–17 15–18
Girls

Age in years

Source: USDA Nationwide Food Consumption Survey, 48 States, Spring 1977 (preliminary);
USDA Household Food Consumption Survey, 1965–66, Report No. 11, 1972.

their vitality, stamina, and ability to learn and intensifying their difficulties with emotional adjustments.

Calcium deficiencies during the teen years are readily traced to the widespread substitution of carbonated and other soft drinks for milk. Lured by the sweet taste and the seductive advertising that links drinking pop with having fun and being part of the crowd, many adolescents have all but abandoned milk as a drink. To make matters worse, the large amounts of phosphorus in soft drinks distort the ratio of calcium to phosphorus in the diet and reduce the body's ability to use what little calcium may be consumed. Calcium requirements are higher during adolescence than at any other time of life, except during pregnancy and lactation. An adolescent's recommended daily calcium intake—1,200 milligrams—could be satisfied by four 8-ounce servings of milk (whole, low-fat, or skim) or yogurt. Ice cream and fast-food shakes are poorer sources of calcium and contain far more calories than plain milk. Cheese, another adolescent favorite, is a good calcium source, but again it's much higher in fat and calories than milk.

Since *vitamin D* is needed for the absorption of calcium, milk fortified with this vitamin remains the best calcium source and is also a good source of vitamin A. Teenagers who simply hate milk or who have difficulty digesting it because of lactose (milk sugar) intolerance should see Chapters 13 and 20 for suitable alternatives.

Iron deficiency is especially common among teenaged girls, but can also be a problem for boys, particularly in the early years of adolescence before appetite increases significantly. The body's need for iron is especially high during growth periods, both for the development of new muscle tissue and for increased hemoglobin, the blood pigment that carries oxygen to body tissues. After menstruation begins, girls also need to replace the iron lost in the menstrual flow. Inadequate iron in the adolescent diet can interfere with growth and produce symptoms of iron-deficiency anemia, including lack of energy, quick fatigue, pale complexion, and an increased susceptibility to infection.

Throughout adolescence, both boys and girls are advised to consume 18 milligrams of iron a day, as much as an adult woman needs during her childbearing years. Good sources of iron include liver, meat, eggs, iron-fortified cereals, whole grains, dried beans and peas, and nuts. Iron supplements may be recommended during the adolescent growth years.

To prevent shortages of various *B vitamins* and *vitamin C,* daily consumption of whole-grain or enriched breads and cereals, vegetables, and citrus fruit or fruit juice is advisable.

If you are a growing adolescent, your daily diet should look something like this (see Table 1.2 on page 18 for details):

- Milk—four or more servings.
- Meat or meat substitute—three or more servings.
- Vegetables and fruit—four or more servings.
- Bread and cereal—four or more servings.

These are the basics, to be consumed as part of your meals and as snacks. If you need more calories, simply increase the number or size of the servings. You can also supplement your diet with some calorie-laden "no-nos" as long as they're not consumed in place of the recommended nutritious foods listed above. If you're trying to lose weight or slow your rate of gain, choose the lower-calorie foods in each of the categories—for example, skim milk instead of whole milk, shakes, or cheese; fish or poultry (but not fried) in place of hamburgers, pizza, and peanut butter; or whole-wheat flakes instead of granola. But don't assume you can get away with cutting out whole categories of foods, such as all carbohydrates or all fats, without ill effect. Distorted diets can threaten your mental and physical development.

Fast Foods: More Nourishing Than You Think

Probably nothing causes more parental concern about the eating habits of teenagers than teenagers' seeming addiction to fast foods—pizza and cola; hamburgers, French fries, and shakes; fried chicken and slaw; fish and chips; roast beef sandwiches; tacos; hot dogs; and other such mass-produced and mass-served quickie meals. Whether parents themselves hate such fare or secretly love it, most adults have been conditioned to think of fast food as nutritionally disastrous "junk food."

Certainly, it's a far cry from gourmet cooking or the "balanced" meals we've been told we need. There's a striking absence of fresh fruits and vegetables with a seeming overabundance of fats and carbohydrates. But is fast food really all that bad? No, say a number of specialists who've analyzed the nutritional composition of fast-food meals. While not recommended as a steady diet, they're better than you might be inclined to think.

To take an extreme and not-to-be recommended example, let's say a teenager consumed a cheeseburger, French fries, and a shake four times a day. Dr. Laurence Finberg, professor of pediatrics at Albert Einstein College of Medicine in New York, believes the average teen-aged male could do a lot worse. Such a menu, he's calculated, would provide 4,100 calories, with 17 percent of the calories from protein, 39 percent from fat, and 44 percent from carbohydrate. The protein content is surprisingly good, Dr. Finberg concluded, and the fat content —although higher than the recommend maximum of 30 percent of calories—is lower than you might have guessed. Furthermore, such a diet would supply all the needed minerals and most of the essential vitamins, except enough A, D, C, and folacin. To make up for the missing nutrients, the shake should be made with milk, fish and liver should substitute for the burger once a week, a citrus fruit or juice can replace the fries once a day, and carrots and leafy green vegetables can be eaten every other day.

Cutting consumption of the fast-food meal to three times a day would reduce calories to a more reasonable 3,075 (but also reduce vitamin intake somewhat). If in place of the cheeseburger the teenager ate pizza, no nutritional disaster would result. In fact, pizza has been described as "the ideal McGovern food" since it supplies the basic nutrients in approximately the amounts recommended in the Dietary Goals established by Senator George McGovern's nutrition subcommittee. A typical slice of pizza has 15 percent protein, 27 percent fat, and 58 percent carbohydrate. Thus, either as a snack or as part of a meal, it's a reasonably well-balanced food.

Nonetheless, overdependence on fast foods can have some serious shortcomings. Many fast-food menus are filled with nutritional booby traps. But if you know where they are and how to compensate for them, you can certainly dine several times a week and perhaps even once a day on fast-food meals without compromising your nutritional well-being, whether you're 6, 16, or 60.

A major disadvantage is *cost,* since a comparable meal prepared at home costs half of what you pay at a fast-food establishment. For example, according to an analysis by the U.S. Department of Agriculture, in February, 1979, a fast-food meal for a family of four consisting of a specialty burger, fries, and a soft drink added up to $6.80. Preparing the same meal at home would have cost only $3.32. So for a family on a tight food budget, overreliance on fast foods may result in "eating cheap" the rest of the time and shortchanging the family's nutritional requirements at other meals.

Here's what a fast-food "freak" should know about the nutritional advantages and disadvantages of the various choices available:

Calories add up quickly. For the amount of nutrients supplied, fast-food meals are usually too high in calories. This is not a problem for the high-school athlete or anyone who's very active, but it could be for a more sedentary teenager or adult. A "simple" fast-food meal can easily total more than half your daily calorie needs. For example, a Kentucky Fried Extra Crispy Chicken dinner (three pieces of chicken, mashed potatoes and gravy, coleslaw, and a roll) contains 950 calories, not including the drink. With a 12-ounce soft drink, the total is about 1,100 calories. Table 21.2 shows the calories in other fast foods. See how "fast" they add up.

Many have too much fat. Fat is usually the main source of calories in a fast-food meal, and not just those parts of the meal that are fried. Surprisingly, most of the burgers served by national chains are reason-

Table 21.2 • WHAT'S IN FAST FOODS?

Item	Calories	Protein (g)	Carbohy-drates (g)	Fats (g)	Sodium (mg)
McDonald's Big Mac	541	26	39	31	962
Burger King Whopper	606	29	51	32	909
Burger Chef Hamburger	258	11	24	13	393
Dairy Queen Cheese Dog	330	15	24	19	N.A.*
Taco Bell Taco	186	15	14	8	79
Pizza Hut Thin 'N Crispy Cheese Pizza (½ of 10-inch pie)	450	25	54	15	N.A.*
Pizza Hut Thick 'N Chewy Pepperoni Pizza (½ of 10-inch pie)	560	31	68	18	N.A.*
Arthur Treacher's Fish Sandwich	440	16	39	24	836
Burger King Whaler	486	18	64	46	735
McDonald's Filet-O-Fish	402	15	34	23	709
Long John Silver's Fish (2 pieces)	318	19	19	19	N.A.*
Kentucky Fried Chicken Original Recipe Dinner	830	52	56	46	2,285
Kentucky Fried Chicken Extra Crispy Dinner (3 pieces chicken)	950	52	63	54	1,915
McDonald's Egg McMuffin	352	18	26	20	914
Burger King French Fries	214	3	28	10	5
Arthur Treacher's Coleslaw	123	1	11	8	266
Dairy Queen Onion Rings	300	6	33	17	N.A.*
McDonald's Apple Pie	300	2	31	19	414
Burger King Vanilla Shake	332	11	50	11	159
McDonald's Chocolate Shake	364	11	60	9	329
Dairy Queen Banana Split	540	10	91	15	N.A.*

Source: Data supplied by the companies to the Senate Select Committee on Nutrition and Human Needs.
*N.A. = not available.

ably lean, but when cheese and sauce are added, you're adding mostly fat. *Fast-food shakes* are also high in fat, although usually not butterfat. *Rather, these shakes are prepared from vegetable oils—sometimes highly saturated coconut oil.* You may have noticed that they're not called *milk* shakes. Nonetheless, with regard to nutrients, a shake is still a better choice than a soft drink since shakes are made from dried-milk products and supply significant amounts of protein, calcium, riboflavin, and niacin.

When foods are deep-fried, the additional fat can more than double the caloric value of the basic food. Potatoes, for example, are a low-fat nutritional bargain as they come from the ground, but when French-cut and fried they become a high-fat, high-calorie food. You can greatly reduce the fat content of fried chicken by removing and discarding the skin. In eating fried fish, stick to the large pieces of fish rather than tidbits like clams, shrimp, and oysters, which have far more greasy batter in proportion to "real" food. Several fast-food chains have recently introduced broiled fish.

A bad shake on salt. The sodium content of most fast-food fare is extremely high—900 to 1,100 milligrams for specialty burgers, 700 to 900 milligrams for fish and roast beef sandwiches, 1,100 to 1,300 milligrams for chili and pizza, 600 to 700 milligrams for chicken (two pieces). Even the shakes (300 milligrams) and pies (400 milligrams) are quite high in sodium. The fries as they come from the oil are low in sodium, but sprinkled with salt and doused with ketchup, they quickly become a high-sodium food. A typical fast-food meal could easily contain three-fourths of the day's recommended sodium allotment of about 2,200 milligrams a day. If you're watching your sodium intake, stick to plain burgers (without pickles) and the sparest sprinkling of salt on your fries. Better yet, don't eat fast foods.

Few fibers in fast foods. In the absence of fresh fruit, salads, whole grains, and beans, most fast-food restaurants supply little fiber to keep your digestive tract working efficiently. A few establishments serve coleslaw, and many have recently introduced salad bars, useful as a low-calorie alternative and a source of fiber and vitamins otherwise absent in fast-food meals. Beware, though, of fatty dressings and salad-bar ingredients already well-dressed. Most offer reduced-calorie dressings, which means less fat.

Short on some micronutrients. Most fast-food meals are deficient in vitamins A and C, several B vitamins, and iron. Salads or slaw can help to correct these deficiencies. Some fast-food chains, including Burger King and Dairy Queen, fortify their shakes with iron. But to assure a reasonable nutrient balance on the days you dine on fast foods, you should include fruit, salad, green or yellow vegetable, whole or enriched grains, and milk at your other meals.

High marks on protein. If there's one good thing you get in ample amounts in most fast foods, it's protein. A meal of a regular burger, fries, and a shake supplies 42 percent of the recommended daily allowance for protein, with even higher percentages for meals based on cheeseburgers, jumbo burgers, chicken, and fish.

Not too sweet on sugar. Save for the drinks and desserts, fast-food meals are low in sugar. Most of the carbohydrates they contain are the desirable complex starches. A fast-food shake, however, may harbor as many as 8 to 14 teaspoons of sugar; in regular soft drinks all the calories come from sugar—more than 5 teaspoons' worth in 8 to 12 ounces, 8 teaspoons in 12 ounces. Diet sodas lack sugar but contain saccharin, which causes cancer in laboratory animals, or aspartame, which may have unwanted brain effects. A better bet is milk or fruit juice (not fruit drink) for youngsters; milk, juice, coffee, or tea for adults. If no better choices are available, ask for water.

You Can't Tell a Teenager What to Eat

"Teenagers are not fed; they eat," note Florida State University nutritionists Eva May Hamilton and Eleanor N. Whitney. "For the first time in their lives, they assume responsibility for their own food intakes." And, as many parents know, this often means total rejection of everything children were ever taught about how and what and when to eat. *Erratic eating habits are normal among adolescents,* and no amount of wheedling, nagging, scolding, or threats will get teenagers back into the family fold when it comes to food—or anything else, for that matter.

But all is not lost. While parents cannot control what a teenager may eat on the outside, many nutritional sins can be forgiven if the right kinds of food are available at home. *Don't buy any junk food*—including cookies, candy, cake, chips, pretzels, and soft drinks. Instead, stock your refrigerator and cupboard with milk, fruit juice, yogurt, whole-grain breads, cut-up fresh vegetables, fruit and fruit salads, whole-grain crackers, cheese, nuts, raisins, popcorn, and the like. Leftovers— chicken, sliced beef, meat loaf, meat balls, fish cakes, boiled or roasted potatoes, stir-fried green beans, steamed broccoli (makes a delicious snack cold with vinaigrette or Italian dressing)—will be gobbled up by a foraging adolescent with a voracious appetite, much to his or her nutritional benefit. Such foods should be the only choices the adolescent diner-on-the-run has at home.

Remember, *snacking* is the adolescent way of life; about a quarter of a teenager's calories come from snacks. Since you can't really fight it, you might as well support it with snack foods worth their caloric weight in essential nutrients.

Sometimes teenagers latch onto philosophies that involve a radical departure from the dietary customs of the rest of the family. *Vegetarian diets* are especially popular these days among idealistic youngsters who wish to help save the world from starvation, or who think it's wrong to eat animals, or who want to avoid the "poisons" they believe exist in animal food. There's nothing wrong with a vegetarian diet (see Chapter 24). As long as it's nutritionally balanced, a teenager can grow well on it. If your son or daughter is determined to be a vegetarian, make sure you both are knowledgeable about the subject and your larder contains every type of food necessary to provide essential nutrients. Strict vegetarian diets that spurn dairy products and eggs are difficult to balance nutritionally for a growing adolescent. Another popular diet, the restrictive macrobiotic regimen that excludes nearly everything but grains, is extremely unbalanced and hazardous for everyone, especially for someone who's still growing.

Overweight, Underweight, and Acne

The most common form of malnutrition among teenagers is over-nutrition, resulting in overweight. Since adolescence is the last opportunity a body has to acquire new fat cells, *excessive weight gain during the teen years can set the stage for a lifetime battle against the bulge.* Furthermore, overweight during adolescence can add significantly to the turmoil of an already turbulent time of life.

Overweight can cast a lasting pall over a teenager's self-image and sense of worth. About 10 percent of adolescents are significantly obese, and a much larger proportion are overweight. Oddly, youngsters who were chubby through most of childhood often slim down and lose their "baby fat" during adolescence, whereas others who had always been slim may suddenly start putting on extra pounds. Girls usually have more of a problem with adolescent obesity than boys, whose hormones encourage muscle development. Teenaged boys also do more growing the long way and tend to be far more active than their female age mates. Even among teenagers who participate in athletic activities, those who are overweight run around less and expend less energy than those of normal weight.

Most teenagers who are reasonably well adjusted emotionally can lose weight on their own by eating carefully and increasing their exercise. Crash diets should be avoided since they deprive a growing young-ster of essential nutrients for normal body development. Skipping meals (breakfast, usually) is also a bad idea since this causes low energy and inability to concentrate on schoolwork. Besides, the calories missed in a skipped meal are almost always regained and then some by eating a high-calorie between-meal snack or by overeating at the next meal.

It's usually wise to consult your family physician, or a nutritionist, or a specialist in adolescent medicine for guidance on a reasonable weight-loss diet that won't interfere with development and that will teach the youngster sensible, life-long eating patterns. (A serious weight problem in a youngster who is having emotional or social difficulties is best handled by a professional counselor such as a psychologist, since psychological as well as nutritional adjustments may be needed.)

A teenager who's trying to lose weight need not become a social outcast when friends stop at their favorite fast-food hangout for a late-night snack. A plain burger, hot dog, or one slice of pizza, with a salad, tea, water, or a diet soft drink, can allow a dieting teenager to eat with friends without calling attention to his or her problem and without spoiling the diet.

While most girls are worried about shedding extra pounds, many boys fret about being underweight. They struggle to put on weight—especially pounds of muscle—lest they look like the proverbial 98-pound weakling. However, many boys are under the misimpression that to build strong muscles they must eat lots of protein and little or no carbohydrates. Nothing could be further from the truth (see Chapter 23). The normal recommended amounts of protein are more than ade-quate to cover the growth requirements of an adolescent body, and most Americans, including teenagers, already consume twice as much protein as the recommendations call for. Unbalancing the diet by favor-ing one category of food over others can only compromise normal development, not enhance it. Besides, without carbohydrates, those new muscles won't have proper fuel to work on.

Teenagers often exclude one or another food from their diet be-cause they've heard it makes them "break out." Careful studies have shown that such teenage favorites as chocolate, potato chips, nuts, cola, shellfish, pizza, and "greasy" foods do not cause *acne* and rarely aggra-vate it. (Hormones do.) However, about one in a hundred acne sufferers finds that certain foods—usually one of the above items—seems to aggravate the condition. If so, it would make sense to eliminate that food for several weeks to see if any improvement occurs. Vitamin A in normal recommended amounts is certainly important to healthy skin. But consuming excess amounts of vitamin A is of no help to acne. In fact, it is a poison in large doses. External treatments with a special derivitive of vitamin A (vitamin A acid) are tricky and best administered only by a physician.

Teen Dieting Can Be Disastrous

Adolescence is characterized not only by the most bizarre eating habits, but also by some of the strangest schemes not to eat. This is particularly true for adolescent girls, and *the consequences are occasionally life-threatening.*

Typically, a teenaged girl cannot be too thin, at least not in her own eyes. In one study of teenagers, 70 percent of the girls said they wanted to lose weight, although only 15 percent were overweight by adult standards. It does little good to tell such a youngster "you look fine just the way you are." Not to her, she doesn't. The combination of self-determination and self-consciousness has led many an attractive adolescent to attempt to live on carrots and celery, diet pop, grapefruit and eggs, or nothing at all. After a few spartan days on such a regimen, a splurge on potato chips and ice cream, pizza and a shake, or some other calorie-laden fare is *de rigueur.* Such a slip from grace is often followed by an even more rigorous diet, intensive exercise, or sometimes induced vomiting.

Of course, such crash diets are nutritionally unsound and almost always doomed to failure. But just try to tell that to an adolescent! The best parents can hope for is that their daughter will discover it on her own. You can try through calm, rational discussion to point out the effects of such unbalanced diets on one's energy (important to most teenagers) and complexion (even more important) and chances for normal linear growth, which is delayed by malnutrition during adolescence.

You can also make sure that tasty, nutritious "diet" foods are readily available—skim milk, lean meat, chicken breasts, salads, fresh fruit, thin-sliced whole-grain bread, eggs, steamed vegetables, and the like—and that tempting high-calorie treats like ice cream, cake, cookies, chips, nuts, and candy are kept out of the house. You can keep mayonnaise, jam, and syrup off the table during meals and avoid cooking with rich gravies and sauces. And you can pray a lot! Just remember that most adolescents pass through this period of "I'm too fat" with no permanent scars.

A few, however, do not escape unharmed. Experts in adolescent medicine are becoming increasingly alarmed about the growing number of young teenagers who are developing eating disorders called *anorexia nervosa* and *bulimia.* These problems afflict ten times as many girls as boys, and are characterized by zealous dieting (sometimes interspersed with gorging), rapid weight loss beyond what everyone (except the dieter) would consider attractive, and the conviction that no matter how thin the dieter gets, she's still too fat. Pleas or threats do not put a stop to the syndrome, which can lead to extreme emaciation. Self-induced vomiting and use of laxatives and diuretics may be part of an anorexic's relentless pursuit of thinness. Such purges are daily affairs for girls with bulimia, whose problem usually goes undetected for years because they do not become emaciated like anorexics and because they are usually able to hide their purge activity.

Anorexia, which has a psychological and probably also a physical basis, is most effectively treated in the early stages. Psychotherapy may involve the parents as well as the anorexic child. If malnutrition becomes too severe, hospitalization may be necessary to correct the life-threatening effects of starvation and to start the patient eating again. In a few severe cases, death may result. Therefore it's extremely important to seek professional help for your child promptly if you detect signs of anorexia.

22 ⌘ EAT WELL, LIVE WELL IN YOUR LATER YEARS

Eᴍᴍᴀ had been married to Jack for 45 years, and together they raised three children. It had been a good life, and except for a long-standing battle with overweight and moderately high blood pressure, Emma had been strong, healthy, and active. Then, just after her sixty-eighth birthday, Jack died suddenly and the bottom dropped out of Emma's world. Lonely and depressed, she lost interest in preparing the "real meals" she and Jack had shared. There was no one to appreciate the effort, and anyway she had no appetite.

Instead of hearty breakfasts, and dinners of meat or chicken, fresh vegetables, and salad, she took to eating largely "off the shelf." Breakfast, when she had any at all, became juice, coffee, toast and jelly or a sweet roll, rather than the hot cereal or omelet with homemade oatmeal bread she and Jack used to enjoy.

Lunch, which usually was a hearty sandwich or leftovers from dinner the night before, was now canned soup, salted crackers, coffee or tea, and a cookie. Supper was also usually ready-made—either a TV dinner, tuna and canned vegetables, packaged noodles and cheese, or hot dogs and beans—with instant pudding and coffee for dessert. Her bedtime snack was usually tea and another cookie.

At first, Emma had been pleased to see her weight dropping. But now, after a year of this routine, people were saying she looked too thin and she wasn't feeling very well. She slept poorly and seemed to catch one cold after another. She had little energy for any of the activities she had previously enjoyed; she suffered from constipation, severe headaches, and occasional dizzy spells. Emma's daughter, fearing her mother might have cancer or some other horrid disease, finally convinced her to see a doctor.

After a thorough examination and laboratory tests, the doctor questioned Emma at length about her living pattern and eating habits. When he was through, his diagnosis both relieved and surprised everyone, especially Emma.

As Emma tells it, this is what the doctor said:

"What's wrong with you is what's wrong with a third or more of the elderly in this country. You're malnourished. Your weight is down because you're not consuming enough calories. Your blood tests show you're anemic, which—in addition to your depression and loneliness—is contributing to your low energy level and poor appetite. You're not consuming enough iron to keep your blood healthy, and you're probably deficient in a number of other vitamins and minerals as well. That's partly why you're a sitting duck for all those cold viruses. And your headaches and dizzy spells are probably the result of your blood pressure, which is way too high even though you've lost weight. In addition to the stresses of being a recent widow, the large amount of salt in those processed foods you've been living on has played havoc with your blood pressure. All that coffee and tea you drink probably contributes to your sleeping problems. People's tolerance for caffeine declines with age, so a little can have a big stimulating effect. In short, you may live in a nice house in a nice neighborhood, but you're eating worse than people who live in the slums."

Emma is one of millions of poorly nourished elderly Americans whose health and productivity may be limited more by their diet than by age itself. Gone are the days when most old people lived with their children in extended families. Like Emma, today many elderly persons live alone and are too lonely and depressed to have much of an appetite or to want to bother fixing meals for themselves. Others are semi-invalids who have a hard time getting out to shop for food or find it too difficult to prepare meals "from scratch." For some, lack of teeth or poorly fitting dentures limit what they can eat to soft, overly refined, and often nutrient-deficient foods. For others, chronic disorders like diabetes, heart disease, or digestive problems restrict their diets, sometimes depriving them of the very foods they like the most.

Socioeconomic factors can also interfere with good nutrition. The elderly may live in "rough" neighborhoods and fear going out to shop lest they be mugged. Many live on a fixed income, most of which is needed for rent, utilities, and medical bills. With a shrinking budget, they're increasingly limited to foods that are "cheap" both in monetary cost and in nutrient value. And because most are shopping for only one or two persons, they usually purchase the smallest food packages, which have the highest unit cost.

But as Emma's case demonstrates, malnutrition among the elderly is hardly limited to the poor. The families of the "affluent" elderly may never think of poor nutrition as a possible cause of the physical and mental disorders plaguing their aging relatives. Older persons are also likely to put out a "good spread" when company comes, so no one may realize how different their eating pattern may be when they're alone.

In the 1970s a dietary study was done among 529 persons aged 60 to 102 who were living independently in central Tennessee. "Satisfactory" nutrient intake was defined as being two-thirds or more of the Recommended Dietary Allowances established in 1974 by the National Academy of Sciences. In other words, the measurements were based on levels close to minimum nutritional requirements, with the built-in safety factor of the RDAs discounted. Even so, the researchers found that large proportions of the elderly persons studied were below this minimum standard. Fifteen percent of the group had "unsatisfactory" intakes of protein, with black women having the lowest average protein intake. For vitamin C and calcium, intakes were unsatisfactory for 23 percent of the group; for iron, 45 percent; for vitamin A, 56 percent; thiamin, 57 percent; and riboflavin, 63 percent. These deficiencies in nutrient intakes were found even though the persons studied subscribed to no faddist food habits and beliefs, had relatively few food dislikes, had good appetites, tended to choose foods of high nutritive value, and were not big snackers. Furthermore, most ate three meals a day.

No adequate nationwide survey has yet been made of the nutritional well-being of older Americans. However, according to Dr. Robert N. Butler, director of the National Institute on Aging, "The principal Federal food consumption studies, including those of the U.S. Department of Agriculture and the Health and Nutrition Examination Survey of the National Center for Health Statistics, confirm that the diets of older Americans are often below standard both in quantity and quality."

The problem is likely to get worse, not better, as both the life expectancy and number of older Americans continue to increase. In 1986 there were 28 million Americans age 65 and older; by the year 2000 there'll be more than 34 million. A child born today can expect to live nearly 75 years, 27 years longer than a child born at the turn of the century. But most of this increase in life expectancy is the result of fewer deaths among infants and children from infectious diseases; relatively little gain has been made at the upper end of the life span. Nonetheless, those who make it to age 65 can look forward to a good number of years remaining—14.5 for men and 18.8 for women. For many, these years could be spent productively and happily if ill health caused by nutritional deficiencies were avoided.

A Poor Diet Can Have Devastating Effects

Emma was lucky. The reversible diet-caused disabilities she had were diagnosed and corrected before they caused permanent damage. Within three months she had put back some of the weight she'd lost, her headaches and dizziness were gone, and she had regained her energy.

Her doctor gave Emma an iron supplement to help build up her blood, instructing her also to increase the iron content of her diet by eating more red meat, liver, and iron-enriched cereals. (The meat also boosted her consumption of vitamin B_{12}, in which her previous diet had been sorely deficient.) He put her on a low-salt diet to help reduce her blood pressure and advised her to stay away from canned and packaged foods that have a high sodium content. Instead, she ate more salads and fresh vegetables, which she flavored with herbs and spices rather than salt. She switched to decaffeinated coffee during the day and warm milk before bed. Last but not least, the doctor put Emma on a daily exercise regimen that included a mile-long walk before lunch and again before supper. This helped her to relax and increased both her energy and her appetite.

The attention Emma was now forced to pay to herself also helped to lift her year-long depression. She saw more of friends and relatives, often sharing meals with them, and became more involved in community activities, her favorite being weekly visits with persons living in a nearby retirement community where she often talked about nutrition. "Better living through better eating," she called it, and most of what she had to say was news—welcome news—to the people she talked to.

No one knows exactly how many Emmas there are in America today. Experts like Dr. Butler believe that the number of nutritional casualties among the nation's elderly is far greater than most people imagine. Both families and physicians tend to accept the physical and mental decline of elderly persons as the inevitable consequences of advancing age, not realizing that much of this decline is potentially avoidable.

As Dr. Butler pointed out at a hearing of the Senate Select Committee on Nutrition and Human Needs, "Proper nutrition throughout life, including in late life, is an effective means of maintaining good health and minimizing degenerative changes in the later years. . . . It is only through adequately nutritious diets that old people retain the capacity to remain active and productive."

To be sure, good nutrition does not provide immunity from the aging process; no matter how well you eat, you can't live forever! But you may be able to delay or avoid entirely some disorders commonly caused by nutritional deficiencies, including fragile bones and fractures, some forms of senility, chronic constipation, and what could best be called a lack of zest for living. What's more, an improved diet may diminish the older person's risk of developing diabetes, high blood pressure, heart disease, cancer, and stroke.

Dr. Butler notes, for example, that "reversible brain conditions [symptoms of senility] can result from malnutrition and, unless treated in time, often cause the permanent disability that requires long-term care." He said that some people, put in nursing homes because they are confused, delusional, or have serious memory lapses, are really suffering from malnutrition and anemia. Their disorientation often disappears after some "TLC" and nutritious food.

Nutritional Needs Change with Age

You don't need an expert to tell you that the body you're feeding at 70 is hardly the same one you nourished at 20. With increasing age, changes take place in the body's physical composition and metabolic needs and abilities. Your body gets flabby, your sense of taste becomes dulled, your digestive system is fussier and less efficient, your kidney function declines, your metabolism slows. But while these and other changes have been well documented, it's not known whether they are always inevitable consequences of age or merely symptoms of avoidable deterioration.

When it comes to studies of nutritional needs, the elderly have been all but ignored. So few data are available that the National Academy of Science's Food and Nutrition Board had no choice but to lump all people past the age of 51 into one category when devising the Recommended Dietary Allowances for various nutrients.

Calories. The most obvious change occurs in the proportion of the body that's made up of lean tissue—muscle and bone. With age, lean body mass declines and the percentage of body fat increases. Thus, even if you weigh no more at 70 than you did at 20, you're "fatter" at 70. If you maintain a youthful level of exercise as you get older, you can probably slow this trend by keeping your muscles and bones in good shape.

A body having a larger proportion of fat needs fewer calories to maintain itself since fat tissue uses less energy than the same weight of muscle tissue would use. This fact, combined with the tendency of most people to become less active as they grow older, leads to a decreased caloric requirement of 2 to 8 percent for each decade of life past 20. This is why so many people gain unwanted weight in middle age. They may eat no more at 50 than they did at 25, but they're less active now and their bodies contain more fat, so they burn fewer calories. If you were maintaining a normal body weight at age 20 on about 2,500 calories a day, by the time you reach 50, you may need only 1,950 to 2,300 to maintain the same weight.

But although you need fewer calories, your need for vital nutrients doesn't diminish significantly. Therefore, you have to pack the same amount of nutrients into fewer and fewer calories as you get older. This means there's less room in your diet for foods that are overly refined, calorically dense, and nutritionally deficient—that is, junk foods. As you grow older it's critically important to make all your calories count, nutritionally speaking. Too often, however, exactly the opposite occurs. As elderly people develop problems chewing and digesting their food, they lean more and more heavily on soft foods of uniform texture— usually foods high in sugar and/or fats and low in proteins, vitamins, minerals, and fiber.

It's not a good idea, on the other hand, to overeat just to consume the required nutrients. Keeping your weight down as you age is especially important because extra pounds cause unnecessary stress on your bones, adding to the risk of fractures. Also, obesity contributes to the development of diabetes, heart disease, and high blood pressure, and is an indirect cause of accidents.

Protein. Theoretically, you should need less protein as you get older since your body has less lean tissue, makes fewer new tissues, and does less repairing of old ones. However, your ability to digest and absorb protein can also decrease with age, so you may have to consume as much or more protein to provide your body with less. Changes also seem to take place in requirements for certain amino acids, including methionine and lysine, substances that are in relatively short supply in certain vegetable sources of protein. Therefore, elderly persons who depend heavily on vegetable proteins must take great care in balancing them (see Chapter 2). Otherwise, meat, which is more costly, may be needed to ensure that protein and amino-acid requirements are met.

Poultry is a good, inexpensive, low-fat source of high-quality protein; fish is also okay, though it costs more. But avoid processed meats and cheap fatty cuts. They may seem like a bargain, but you actually end up paying a higher price for the protein in such foods than you would if you bought more expensive lean meats (see page 53). Animal protein foods are also an important source of iron and vitamin B_{12}.

Fiber. Many older people are caught in a vicious dietary circle. As their ability to chew diminishes, they tend to eat less and less "roughage"—fibrous foods like fresh fruits and vegetables and whole grains. The absense of roughage slows the activity of their bowels, which may already be functioning inefficiently because of age and inactivity. To correct the resulting constipation, many elderly persons rely on laxatives such as mineral oil, which prevent their body from absorbing the fat-soluble vitamins A, D, E, and K. Laxatives also speed the passage of food through the digestive tract, which decreases absorption of vitamins and minerals and possibly other nutrients as well. Thus, *one dietary deficiency—the lack of fiber—can lead to several others.* What's more, a shortage of vitamin D can worsen the deterioration of bones and teeth, further impairing the individual's ability to chew.

Generally, laxatives should be avoided because they interfere with the normal muscle action of the bowel, eventually causing it to stop working on its own. If for some reason you can't eat fibrous foods, stick to stool softeners like Colace and Metamucil as a medicinal aid to bowel function. And be sure to drink enough liquid—six to eight glasses a day.

Sugar. As you age, your body's ability to process blood sugar decreases. A large proportion of older people have what is called "chemical diabetes,"—that is, their bodies flunk the glucose-tolerance test. This doesn't mean they actually have the disease diabetes, but it suggests that a diet high in simple carbohydrates (sugars) may overwhelm their body's ability to remove sugar from the blood. Too much sugar in the diet also raises the level of fats in the blood and may contribute to atherosclerosis and heart disease. So unless you have a problem keeping enough weight on, sweets should be, at most, an occasional treat.

Fats and cholesterol. For the most part, fat is an expendable part of the diet of older persons, who need to concentrate on more nutritious sources of calories. Although many people believe that after decades of consuming a diet high in fats and cholesterol, it's too late to change, the available evidence shows otherwise. Studies in both monkeys and humans strongly suggest that even if arteries are badly clogged, a switch to a more prudent diet can result in a partial reduction of accumulated fatty deposits.

Calcium. The strength of your bones very much depends on the composition of your diet. Without adequate amounts of vitamin D, calcium, and phosphorus, your bones slowly "dissolve," become weakened, and break easily. Not only do you need to consume enough calcium and phosphorus, these nutrients also must be present in your diet in a certain proportion, with calcium at least as prominent as phosphorus. The diets of most American adults, however, contain up to three times as much phosphorus as calcium, causing inexorable loss of bone as people age. This bone loss, called osteoporosis, is one of the most common health problems among older Americans. It is the primary cause of "shrinkage" in stature and bone fractures among the elderly. Past 50 years of age, 25 to 30 percent of women and 15 to 20 percent of men suffer a shortening of the spinal column as a result. Some evidence indicates that periodontal disease—loss of the bone that supports the teeth and consequent loss of the teeth themselves—is an early sign of osteoporosis. Once the disease is well established, dietary change can't do much more than slow bone loss. Thus, prevention is all important.

Foods that are relatively rich in calcium include milk, sardines and canned salmon (with the bones), yogurt, cottage cheese, sesame seeds, molasses, seaweed, collard greens, and broccoli. Few of these foods are commonly consumed by Americans in their middle and later years. Therefore, some experts recommend supplementing the diet of persons past middle age with a combination of vitamin D and calcium and possibly fluoride, which also helps to keep bones strong. Don't try this regimen on your own, though, since each of these substances can cause serious health problems (fluoride and vitamin D are poisonous) if consumed in excessive amounts. Consult your physician first; if prescribed, take no more than the medically recommended amounts.

Vitamins and minerals. Despite their tight food budgets, many elderly people fall prey to costly and wasteful nutritional quackery—supposed elixirs of youth and magical healers in the form of pills, potions, and special supplements that are loaded with various vitamins and minerals. Megadoses of nutrients, and substances claimed to be nutrients, are of no known value to the elderly or to anyone else. They represent a cruel diversion of money and attention away from the truly useful foods that contain needed nutrients in more reasonable and balanced amounts. If you're nutritionally wise, you won't take vitamin or mineral supplements unless they are prescribed or recommended by your physician.

With increasing age, the levels of vitamins in the body tend to fall, even among people eating a good diet. But currently there are no data to indicate either that this drop is of any health or nutritional significance or that supplementing the diet with a multivitamin pill does any good. Neither is there evidence that taking a one-a-day multivitamin and mineral supplement does any harm, if you can afford it. But stay away from megadoses of single nutrients, or combinations of nutrients, without a doctor's advice. And don't assume that if you do take a supplement, you can afford to skimp on the quality of your food.

Persons most likely to need a vitamin-mineral supplement are those consuming fewer than 1,500 calories a day; those who, for health reasons, must eliminate a major category of food from their diets (for example, all dairy products or fresh fruits and vegetables); or those taking medications that interfere with the body's ability to absorb or use certain vitamins or minerals. Chronic use of laxatives, antibiotics, antacids, diuretics, oral diabetes drugs, some anti-inflammatory drugs, and certain cancer drugs, among others, can result in a depletion of essential vitamins and minerals. If you are taking any medication on a regular basis, ask your doctor if you need a vitamin or mineral supplement or whether a dietary adjustment can correct any deficiency.

There is some evidence that older persons use the B vitamin thiamin less efficiently than younger adults do, so the Food and Nutrition Board recommends a doubling of the usual intake of this vitamin. It is plentiful in pork, liver, whole-grain and enriched cereals, bread and pasta, wheat germ, oatmeal, peas, and lima beans.

Iron supplements, commonly prescribed for older persons if they're not already taking them on their own, are rarely necessary. Before iron is prescribed for an adult who is anemic, the cause of the anemia must be determined. Often it is not a nutritional deficiency but due instead to internal bleeding from a tumor or other disorder.

Solving Special Problems

Many old people with economic, social, or medical disabilities suffer needlessly from malnutrition because they don't take advantage of special foods and services available in their communities. Among the alternatives are:

Baby foods. The preferred solution for people who have difficulty chewing ordinary foods is to obtain dentures that fit well. But if this is not possible, baby foods may be the answer. Baby foods are not the most interesting way for an adult to eat, but they can provide balanced nutrients for elderly persons if the right ones are consumed in adequate amounts. Select those of "pure" ingredients—jars of meat, jars of vegetables, jars of unsweetened fruits—rather than combination dinners or soups or puddings. Round out the meal with dairy products and bread. For breakfast, try iron-fortified hot cereal (baby or regular) prepared with milk.

Communal meals. Many communities offer meal programs for elderly persons in which groups are brought together (in some cases transportation is provided) to some central location, such as a church or school cafeteria, for lunch or dinner. This helps to make eating fun for those who otherwise must dine alone. These programs are sponsored by the federal government under the Nutrition Program of the Older Americans Act, and are open to all persons over 59 years old and their spouses, regardless of income level. To find out about this program, contact your state or local Office on Aging or Department of Welfare, Human Resources, or Social Services.

Meals on Wheels. Another service available in some communities for homebound elderly persons is a hot meal brought to the individual's home once a day. Check with your local Health Department, Visiting Nurse Association, or other community service organizations to find out if there's a Meals on Wheels program in your community.

Food Stamps. Many economically strapped elderly persons are reluctant to take advantage of this federal program to help assure that every American can afford a nutritious diet. Food Stamps are not "welfare." The individual pays for his or her stamps according to income. The stamps can extend your budget and enable you to purchase healthful foods that you might otherwise consider too costly. Don't let pride stand in the way of good nutrition. To apply for the Food Stamp program, contact your local Social Services Department.

Family and friends. Friends and relatives can make an important contribution to the nutritional well-being of elderly persons by providing transportation to the supermarket, doing the shopping, carrying heavy bundles, or bringing over a cooked meal, fresh fruit (better than cookies), or even a rice pudding now and then. When cooking for your own family, you can easily make extra portions for the older person in your life. Single-portion servings can be sealed in plastic bags, frozen, and then reheated in boiling water. Heat-and-serve bags of homemade stew, chicken and vegetables, or hearty soup is a gift of love to an elderly person living alone. If your gift is of several such meals, be sure to check on the person's available freezer space first. For those with only a tiny freezer compartment in the refrigerator, you might consider pooling resources from family and friends and buying the elderly person a small freezer on the next appropriate occasion.

Cooking Hints for Older Folks

• Buy small quantities of fresh produce at a time. If your market has only large prewrapped packages, ask the produce manager to break them open for you and weigh and bag three apples or two tomatoes separately. (In most localities, stores are required by law to do so at your request.) If you have to buy larger quantities because you shop only once a week, be sure to select some produce that is underripe to reduce chances of spoilage by week's end.

• Buy half a dozen eggs, instead of a whole carton, and pints of milk instead of quarts. Even better, keep nonfat dry milk on hand and use it as a protein supplement in casseroles, drinks, soups, etc., as well as for mixing with water to drink "straight."

• If you have freezer space, large bags of frozen vegetables are ideal for one-person cooking. You can shake out as much as you want at one time and return the rest to the freezer where they will remain in good condition for months.

• When freezer space is limited, you may want to buy small-size cans of fruits and vegetables containing only one or two servings. But since these are more expensive (per serving) than large-size cans, a better approach is to buy the big ones and plan to use them for two or three meals within a few days. Put a date on any leftovers you store in the refrigerator so you won't have to rely on your memory and worry about whether they're "still good."

• When you cook a complicated or time-consuming dish, double or triple the recipe. Then package individual servings and store them in the freezer to be reheated at a later date.

• Again, if you have a large enough freezer, you can take advantage of meat specials in "family size" packages, repackaging them at home into meal-sized portions individually wrapped in foil or plastic. Put the individual packages together in one paper bag and label it clearly with contents and date. Then put the whole thing into a clear plastic bag for freezer storage. This makes the food easy to find and protects it from freezer burn.

• Make sure the food items you use regularly are stored on shelves you can easily reach. You may want to hang your pots and pans on the wall and use the pot cupboard for handier food storage. Glass or Lucite storage containers are ideal for staples like rice, beans, flour, noodles, powdered milk, etc., and can be lined up, well labeled, on a kitchen counter or in a cupboard.

• Sit while you work in the kitchen, preferably on a high chair that brings you within easy reach of your countertop or sink, and keep a stool under your feet.

• Wear safe and suitable clothing—no loose sleeves or filmy robes that could catch on fire. Comfortable, sturdy shoes are important.

• A divided skillet, in which an entire meal can be prepared, is excellent for cooking for one, leaving only one pot to wash! If you can afford it, treat yourself to a toaster-oven in which you can broil without having to bend to the floor.

• A number of cookbooks have been published with recipes specially designed for one- or two-person dining. Among them are *Cooking for One,* by Elinor Parker (New York: Crowell, 1976) and *Cooking for One Is Fun,* by Henry Lewis Creel (New York: Times Books, 1976). Check your local library or bookstore for other titles. The federal government offers *Cooking for Two,* for sale as Program Aid No. 1043, from the Superintendent of Documents, U.S. Government Printing Office, Washington, D.C. 20402. You may also find useful the *Mealtime Manual* designed for people with disabilities as well as for the aged, prepared by the Institute of Rehabilitation Medicine at New York University Medical Center, and published in 1978 by Campbell Soup Company, Box (MM) 56, Camden, New Jersey 08101.

• If your appetite is small and you can't eat a big meal all at once, divide your day's food into three small meals with substantial snacks between them and another big snack before bedtime.

• You can organize your own potluck "communal meal" one or more times a week by getting together with a small group of friends, each of whom brings one course. That way you can dine on "only the best" with pleasant company, and no one person has to do all the work. You can set it up on a rotating basis in a different person's house each week, perhaps with the host or hostess for the day preparing the main dish while others bring such items as soup, salad, bread, or dessert.

23 ⚜ ATHLETES:
CAN YOU EAT TO WIN?

MYTHS OR FACTS?

An athlete who works up a good sweat needs to take salt tablets. *Athletes perform best on a salt-restricted diet.*

If you want strong muscles, you've got to eat lots of red meat. *Many of the best athletes eat little or no meat of any kind.*

Don't swallow drinks before or during play—just rinse your mouth or suck on ice cubes. *If you don't drink enough during an event, you can seriously impair your performance and your health.*

To keep up with the demands of heavy exercise, you need to take protein supplements. *Excess protein is unnecessary and potentially harmful to an athlete.*

You need lots of vitamin and mineral supplements to maintain top form and peak energy levels. *If you eat properly, you shouldn't need any extra vitamins or minerals no matter how active you are.*

Carbohydrates make you fat, not strong. *Carbohydrates are the primary fuel for muscles and should be the main ingredient in an athlete's diet.*

The list of contradictory beliefs about what an active person should and should not eat could fill a play-by-play scorecard at a doubleheader. In each pair of the above statements, one is right and one is wrong. Chances are you're not sure which is which. (Actually the second statement in each pair is the correct one.) But don't be embarrassed by your confusion. Many professional athletes and even coaches and trainers are equally uncertain. And now with tens of millions of Americans taking up exercise for the first time, by and large without professional guidance, confusion reigns about a proper diet for good performance and good health.

Even if you're just an occasional weekend hiker, biker, or tennis buff, how you fuel your body can affect your performance, your enjoyment, and the physical benefits you derive from your activity.

"There is no scientific evidence at the present time to indicate that athletic performance can be improved by modifying a basically sound diet," says Dr. Herbert A. deVries, exercise physiologist at the University of Southern California in Los Angeles.

The nation's athletes spend millions of dollars on all kinds of dietary supplements—from energy pills and protein supplements to bee pollen and seaweed. They're all wasting their money because no matter how demanding your sport, you don't need a special diet or a particular food or supplement to keep your body in top condition. Countless studies of extremely active people, both young and old, have shown that *a normal, well-balanced diet best meets the daily demands of any athlete.* This means that, like everyone else, about 10 to 15 percent of your calories should come from protein, no more than 30 percent from fat, and 55 to 60 percent from carbohydrates.

There are many ways to achieve a balanced diet. As an athlete you can be a meat eater or a vegetarian and can enjoy lots of variety in your diet. Also, like other people, you should avoid excessive amounts of saturated animal fats and unnourishing sweets. But unlike your more sedentary neighbors, you can eat more because you expend more calories.

The Protein Propaganda

Muscles are constructed primarily of protein, and many athletes think they've got to eat lots of protein if they want big, strong, dependable muscles. Right? Wrong. As a rule, the well-developed, muscular athlete does not need a greater proportion of protein in his or her diet than someone who runs only to get in out of the rain or who lifts nothing heavier than a pen all day. Using your muscles does not cause them to deteriorate, so no extra protein is needed to rebuild them. What's more, muscles do not require protein for fuel. A study done as long ago as 1866 clearly showed that *strenuous physical activity involves no increased use of protein.*

Only if you were on a starvation or semistarvation diet and had exhausted your carbohydrate stores and easily mobilized fat reserves would your muscles turn to protein for energy. Even then, protein is an inefficient fuel, and when used for energy rather than for tissue building, it forces the body to get rid of the nitrogen that's left over. That means extra work for the liver and kidneys, possibly leading to dehydration (since the kidneys need to dilute the nitrogen with water to excrete it), loss of appetite, and diarrhea. Any time you consume more protein than your body needs as protein, this problem of getting rid of the extra nitrogen comes up. That's why unneeded protein supplements are a bad idea for athletes and sedentary folks alike.

There are just a few instances in which sports and exercise enthusiasts may need more than the usual amounts of protein—when a very young athlete is still growing and putting on new muscle and other tissues; when an adult is building up a significant amount of new muscle (for example, by taking up weight lifting); and when muscle tissues are frequently injured, such as in football or soccer, and must be repaired. But in each of these situations, protein or amino-acid supplements are not needed. The extra protein can easily be obtained through a normal diet that meets the athlete's energy requirements.

There is no mystique about the types of protein athletes require. Red meat in general, and steak in particular, has come to be identified with strength of steel, but the body is not nearly so selective. It can make good use of protein from many kinds of foods—plant and animal. *As a protein source, steak is no better than poultry, fish, pork, lamb, cheese, eggs, or balanced combinations of vegetable protein* (see Chapters 2 and 24). Some of the world's top athletes—including an impressive list of Olympic gold medalists—are vegetarians (see Chapter 24). One vegetarian, Siegfried Bauer, ran the length of New Zealand—a total of 1,350 miles—in just eighteen days. That's an incredible average of 75 miles a day, and he needed not a scrap of red meat to do it.

What Your Muscles Really Run On

The main and most efficient fuel for muscles during vigorous activity comes from carbohydrates. This carbohydrate fuel is stored in your muscle tissue as *glycogen,* with an extra supply housed in the liver. Glycogen, a large molecule, is readily broken down into many molecules of the blood sugar *glucose,* which is the ultimate fuel for muscle cells.

But body stores of glycogen are limited, amounting to only about half a day's supply for a sedentary person. That's why someone who's active should be sure to replenish the body's supply of muscle fuel by eating carbohydrates several times throughout the day. Although the body can make glycogen from fats and protein, this is desirable only if the athlete is trying to lose weight and is not involved in an intensive training program or competition. *A high-protein, high-fat, low-carbohydrate diet is a sure path to quick fatigue and poor performance.* This doesn't mean that the athlete should snack on candy bars or gulp sweetened soft drinks all day. It *does* mean eating nutritious carbohydrates like bread, cereals, pasta, potatoes, rice, and fruit as a regular part of meals and snacks.

In his excellent book *Food for Sport,* Dr. Nathan J. Smith relates what happened to a freshman college basketball player who otherwise ate well but who skimped on his supply of carbohydrate fuel when he most needed it. The student ate a large dormitory breakfast at 8:30 each morning, a generous lunch when the dining room reopened three hours later, and then had nothing more to eat until dinner. Midway through afternoon basketball practice, he'd start to fade. He lacked endurance and had difficulty concentrating. Quite simply, his muscles were not getting enough carbohydrate fuel to keep him going through the strenuous routine. His problem was readily solved. Just before the dining room closed at 2:00 P.M., he went back for a sizable high-carbohydrate snack, and his performance picked up rapidly.

The exact "mix" of fuel used by your muscles depends on how hard you're working them. During light and moderate exercise, the muscles run on free fatty acids as well as on glucose from glycogen. During more demanding exercise—for example, the type involved in strenuous conditioning exercise like running or hard cycling—the muscles draw on their own store of glycogen. When this runs out, you become exhausted. Muscle glycogen becomes the limiting factor in any rigorous activity that requires sustained effort for more than 15 minutes without a rest. It is the crucial factor in endurance sports of all kinds.

When the exercise is extremely intense, such as in sprinting or other activities that cannot be sustained for more than about five minutes, you become exhausted before all your muscle glycogen is used up. At such intense levels, the muscle cells work anaerobically—that is, without the benefit of oxygen. Fatigue results from the rapid build-up of waste products, especially lactic acid, in the muscles.

Carbohydrate Loading

Glycogen stores are vital to an endurance activity, and several studies have shown that the contents of your diet can influence how much glycogen your muscles hold. In one study, ten athletes ran the same 30-kilometer (18.6 miles) race twice, three weeks apart, once after consuming a mixed diet of fats, protein, and carbohydrates for the three previous weeks and once after consuming a high-carbohydrate diet. Every athlete performed better after the high-carbohydrate diet, and the researchers were able to demonstrate that the amount of glycogen in the runners' thigh muscles was doubled by the high-carbohydrate diet.

Dr. Per-Olof Åstrand, a world-renowned exercise physiologist from Stockholm, describes a series of studies that demonstrates the ability of muscles to accumulate extra glycogen by increasing the proportion of carbohydrates in the diet. The most dramatic study involved a test of nine men who were worked to exhaustion on a stationary bicycle after eating different types of foods for the three previous days. After a normal mixed diet of fat, carbohydrates, and protein, the thigh muscles contained an average of 1.75 grams of glycogen per 100 grams of muscle tissue, and the men were able to pedal for an average of 1 hour and 54 minutes. They did only half as well after a diet containing only fats and protein. The best performance was turned in following the carbohydrate-rich diet. The starting level of muscle glycogen was 3.51 grams per 100 grams of muscle (double that following the mixed diet), and the men lasted an average of 2 hours and 47 minutes on the bicycle.

From these and related experiments, Dr. Åstrand and his colleagues developed a diet-exercise scheme for maximizing muscle glycogen in preparation for special endurance events, such as marathon running, cross-country skiing, mountain climbing, hiking, or long-distance swimming. The technique, called carbohydrate loading, can increase an athlete's ability to do hard work by 300 percent, the researchers showed. Their precise method has been modified as a result of recent studies. Here's what sports-medicine specialists now recommend as a safe and effective means of increasing your muscles' energy supply for prolonged endurance events.

Starting three days before the event, decrease the intensity and amount of your exercise program. At the same time, increase your consumption of carbohydrates, concentrating on starchy foods like pasta, perhaps washed down with sugary soft drinks and with ice cream for dessert. Carbohydrates should supply about 70 percent of your day's calories, with the remaining calories fulfilling your daily need for protein along with some fat. This kind of menu, consumed as two or three large meals a day, has been shown to superload the muscles with glycogen in time for the big event.

Carbohydrate loading is recommended *only for occasional prolonged endurance events,* not as a regular dietary pattern. It is of no known benefit to those whose strenuous activity lasts for only 30 to 60 minutes, nor can it possibly help those who do very-high-intensity but brief activities, such as sprinting, where achievement is not limited by lack of fuel.

Some experts say carbohydrate loading should only be attempted by professionally trained athletes under the guidance of a professional nutritionist. Others point out that well-trained athletes are least likely to benefit from overloading their muscles with glycogen because these athletes rely on fatty acids for muscle energy. For them, an ordinary high-carbohydrate diet should do just as well. Possible side effects attributed to carbohydrate loading include stiffness and a heavy feeling in the muscles.

Small spurts of carbohydrate in the form of sugar are of no help during activities that last an hour or less. However, periodic doses of sugar can help improve endurance if consumed at intervals during a prolonged event, such as a Channel swim or a long bicycle race which lasts more than three hours. The sugar you eat is rapidly converted to glucose and carried through the bloodstream to the glycogen-depleted muscles. It matters little what kind of sugar—honey, table sugar, syrup, dextrin, or what have you—as long as it's not consumed in too concentrated a dose. *Avoid taking the sugar straight.* Large, concentrated doses of sugar draw water into the intestinal tract and can cause bloating, cramps, nausea, and diarrhea during vigorous exercise. It's better to get that extra glucose by consuming *lightly sweetened drinks* that also provide the hard-working body with much-needed fluids.

Water: The Athlete's Drink

Few people, including many athletes, appreciate the critical importance of water in keeping the body's machinery operating at peak efficiency. *Inadequate hydration is a major cause of poor performance, fatigue, illness, and occasionally even death during vigorous activity,* especially in hot weather. The body needs water to regulate its temperature through perspiration, to get rid of toxic wastes through urination, to maintain the proper volume and pressure of blood, to supply oxygen and nutrients to muscles and vital organs, and to permit the energy-producing chemical reactions in muscle cells to take place. If muscles are not well hydrated, they'll feel weak and tired; eventually, they'll simply stop working.

The most important thing to realize is that *thirst is not an adequate indication of the amount of water your body needs.* Your thirst can be satisfied long before you've consumed enough liquids to maintain your body in top form during strenuous physical activity. Rather, you have to think actively about drinking and actually "force" fluids to be sure you get enough. As a general rule, you should consume 1 quart of water for every 1,000 calories of food you eat. For the typical athlete who eats 3,000 to 6,000 calories a day, that means 3 to 6 quarts of liquid daily.

Start monitoring your state of hydration for at least two or three days before an event. Not only should you begin your activity with a well-hydrated body, you must also replenish lost water periodically during a prolonged event. A good rule of thumb is to start out with three or more glasses of liquid consumed about three hours before the event. *Never wait to drink until you're thirsty.* Water is far and away the best drink, but pre-event drinks might also include skim milk, fruit juice, lemonade, diluted pineapple juice, clear beef or chicken broth, bouillon, or consommé. Then take another two glasses of water about an hour and a half before (some suggest this amount be taken 15 minutes before). *Continue to drink during the event itself, at least two glasses of water every hour,* best consumed a few ounces at a time every 10 to 15 minutes. It is not enough merely to rinse your mouth or suck on ice. *Don't drink carbonated drinks* since they bloat you with gas. *Ice-cold beverages are okay* and especially useful in cooling the body, but be sure to drink them slowly to avoid gastrointestinal upset.

A good way to assess your body's need for water is to weigh yourself before and after a regular workout. For every pound of weight you lose, you need to replace at least two cups of water. An athlete who loses 3 or more percent of body weight (that means 4 to 5 pounds for the average male) during a strenuous workout or event is likely to perform at less than peak efficiency.

A dramatic example of how the body's supply of water can make or break an athlete's success involved an unsuccessful attempt by a Swiss team to climb Mount Everest. The team carried only enough fuel to melt snow to provide each climber with a pint of water a day during the last three days of the ascent. Not surprisingly, given the extraordinarily hard work of climbing and the low humidity on the mountain, the climbers became increasingly dehydrated and developed such severe fatigue that they had to turn back. When Sir Edmund Hillary's party later succeeded in their conquest of the world's highest mountain peak, they had enough fuel to provide each climber with a full 7 pints of water a day!

Coffee, tea, and colas are dehydrating and, according to some experts, best avoided during practice and competition. But others say coffee and tea are okay in limited amounts because the caffeine they contain reduces fatigue of the muscles. However, caffeine also makes the heart work harder and can aggravate nervous tension during athletic competition. Furthermore, caffeine is a diuretic; it washes water from your body through increased urination, and takes with it vital body salts. Colas contain too much sugar to be used as sources of liquid just before and during vigorous exercise.

Alcohol is also on the no-no list for competing athletes. Although the body metabolizes alcohol as if it were a carbohydrate, the muscles cannot use alcohol as a direct source of energy. Rather, alcohol can dehydrate cells and impair muscle efficiency. And, obviously, it can also interfere with judgment and coordination.

WHAT THE ENDURANCE ATHLETE SHOULD DRINK

The following advice on the best sources of fluids before, during, and after prolonged athletic events was compiled by William J. Fink, physiologist at the Ball State Human Performance Laboratory, at the request of *The Runner,* a magazine on running. It is reprinted with their permission. In the table, "before" means less than half an hour prior to the events, "during" means at any time during the event, and "after" means soon after the event.

WHAT TO DRINK, WHEN, AND WHY

Drink	Before	During	After	Reason
Tap water	Yes	Yes	Yes	The basic liquid your system needs.
Carbonated mineral water	Yes	No	Yes	Carbonation can cause problems during event.
"Athletic" drinks (such as Gatorade, ERG, and the like)	Yes	Yes*	Yes	Only if 10 to 15 minutes before because of possible insulin reaction to sugar.
Cola	No	No	Yes	Has twice as much sugar as athletic drinks and may retard emptying of fluids; good after for carbohydrate replacement.

Table continues on next page

Table continued

Drink	Before	During	After	Reason
Diet cola	Yes	No	No	Carbonation is a problem during and lack of carbohydrates limits value after.
Defizzed cola	No	Yes	No	Properly diluted, a good fluid during but lack of palatability may make it undesirable at other times.
Beer	No	No	Yes	Controversial; alcohol does not help performance; mellowing effect after.
Wine and liquor	No	No	No	Alcohol content is undesirable.
Fruit juices	No	No	Yes	Sugar concentration is high; after, when fluid emptying speed not a factor, okay.
Coffee	Yes	No	No	Caffeine may provide pre-event stimulation.
Iced tea	Yes	Yes	Yes	Plain (without sugar) iced tea is a good source of fluid, plus its caffeine content can be pre-event stimulant.
Milk	No	No	No	More a food than a drink.

*Qualified "yes" during the event because if not well diluted, sugar may retard the emptying of fluid from stomach to intestine.

Salt Tablets Are Dangerous

When you sweat, you lose salt. Many athletes assume that if you work up a good sweat on a regular basis, you've got to replace that salt by taking salt tablets. While this may seem logical, in fact it is unnecessary and potentially dangerous and more likely to hinder than enhance athletic performance.

To operate efficiently, your body depends on water and electrolytes —sodium, potassium, and chloride—that regulate the transport of water into and out of cells and in body fluids. (Salt is sodium chloride, and once in the body it separates into its component parts, sodium and chloride.)

Sodium resides in the fluid outside of cells; potassium regulates fluid within cells. If there is excess sodium in extracellular fluids, which can result from consuming too much salt and other sodium-containing substances (see Chapter 10), water is drawn out of the cells and out of the blood to dilute it. This dehydrates the cells and causes them to work less efficiently; inefficient muscle cells make for poor athletic performance. By lowering the level of water in blood, excess sodium can interfere with the transport of nutrients to muscle and other cells, with the elimination of toxic wastes, and with sweating, which cools the body during exercise. Concentrated doses of salt also increase the loss of potassium, which is essential to the proper working of muscle cells, including those in the heart.

Although salt is lost along with sweat, the concentration of salt in sweat is less than that in the blood, so proportionately more water than salt needs to be replaced if you sweat heavily. According to Dr. Smith, *the safest way to replace lost sweat is with plain water.* Rarely is it necessary to specifically replace the salt, unless you lose 5 to 10 pounds during a workout or event. Then the best way to get the extra salt is by sprinkling a little on your food or by consuming a cup of bouillon or drinking a very diluted salt solution containing ⅓ teaspoon of salt per quart of water.

Taking salt tablets greatly distorts the desirable ratio of salt to water. In addition to impairing performance by dehydrating your cells, this salt excess can actually contribute to heat prostration by interfering with your sweating mechanism. *Salt tablets are dangerous substances that every athlete should avoid, unless the tablets are prescribed by a knowledgeable physician for a specific problem.*

Dr. Gabe Mirkin, a sports-medicine specialist and competitive athlete from Silver Spring, Maryland, and coauthor with Marshall Hoffman of *The Sportsmedicine Book* (Boston: Little, Brown, 1978), states that, rather than loading an athlete with salt, restricting salt is the best way to improve athletic performance during hot weather. Through repeated workouts during warm weather, the body gradually learns to conserve salt. As summer approaches, the sweat gets less and less salty and the kidneys also retain salt. Several studies of accomplished athletes have shown that some athletes consistently perform better in hot weather following a long-established salt-restricted diet.

B_1, B_{12}, Bee Pollen, and Other Fads

Although the public image of athletes is of pure and simple folk who are careful to preserve their health and eat only what's good for them, many in fact are pill poppers. In all fairness, most of it is well intentioned and primarily involves vitamin and mineral preparations that athletes hope will preserve their health and improve their performance. Unfortunately, it's all a waste of time and money, and some of it is downright dangerous.

In Dr. Mirkin's view, the prize for the most pills goes to Bob Scharf, a marathoner of the 1960s who gulped down fifty-one food supplements each day, including vitamins C, E, and B complex, iron, zinc, phosphates, lecithin, bone meal, dessicated liver, yeast, wheatgerm oil, kelp, garlic, bee pollen, and ginseng.

There is no evidence that any of these supplements, or any other nutrient concoctions purported to promote athletic prowess, improves performance, strength, or endurance or prevents illness or injury. Unless an athlete is suffering from a shortage of a particular vitamin or mineral, supplements can do him or her no good. If athletes eat a reasonably well-balanced diet, given the number of calories they consume, the likelihood of a shortage of a micronutrient is slim.

The one possible exception is *iron* for adolescent girls and women. Iron deficiencies are common among menstruating females, a combined effect of lost menstrual blood and low food intake in an attempt to keep body weight as low as possible. While it is certainly best to get needed iron from your regular diet—say, by eating liver or kidneys once a week and by daily consumption of such iron-rich foods as beef, dark-green leafy vegetables, dried beans and peas, or iron-fortified cereals—some female athletes may need to take an iron supplement.

Athletes of both sexes should pay particular attention to two micronutrients important to the proper functioning of muscle cells. One of these is the mineral *potassium,* which helps to regulate water balance and catalyzes the release of energy and other activities within muscle cells. Some potassium is lost to the blood and urine in your body's effort to prevent overheating, but even more serious losses occur following the use of diuretics and cathartics. Insufficient potassium in the muscles causes weakness and fatigue. If you include such potassium-rich foods as bananas, orange juice, dried fruits, and nuts (unsalted) in your daily diet, no potassium supplement is needed or desirable. In fact, potassium supplements can be dangerous.

Magnesium can also be lost to the detriment of athletic performance. It is necessary for proper contraction and relaxation of muscle fibrils and for releasing the energy in carbohydrates. Good sources of magnesium include nuts (especially almonds and cashews), meat, fish, milk, whole grains, and fresh dark leafy greens.

Athletes also need more *thiamin* and *riboflavin* than nonathletes to help them burn the extra carbohydrates they consume, but they get all they need from their diet because they eat more calories than nonathletes. Thiamin-rich foods include whole-grain and enriched breads and cereals, milk, eggs, organ meats, and pork. Foods rich in riboflavin include liver, milk, meat, dark-green vegetables, eggs, whole-grain and enriched cereals and bread products, mushrooms, and dried beans and peas. There is no evidence that supplements of thiamin or other B vitamins improve athletic performance.

As for other highly touted supplements for athletes, the evidence shows that none is necessary or helpful to athletic performance.

Vitamin C. Large doses don't prevent colds or speed the healing of athletic injuries. Possible side effects of megadoses of C include diarrhea, kidney and bladder stones, destruction of vitamin B_{12}, and iron poisoning (from the increased absorption of iron caused by too much C).

Vitamin E. Scientific findings do not support the belief that vitamin E increases stamina or improves the delivery of oxygen to the muscles. More than adequate amounts of this vitamin are obtained in diets that include vegetable oils and whole grains.

Vitamin B_{12}. Deficiencies of this vitamin are extremely rare and limited to persons with a disorder in which the protein needed to absorb B_{12} through the gut is lacking. Vegetarians who consume no animal foods also need B_{12} supplements. For the rest of the population, Dr. Mirkin says, B_{12} supplements do nothing to counter fatigue.

"Energy" pills. These are a waste of time and money. As Dr. Smith points out, if you take six tablets a day as the package prescribes, you consume only 84 calories—less than the caloric content of a glass of soda or a slice of buttered toast. Nor can large doses of any vitamin, either alone or in combination, increase your energy. Vitamins are merely regulators of metabolic activity, not sources of energy.

Aspartate salts. Studies by the United States Army of both animals and men found no support for the claim that the magnesium and potassium salts of aspartic acid increase endurance by reducing muscle fatigue.

Gelatin. Endurance tests have shown no benefit from eating gelatin or the amino acid glycine found in it (and in many other protein foods). In fact, gelatin by itself is a useless form of protein for the body because it lacks two essential amino acids.

Weight Control

Except for fashion models and professional dancers, athletes worry more about their weight than any other group of people. An overweight athlete tends to be slower and to tire more readily than his slimmer rival. One who is too thin may lack needed energy reserves to meet the demands of sports. Yet for someone in intensive training who's burning 6,000 to 10,000 calories a day, eating enough to maintain body weight can be a problem.

You've already seen that exercise is important to weight control, giving you more caloric leeway in your diet and suppressing appetite (see Chapter 17). The number of calories burned during physical exercise depends on many factors—how big you are (thinner and smaller people burn less calories at the same activity level than heavier or larger people), how hard or fast you work out (the harder the labor or faster the speed, the more calories burned per minute), the air temperature (you burn more calories in colder weather), the clothes you wear, the type of surface you play on, as well as the particular activity you're involved in and how you carry it out. For example, you can burn 600 calories an hour playing tennis if you play a fast-paced game and run after every ball, but only half that amount if you're a lackadaisical player.

Table 23.1 provides an estimate of caloric expenditure involved in various athletic activities for the average person at various weights. It should be used only as a rough guide to the amount of calories you may be burning at your sport.

As a rule, an athlete in training needs to consume at least 2,000 calories a day—even while on a weight-reducing diet—to have enough of a ready energy supply to get through workouts and events. Since the typical athlete burns more than 3,000 calories a day, such a diet means a daily caloric deficit of at least 1,000 calories, resulting in loss of 2 pounds a week since each pound of body fat contains about 3,500 calories. It is unwise for a physically active person to try to lose weight

Table 23.1 • HOW MANY CALORIES DO YOU BURN?
CALORIES USED PER MINUTE ACCORDING TO YOUR WEIGHT

Activity	Weight in Pounds						
	100	120	150	170	200	220	250
Badminton	4.3	5.2	6.5	7.4	8.7	9.6	10.9
Bicycling, 5.5 mph	3.1	3.8	4.7	5.3	6.3	6.9	7.9
Bicycling, 10 mph	5.4	6.5	8.1	9.2	10.8	11.9	13.6
Calisthenics	3.3	3.9	4.9	5.6	6.6	7.2	8.2
Canoeing, 4 mph	4.6	5.6	7.0	7.9	9.3	10.2	11.6
Golf	3.6	4.3	5.4	6.1	7.2	7.9	9.0
Handball	6.3	7.6	9.5	10.7	12.7	13.9	15.8
Mountain climbing	6.6	8.0	10.0	11.3	13.3	14.6	16.6
Jogging, 11-min. mile	6.1	7.3	9.1	10.4	12.2	13.4	15.3
Running, 8-min. mile	9.4	11.3	14.1	16.0	18.8	20.7	23.5
Running, 5-min. mile	13.1	15.7	19.7	22.3	26.3	28.9	32.8
Racquetball	6.3	7.6	9.5	10.7	12.7	13.9	15.8
Skating, moderate	3.6	4.3	5.4	6.1	7.2	7.9	9.0
Skiing, downhill	6.3	7.6	9.5	10.7	12.7	13.9	15.8
Skiing, cross-country	7.2	8.7	10.8	12.3	14.5	15.9	18.0
Squash	6.8	8.1	10.2	11.5	13.6	14.9	17.0
Swimming, breaststroke	4.8	5.7	7.2	8.1	9.6	10.5	12.0
Swimming, crawl	5.8	6.9	8.7	9.8	11.6	12.7	14.5
Table tennis	2.7	3.2	4.0	4.6	5.4	5.9	6.8
Tennis	4.5	5.4	6.8	7.7	9.1	10.0	11.4
Volleyball, moderate	2.3	2.7	3.4	3.9	4.6	5.0	5.7
Walking, 3 mph	2.7	3.2	4.0	4.6	5.4	5.9	6.8
Walking, 4 mph	3.9	4.6	5.8	6.6	7.8	8.5	9.7

Note: To calculate the approximate number of calories you burn at a given activity, find the figure in the table closest to your weight and multiply by the number of minutes of continuous activity. These numbers were developed under standardized conditions at the Human Performance Research Center at Brigham Young University in Provo, Utah. Many factors, such as air temperature, clothing, and the vigor with which you participate, can result in an increase or decrease in the number of calories you burn.

much faster than this. A more stringent diet can result in fatigue and weakness and compromise the training program.

Diuretics (water pills) or cathartics should never be used to achieve a quick weight loss. They wash potassium and water out of your body and can impair the workings of your muscle cells. If you must take medically prescribed diuretics because of high blood pressure or some other illness, be sure to consume an adequate amount of potassium-rich foods (see page 185) and drink plenty of water to avoid dehydration.

Female athletes, as well as some male wrestlers, jockeys, and oarsmen, sometimes attempt to maintain weights that are too low for their body types, shortchanging themselves on stamina in the process.

A girl with a large bone structure cannot expect to weigh the same as her companion who is slightly built, even if they're the same height. The amount and distribution of body fat determine desirable body weight, and body fat is something most athletes have very little of. Their weight is determined mainly by muscle, water, vital organs, and bone. At any given weight the well-conditioned person will look and measure thinner than someone who is not active and has a higher percentage of body fat.

The average American male carries around 15 to 20 percent of his weight as fat, and the female 25 to 30 percent. Athletes, including football players who weigh over 200 pounds and weight lifters who may approach 300, have half that percentage of fat or less. Some gymnasts have no body fat stores at all, and marathoners typically carry around only a few percent of their weight as fat. In sports that involve physical contact and potential injury, like football, a higher percentage of fat is desirable since it provides protective padding for the kidneys and other vital organs.

Rather than having to worry about losing weight, some athletes have a problem keeping their weight from dropping too low. For many, it requires a special effort to eat enough to keep up with their daily caloric expenditure. An athlete who burns more than 4,000 calories a day will need substantial snacks several times a day in addition to regular meals (at which second helpings are *de rigueur*). But while it may be easy to pack in calories by consuming foods high in sugars and saturated animal fats, that's no more healthy for the athlete than for anyone else. Better to eat peanut-butter sandwiches, bananas, raisin bread, low-fat milk shakes, or fruit-flavored yogurt to fill out the calorie quota.

One word of warning, though: if and when you stop intensive training and competition, you have to reduce the amount of food you eat or you'll gain weight. Some former athletes actually become obese following retirement because they continue to eat the way they did when they were working off 6,000 calories a day, although as salesmen, coaches, or teachers they are burning only half that. Former athletes should also continue to exercise as they get older, since those who are athletic in their youth and sedentary in middle age appear to be even more susceptible to coronary heart disease than persons who had never exercised strenuously at all! Among football players who made it into *Who's Who in American Sports,* 35 percent died before the age of 50, and the average age of death for the group was 57—10 years younger than for the average American male.

What to Eat before Competition

Athletes are a superstitious bunch when it comes to food. Dr. Smith points out that "many runners regard pizza as a 'fast' food (one that helps them run fast), while soccer players the world over demand bacon and eggs before a game." Football players traditionally down a pregame ceremonial meal of steak, baked potatoes, dry toast, and tea. Then there was the lady swimmer who broke the world's record for the 200-meter butterfly after a prerace meal of two hamburgers with onions, French fries with ketchup, root beer, three brownies, and a candy bar.

However, most athletes would do better on simpler fare. The goals of the pre-event meal are to give your muscles the energy they need, to keep you from getting hungry while you're competing, to make sure your body is well hydrated, and to prevent gastrointestinal upset during the event. You don't want to be exercising strenuously with a stomach and intestinal tract filled with food or waste. Thus, both the timing and the constituents of the pre-event meal must be carefully planned. As with fluids, you should start thinking about your foods a day or two before the event. Avoid foods that produce intestinal gas and bulk for 48 hours before competing. These include raw fruits (except oranges, bananas, and peeled apples, which you should eat), raw vegetables (except lettuce), nuts, popcorn, cabbage, beans, onions, cauliflower, vegetables with seeds (for example, tomatoes and cucumbers), bran, and other whole-grain products.

The pre-event meal should be eaten three to four hours beforehand to give your gastrointestinal tract time to process it before you begin exercising vigorously. The idea is to have your stomach and upper small intestine relatively empty before the event. Thus, the meal should be low in fats and proteins, which take a relatively long time to digest, and high in carbohydrates.

Too much protein can also create a water shortage in your blood and muscle cells. Too little carbohydrate deprives your muscles of needed fuel. But avoid too much sugar, since this can lead to gnawing hunger two to three hours later and may result in cramps and nausea from the water the sugar draws into the stomach and small intestine.

Here are two examples of easy-to-digest pre-event meals:

• Orange juice, cereal with skim milk, lightly buttered toast, banana, two glasses of fluid (but preferably not coffee or tea).

• A small serving (2 ounces) of lean meat or poultry (broiled or roasted, not fried), skim milk, orange or banana, baked or mashed potato or pasta, tomato juice, cooked carrots, two plain cookies, and 2 cups of liquid.

In addition, the experts agree that you can eat any food that you believe helps you to win and that you've consumed before previous events without gastrointestinal mishap. Regardless of the general rules, everyone is an individual. If you think a pickle before a race is a winning food and your system can handle it, eat it. Athletic victories are as much psychological as they are physical, and no sports physician wants to deprive an athlete of that all-important psychological boost.

For those whose stomachs are sufficiently finicky at competition time to prevent solid food from going down or staying down well, there are a number of commercially prepared liquid meals that are easy to digest and that provide adequate pre-event nutrition. They are also useful as a source of fuel and water during prolonged endurance events. These products, developed for hospital patients who cannot eat solid foods, include Ensure, Sustacal, and Sustagen and can be purchased at pharmacies. They are different from powdered meals or instant breakfasts, which contain too much fat and protein to be used before athletic events.

You can also make your own pre-event liquid meal by combining the following:

Pre-Event Liquid Meal

½ cup nonfat dry milk	¼ cup sugar
3 cups skim milk	1 teaspoon vanilla or other
½ cup water	flavoring

Yield: 4 cups.

One cup of this drink provides 200 calories. Two cups consumed on a relatively empty stomach passes through the stomach within about two hours.

Eat well, and may the best person win!

FOR FURTHER READING

Nathan J. Smith, M.D., *Food for Sport* (Palo Alto, Calif.: Bull, 1976).

24 ⟨⟨ IS IT HEALTHY TO BE A VEGETARIAN?

FOR CENTURIES, the few who chose to be vegetarians were considered a little crazy. The domestication and slaughter of animals for food was, after all, one of the great achievements of humankind. Those who shunned animal foods for religious reasons were tolerated. But most people thought (and many still do) that you had to be some kind of nut to exclude such foods on mere dietary grounds.

To be sure, some vegetarians were popular despite their strange diet. George Bernard Shaw became a vegetarian because he refused to eat "corpses." Leonardo da Vinci, Ralph Waldo Emerson, Henry David Thoreau, Benjamin Franklin, Mahatma Gandhi, Albert Schweitzer, and Gloria Swanson also advocated a meatless diet, as did several notable Greeks—Pythagoras, Socrates, and Plato (although they were not strict vegetarians themselves).

Contributing to vegetarianism's bad name were those proselytizing fanatics who raged against the killing of man's fellow beasts and painted gory pictures of animal slaughter. There were also those who adopted bizarre diets repugnant even to their fellow vegetarians. One such diet, "zen macrobiotics" originated by a Japanese named Georges Ohsawa, actually led to the deaths of some adherents who followed the regimen to its "highest" level—a 100-percent cereal diet. Ordinary vegetarians are not nearly so limited in food choices and can live very healthfully without animal foods.

In recent years, however, vegetarianism has acquired a better reputation and a burgeoning popularity. Large numbers of young adults, many of whom as children probably had to be begged to eat their vegetables, have for a variety of aesthetic, health, and moral reasons chosen a meatless way of life. Countless articles, books, and cookbooks now guide vegetarians through the maze of vegetable matter and help to win wider public acceptance for the vegetarian diet and its many converts.

What Is a Vegetarian?

There are different kinds of vegetarian diets, so just knowing that people are vegetarians doesn't really tell you what, in addition to vegetables, may be included in their diet. The following are the three basic types of vegetarian diets:

Strict vegetarians, or vegans. No animal foods of any kind are eaten. All protein is derived entirely from plant sources.

Lactovegetarians. Animal protein in the form of milk, cheese, and other dairy products is included, but no meat, fish, poultry, or eggs are eaten.

Ovolactovegetarians. Animal protein in the form of eggs and dairy products is eaten, but no meat, fish, or poultry.

In addition, many people are "part-time" vegetarians. That is, they rely mainly on plant foods but occasionally eat meat, fish, or poultry. The departures from their regular vegetarian diets are most commonly made when visiting friends or relatives who are not vegetarians. Still others who consider themselves vegetarians are willing to eat fish, but not meat or poultry.

Why People Become Vegetarians

Ancient Hebrew Scriptures contain the earliest written record of a vegetarian diet. God tells Adam in the Garden of Eden about the fruits, nuts, and grains "to you it shall be for meat." After the expulsion from Eden, Adam's diet was extended to include the entire plant. But it wasn't until the Great Flood had destroyed all vegetation that the Hebrew God gave people permission to eat "every moving thing that liveth."

Many Eastern religions, including Buddhism, Brahmanism, Hinduism, and Jainism, extol a vegetarian diet, although there are no penalties for eating flesh. Two religious groups in the United States today also are vegetarian: the Trappist monks of the Roman Catholic Church and the Seventh-Day Adventists. The Adventist Church recommends a vegetarian diet to its followers, but makes it a matter of individual choice.

Others become vegetarians for health and hygienic reasons, spurning meat as a cause of digestive problems and disease and a source of unhealthful chemicals and infectious organisms. In fact, it was the presumed healthfulness of a meatless diet that led to the beginnings of an organized vegetarian movement in England and the United States in the last century. One advocate in this country was Dr. John Harvey Kellogg (of the family that started the cereal company), who, as medical director of the Battle Creek (Michigan) Sanitarium, prescribed an "antitoxic diet" consisting chiefly of fruits, cereals, and fresh vegetables.

In recent years, ecological considerations have attracted large numbers of people, particularly members of the youth counterculture, to vegetarianism. These people reason that it is wasteful of the earth's limited resources to feed plants to animals and then eat the animals. And they are right. Depending on the animal, it takes anywhere from 2 to 10 pounds of grain to produce 1 pound of edible meat. An acre of land can produce ten times as much vegetable protein if planted as it can of animal protein if given over to cattle grazing. Currently, 90 percent of the soybeans, corn, oats, and barley grown in this country is fed to livestock. There would be a lot more protein to go around if these plant sources of protein were eaten by people directly instead of by pigs, cattle, and chickens.

Vegetarians and food economists call this alternative "eating low on the food chain." One potential advantage is that the higher on the food chain you eat, the greater your chances of accumulating large amounts of toxic materials present in tiny amounts in foods at the bottom of the chain. This is, in fact, what has happened to birds of prey like falcons, ospreys, and eagles. They eat big fish that eat smaller fish that eat still smaller fish, and so on down to one-celled organisms. Each creature up the line accumulates the residues of long-lasting pesticides like DDT from the animals it feeds on; the birds at the top of this food chain end up with so much DDT that their reproductive ability is severely damaged. It is not known whether we who live primarily on meat, right at the top of the human food chain, also accumulate dangerous residues. But many ask, "Why take the chance?"

Were We Meant to Be Meat Eaters?

Some believe that eliminating meat as a source of nutrients literally goes against human nature. But the evidence from evolution and comparative anatomy suggests otherwise. While Homo sapiens was not designed exclusively for a herbaceous diet, neither is a human being built like a flesh-eating carnivore. In fact, we have some features of both the herbivore and the carnivore, and on balance our omniverous (both plant- and meat-eating) anatomical equipment strongly leans toward a heavily vegetarian diet.

The teeth of carnivores are designed for killing prey and cutting and tearing flesh. Carnivores have long, strong, pointed canine teeth— the fangs—next to the small incisors in front. The fangs stab and hold flesh. Their upper premolars and lower molars are also large and better designed for cutting than for grinding. They are called "flesh teeth" and serve to slice through flesh like a pair of shears. As a result, the jaw moves very little from side to side, limiting the carnivore's ability to grind food. Carnivores don't chew their food very well, and tend to swallow large chunks after only a few chomps.

Herbivores, on the other hand, have small canines and sharp cutting incisors in front for biting off mouthfuls of food. Their molars have flattened surfaces well suited for crushing and grinding. In addition, the jaws of herbivores can move a great deal from side to side, enabling them to chew well the fibrous vegetable matter they live on. This greatly enhances the digestibility of plant foods.

Our teeth are more like those of herbivores than of flesh eaters. Our front teeth are large and sharp, good for biting; our canines are small—almost vestigial compared to a tiger's; our molars are flattened; and our jaws are mobile for grinding food into the small bits we are able to swallow. Dr. Alan Walker of Johns Hopkins University conducted microscopic analyses of the wear patterns on the teeth of our humanlike ancestors, which indicate that we evolved from fruit eaters, not flesh eaters. The fossil teeth of these early hominids contain none of the scratch marks found on the teeth of animals that gnaw on bones and flesh.

As for the digestive tract, here, too, we are more like the herbivore. Carnivores have a comparatively short, smooth intestinal tract, only about three times the length of their body. Since they eat raw meat that decomposes rapidly, they must digest it fast and get rid of the wastes before toxins accumulate. With the carnivore, food goes in and waste comes out of the digestive tract very fast.

The human digestive tract, while lacking the double stomach of herbivorous ruminants like cattle, bears even less resemblance to that of the carnivores. Our intestines are long—twelve times as long as the torso—and highly convoluted, allowing us to digest substances that take a long time to be broken down and absorbed. Plant foods, with their large amounts of fiber, are just such substances. But whether plant or animal, food takes its merry time passing through the human digestive system. This leaves animal waste in the body for far longer than it remains in carnivores, and (as you will see later in more detail) this fact may be related to the high rates of cancer of the colon and rectum among people who eat a lot of meat.

Early man, anthropologists and archeologists have reason to believe, subsisted mainly on vegetation—fruits, nuts, tubers, berries, and grains. Analyses of fossilized human fecal matter certainly show this. Meat was only occasionally on the menu, following infrequent kills. The invention of agriculture—the cultivation of crops for food—further assured a steady supply of edible plants for our ancestors. But it was a long time before animals were domesticated and raised for food, and even then, they were infrequently consumed. More likely, they served as suppliers of such renewable resources as milk and eggs, and were only eaten for meat when they no longer produced.

The American Dietetic Association notes that "most of mankind for much of human history has subsisted on near-vegetarian diets," and much of the world still lives that way. Until relatively recently Americans did as well. The American love affair with meat is but a century old. The affluence of the twentieth century has led to a dramatic increase in our dependence on animal foods. Consumption of beef (thanks largely to hamburger chains) has increased most dramatically, from 58 pounds per person a year in 1940 to 89 pounds per person per year in 1978. The U.S. Department of Agriculture says that each year, the average American consumes a total of more than 200 pounds of meat, poultry, and seafood. And that's not counting such foods as dairy products and eggs. With meat serving as an international status symbol, eleven developed countries consume about 40 percent of the entire world's meat supply.

In our tendency to consume animal food at every opportunity, we resemble our nearest living evolutionary relative, the ape. Although long considered to be vegetarians, primates like chimpanzees, orangutans, gorillas, and gibbons are now known to eat animal matter whenever they can. Mostly, they eat insects, and usually in small amounts. When no insects or other animal foods are available, the lower primates revert to a vegetarian diet with no ill effects. However, when insects are abundant and easily caught, they may form 90 percent of the primate diet. Sometimes primates kill larger prey, ranging in size from rodents to infant antelopes and the adult females of other primate species.

But while lower primates are limited by natural forces in their dependence on animal foods, for affluent humans there are no such barriers. Faced with constant opportunity, we eat vast quantities of animal foods, more than our bodies were designed to handle.

Do Vegetarians Live Longer?

The notion that big animals like us can't make it without eating meat is patently false. After all, the mammoths of yore were vegetarians, and the elephants, oxen, and horses of today perform feats of great strength exclusively on plant foods.

During World War I, the British blockade of the North Sea effectively cut off Denmark from the sources of imported foods needed to maintain the country's omnivorous diet. Denmark was dependent on imported grains to feed its livestock. Rather than starve, the Danes diverted their livestock food supply to feed themselves. Instead of meat, they lived on potatoes, bran, and barley plus green vegetables and some dairy products. Three million people, although not happy about their meatless, low-protein diet, survived, and, the statistics later showed, fared better than usual. During the year when food was most severely restricted, the death rate in Copenhagen fell dramatically, 34 percent below the level of the previous eighteen years. Although other events, such as wartime limitations on alcohol and tobacco, undoubtedly contributed to the lowered death rate, the dietary change is thought to have been a very significant factor.

World War II foisted a similar situation upon Norway. For five years, only meager rations of meat were available to its citizens, who had to rely heavily on cereals, potatoes, and other vegetables and fish. Deaths from heart and blood-vessel diseases dropped dramatically during the war years, only to rise to their high prewar levels as soon as the restored peace enabled Norwegians to return to their old animal diet.

Then there are the long-lived peoples—the Hunzans of northern Pakistan, the Abkhasians of the Soviet Union, and the Vilcabambams of Ecuador—whose diets contain little animal foods. While many factors, including high levels of exercise and low levels of stress, undoubtedly contribute to the longevity of these people, suffice it to say that their diets do no harm and may do some good.

A Vegetarian Diet Can Protect Your Heart

Some telling statistics:

Seventh-Day Adventists, most of whom eat no meat or poultry (and also don't smoke or drink), have only 60 percent the amount of heart disease that other Americans have.

A comparative study of diet and heart disease in seven countries showed that the death rate from coronary heart disease was highest in those countries that consumed the most animal products. The Finns, who consumed the most animal fats, also had the highest death rate. Americans were next, but the Greeks and Italians, who eat relatively little animal fat, were near the bottom of the death-rate list. In Japan, where very little fat of any kind is eaten, the heart-disease death rate is lower than in any other industrialized nation, despite high rates of high blood pressure and cigarette smoking among the Japanese.

A study of 116 young vegetarians in Boston showed that those vegetarians who consumed dairy products and eggs more than five times a week had higher blood pressures and cholesterol levels than those who ate these animal foods less often or not at all. But all categories of vegetarians had lower blood pressures and cholesterol levels than comparable groups of meat-eating young adults.

The main dietary factors affecting heart-disease rates are believed to be saturated fats and cholesterol derived primarily from animal foods (see Chapter 3), which clog blood vessels with fatty deposits called atherosclerotic plaques and make a heart attack more likely. If this association is correct, as is widely indicated by studies throughout the world, it stands to reason that vegetarians would be spared this disease.

A recent study in Italy suggests that an additional factor—the source of protein—may be at work in protecting vegetarians from heart disease. Scientists at the University of Milan showed that on diets equally low in fat and cholesterol, persons eating animal protein had higher levels of cholesterol in their blood than those fed a diet containing primarily vegetable (soy) protein. Furthermore, recent research has shown that certain types of dietary fibers found in plant foods can help to lower blood cholesterol (see Chapter 7).

Even those vegetarians who eat dairy products and eggs, which contain saturated animal fat and cholesterol, are not likely to come anywhere near the fat and cholesterol content of the typical mixed American diet. This is because vegetarians depend heavily on plant foods, which contain no cholesterol whatever and little or no saturated fat. Thus, a vegetarian could consume a quart of whole milk or several ounces of cheese or one egg a day and not exceed the recommended intake of cholesterol. However, a wise vegetarian would avoid an overdependence on eggs and high-fat dairy products and rely instead on skimmed milk and low-fat yogurt and cheeses. Too many people who have stopped eating red meat have substituted fatty cheeses, which have as much fat and a lot more salt.

It's Hard to Be a Fat Vegetarian

Considering the vast number of weight-conscious Americans, it's surprising that more people have not become vegetarians. The young vegetarians studied in Boston weighed on average 33 pounds less than the meat-eating comparison group. Because a vegetarian diet is bulky and filling, it's hard to eat more calories than your body burns. As a result, most people lose weight when they start a vegetarian diet. A look at the calories eaten by a theoretical meat-and-potatoes man will show why.

A "MEAT AND POTATOES" MENU

Meal	Calories
BREAKFAST	
Juice, 4 ounces	54
2 slices bacon	140
2 eggs, fried	225
2 slices toast and jelly	235
Total	654
LUNCH	
Cheeseburger	390
French fries	170
Beer	150
Total	710
DINNER	
Steak, 6 ounces	700
Potato with 1 tablespoon butter	250
Carrots, ½ cup	25
Salad with blue-cheese dressing	175
Apple pie	350
Total	1,500
Total for day:	2,864.

No wine or martinis, or between-meal snacks have been included. These could easily swell the day's caloric total by another 500 calories. For the average 160-pound man of moderate activity, a daily menu like this would mean an excess of some 150 calories a day and a weight gain of about 16 pounds in a year.

Unless a vegetarian gorges on bread and cakes and cheese, he or she would be hard put to consume this many calories in a day. The calories in two slices of bacon exceed those in a cup of cooked oatmeal. A lunch of vegetable soup, a slice of whole-grain bread, and a cottage cheese and fruit salad has a third fewer calories than the cheeseburger lunch (and far, far less saturated fat and cholesterol). And for the caloric value of a 6-ounce steak, a vegetarian could eat 3 cups of rice or a whole pound of noodles! Or, to be more reasonable, the vegetarian could eat a very generous serving of a casserole of noodles, vegetables, and cheese, which would eliminate the need for the potatoes and carrots in the steak dinner.

Those who are strict vegetarians (vegans) and eat no dairy products or eggs may actually have a hard time consuming enough calories to maintain their weight. A meal of a cup of brown rice and lentils, two slices of whole-grain bread (or a large baked potato) with margarine, ½ cup each of carrots and peas, a lettuce and tomato salad with dressing, and a fruit salad containing one banana, one apple, one orange, 2 tablespoons of raisins, and half a dozen walnuts, would contain about 890 calories (610 less than the steak dinner) and leave the diner positively stuffed. While this is not typical of a meal that might be prepared by an experienced vegan, it does illustrate the huge amounts of food a vegan can consume without exceeding the body's caloric needs.

In addition to the social and psychological rewards of a trim figure, the health benefits of maintaining a normal body weight include a reduced risk of developing heart disease, diabetes, high blood pressure, back troubles, and certain types of cancer (see Chapter 15).

A Vegetarian Diet and Cancer

Tantalizing research findings during the last decade have revealed that hand in hand with a low risk of coronary heart disease goes a low risk of contracting cancers of the colon, breast, and uterus. It seems as if the same kind of diet high in animal fats and cholesterol that sets the stage for heart disease may also contribute to the growth of these cancers. Among the Seventh-Day Adventists and the Japanese, for example, these cancers are quite rare, but they are leading causes of cancer among ordinary meat-eating Americans. (The Japanese get stomach cancer, but that's an entirely different matter.)

There are several possible explanations for this relationship (see Chapters 3 and 7 for greater detail). With regard to colon cancer, diets rich in saturated fats and cholesterol may result in large accumulations of natural cancer-promoting chemicals in the gut. And the relatively low fiber content of such diets may result in slow-moving bowels and prolonged contact of the cancer-promoting chemicals with body tissues.

As for cancers of the breast and uterus, their growth is stimulated by estrogen hormones. Diets high in fat and cholesterol result in the production of estrogenlike hormones in the gut, and similar hormones are produced in body fat.

Another possible source of cancer protection for vegetarians is the finding that a variety of vegetable foods and fruit, including Brussels sprouts, cauliflower, broccoli, turnips, cabbage, spinach, celery, citrus fruits, beans, and seeds, can stimulate the production of anticancer enzymes in the body. In a study by Dr. Saxon Graham, professor of social and preventive medicine at the State University of New York at Buffalo, people who regularly consumed large amounts of vegetables in the cabbage family were found to have lower-than-expected rates of cancer of the colon and rectum. A chemical found in these vegetables is known to block the action of certain cancer-causing substances.

Athletes Don't Need Meat

It has been known for more than a hundred years that muscles use carbohydrates and fats, not protein, for fuel. Yet the myth that athletes need extra protein persists. This is true only for people who are in the process of increasing the size of their muscles, and even then the amount of additional protein needed is ordinarily supplied by a normal diet, which usually contains excess protein to begin with (see Chapter 23 for a detailed discussion). Thus, a vegetarian athlete who is consuming the recommended amounts of protein is not likely to be shortchanging his or her performance potential. In fact, studies show that he or she might be achieving the reverse!

Back in 1904, vegetarian and nonvegetarian students were compared as to how many times they could squeeze a grip meter in quick succession. The vegetarians scored an average of 69 times; the nonvegetarians averaged 38. More recently, nine Swedish athletes tested for endurance on a stationary bicycle lasted nearly three times longer after a three-day diet high in vegetables and grains but low in protein than they did after three days of a high-meat diet (see page 420 for details).

If you're still not convinced that champions can be made on what is sometimes disparagingly called "rabbit food," note these achievements recounted by Vic Sussman in his illuminating book, *The Vegetarian Alternative:*

- Paavo Nurmi (the Flying Finn) trained on a vegetarian diet and set twenty world running records between 1920 and 1932.
- Bill Pickering, a British vegetarian, swam the English Channel in 1956 in record-breaking time.
- Murray Rose, an Australian who had been a vegetarian since the age of 2, at age 17 became the youngest Olympic triple gold medal winner for swimming events in 1956. In later years, he won more medals and set new records in swimming meets.
- Bill Walton, star of the Portland Trailblazers and perhaps the world's best all-around basketball player, is a vegetarian.

It's Easy to Be a "Good" Vegetarian

. . . if you know how. As explained in Chapter 2, there are two important facts that a vegetarian must appreciate to assure an adequate diet. One is that vegetable sources of protein are less complete and less efficiently used by the body than animal proteins. This means that *you must know how to combine vegetable proteins in a way that makes them complete and thus able to fulfill your body's protein requirements.* The second fact is that *if the protein you eat is to be used to meet your protein requirement, your diet must contain enough calories to support your ideal weight.* Otherwise, the body will use the protein for fuel and there won't be enough for growth and rebuilding of body tissues.

These facts are less crucial to a lacto- or ovolactovegetarian than to a vegan. But anyone who relies primarily or exclusively on vegetable protein should keep these needs uppermost in mind. A third fact to remember is that strict vegetarian diets contain inadequate amounts of vitamin B_{12}, unless some B_{12} supplement is included. *A vegetarian diet that is haphazard can lead to serious nutritional deficiencies.* In addition, if you are pregnant or nursing a baby, your requirements for protein, vitamins, and minerals increase significantly. It's difficult to meet these increased needs on an all-vegetable diet. Guidance from a physician and a nutritionist is advisable to avoid shortchanging yourself and your baby.

That said, let's go back to the original statement. It really *is* easy to be a good vegetarian. You don't need a lot of time, a detailed knowledge of nutrition, elaborate charts or formulas, a calculator, or a computer. What you *do* need is to remember how to combine the various groups of vegetable protein foods so that you end up eating complete protein, properly balanced in amino-acid content. As explained in Chapter 2, vegetable proteins have varying strengths and weaknesses in terms of the amount of essential amino acids they contain. The trick is to combine vegetable proteins so that the strengths of one compensate for the weaknesses of the other, and vice versa. Here, in three simple alternatives, is how to do it:

- Combine legumes (dried peas and beans or peanuts) with grains.
- Combine legumes with nuts and seeds.
- Combine eggs or dairy products with any vegetable protein.

Tables 24.1, 24.2, and 24.3 show the amino-acid strengths and weaknesses of various food groups, what kinds of foods you might consume in each group, and some typical combinations.

As for amounts of protein, three things are worth bearing in mind. First, most meat eaters are already consuming twice as much protein as they really need. Second, the protein in milk and eggs is more efficiently used than that in meat, fish, or poultry, so relatively little goes a long way nutritionally. Third, legumes—especially soybeans—contain the largest percentage of protein among vegetable foods and are in the same ballpark as many meats. If legumes play a central role in your diet, you're not likely to shortchange yourself on protein. Thus, one cup of cooked soybeans contains about 20 grams of protein—as much protein as three frankfurters, or ¼-pound hamburger, or 18 ounces of milk, or 3 ounces of cheese! Each would supply two-thirds of a 60-pound child's daily protein needs, nearly half the recommended protein allowance for a 120-pound adult, and a third the amount needed by a 170-pound man.

Table 24.4 gives you some examples of how you can obtain adequate amounts of balanced protein on a vegetarian diet. In each case, the items and the amounts shown add up to 18 grams of usable protein, which represents a third of the recommended daily allowance for protein for a 150-pound adult.

But protein should not be your only concern. As a vegetarian you must also be aware of how to meet your vitamin and mineral needs. A lactovegetarian need not worry very much because dairy products contain the vitamins and minerals—B_{12}, calcium, riboflavin, and vitamins A and D—likely to be in short supply in vegetable foods. An ovolactovegetarian gets the additional benefit of iron from eggs. But even if you eat both eggs and milk products, you should also be certain that

Table 24.1 • BALANCING AMINO ACIDS

Food group	Weaknesses	Strengths
LEGUMES	Tryptophan, Methionine, Cystine*	Lysine, Isoleucine
GRAINS	Lysine, Isoleucine	Tryptophan, Methionine, Cystine*
SEEDS AND NUTS	Lysine, Isoleucine (except cashews and pumpkin seeds)	Tryptophan, Methionine, Cystine*
OTHER VEGETABLES	Isoleucine, Methionine, Cystine*	Tryptophan, Lysine
EGGS	None	Tryptophan, Lysine, Methionine, Cystine*
MILK PRODUCTS	None	Lysine

Note: To achieve balanced protein, combine food groups so that the amino acid strengths of one compensate for the weaknesses of the other.
*Although cystine is not an essential amino acid, its presence in foods spares methionine, which is essential.

Table 24.2 • VEGETABLE PROTEIN FOODS

Grains

Barley	Millet	Rye
Buckwheat	Oats	Triticale
Bulgur	Rice	Wheat
Corn		

Legumes

Beans (black, broad, kidney, lima, mung, navy, pea, soy)	Black-eyed peas (cow-peas)	Peanuts
	Chickpeas (garbanzos)	Peas
	Lentils	

Seeds

Pumpkin	Squash	Sunflower
Sesame		

Nuts

Almonds	Filberts	Pine nuts
Brazil nuts	Macadamia	Pistachio
Cashews	Pecans	Walnuts
Coconut		

Table 24.3 • VEGETARIAN DISHES WITH COMPLETE PROTEIN

Grains with Legumes

Rice with lentils

Rice with black-eyed peas

Peanut-butter sandwich

Bean taco

Macaroni enriched with soy flour

Bean soup with toast

Falafel (chickpea pancake) with pita bread

Grains with Milk

Oatmeal with milk

Wheat flakes with milk

Rice pudding

Pancakes and waffles

Breads and muffins made with milk

Pizza

Macaroni and cheese

Cheese sandwich

Creamed soup with noodles or rice

Quiche

Meatless lasagne

Granola with milk

Legumes with Seeds

Bean curd with sesame seeds

Hummus (chickpea and sesame paste)

Bean soup with sesame meal

Grains with Eggs

Rice pudding

Kasha (buckwheat groats)

Fried rice

Oatmeal cookies

Quiche

Egg-salad sandwich

Spaghetti pancake

Noodle pudding

French toast

Other Vegetables with Milk or Eggs

Potato salad

Mashed potatoes with milk

Eggplant Parmesan

Broccoli with cheese sauce

Cream of pumpkin soup

Cheese and potato soup

Vegetable omelet

Escalloped potatoes

Spinach salad with sliced egg

---

your diet contains a variety of vegetable foods, since different kinds provide different essential nutrients. If you choose your foods properly, you will not have to take any vitamin or mineral supplements. Thus, as a general rule, it's a good idea to select your daily menu from each of the following food groups:

• Legumes, nuts, and seeds, 2 or more servings. (Supply iron, thiamin, riboflavin, and niacin.)

• Whole-grain and enriched breads and cereals, 3 or more servings. (Supply iron, several B vitamins, and, in whole-grain foods, vitamin E.)

Table 24.4 • HOW TO GET ENOUGH BALANCED PROTEIN

Food combination	Amount	Protein (g)
Peanut butter	3 tablespoons	12.0
Whole-wheat bread	2 slices	5.2
Soybean curd (tofu)	1 piece (4.2 ounces)	9.4
Soybean sprouts	1 cup	6.5
Sesame seeds	2 tablespoons	3.0
Lentils	1 cup	15.6
Brown rice	½ cup	2.5
Split-pea soup	¾ cup cooked peas	12.0
Brown rice	½ cup	2.5
Whole-wheat bread	1 slice	2.6
Macaroni	1 cup	6.5
Cheddar cheese	1½ ounces	10.6
Roll (brown-and-serve)	1 roll	2.2
Kasha (buckwheat groats)	1 cup	8.0
Egg	1 large	6.5
Potato (baked)	7 ounces	4.0
Egg noodles	½ cup	3.3
Cottage cheese (creamed)	½ cup	14.3
Oatmeal	1 cup cooked	4.8
Milk (skim)	1 cup	8.8
Whole-wheat toast	2 slices	5.2

• Vegetables and fruits. 1 or more servings of the following: citrus, potato, melon, tomato, raw cabbage, strawberries, broccoli, sweet peppers, spinach, etc. (Supply vitamin C.)

2 or more servings of dark-green and deep-yellow vegetables and fruits. (Supply vitamin A.) Dark-green leafy vegetables also supply iron and vitamin C, and dried fruits supply iron.

• Fats (vegetable oil or margarine), 1–2 tablespoons daily. (Supply essential fatty acids and vitamin E.)

Vegans must pay very close attention to vitamin sources. They should be certain to include a source of vitamin B_{12} in their daily diet. Since B_{12} is found only in foods of animal origin, a strict vegetarian should get this essential vitamin from fortified nutritional yeast, B_{12}-fortified soymilk, or B_{12} tablets. Brewer's yeast, baker's yeast, and live yeast have almost none of this vitamin. B_{12} deficiency can be sneaky—symptoms, like anemia, may take a long time to develop, sometimes years—but it can result in impaired blood-cell formation and nerve damage.

Without milk in the diet, it's also difficult to get enough calcium. However, the following vegetable foods do contain worthwhile amounts of calcium: collards, dandelion greens, kale, mustard greens and turnip greens, broccoli, spoon cabbage (bok choy), okra, rutabaga, soybeans and other legumes, black-strap molasses, most dried fruits, and almonds. Calcium is essential to the formation of strong bones and teeth, the clotting of blood, and the functioning of muscles and nerves.

Vitamin D can be obtained from fortified margarines and by exposing your skin to sunlight. Riboflavin sources include green leafy vegetables, asparagus, broccoli, Brussels sprouts, okra, and winter squash. In areas distant from the seacoast, use iodized table salt to obtain needed iodine.

Your Baby Needs Animal Protein

Despite the foregoing evidence that adults can live healthfully on a strict vegetarian diet, *infants and very young children need animal sources of protein to grow properly.* A baby can be properly raised on a lactovegetarian or ovolactovegetarian diet. But some of those fed as vegans suffer growth retardation and even evident malnutrition. In recent years there have been several reports in the medical literature describing young children suffering from rickets (vitamin D deficiency), vitamin B_{12} deficiency, or severe protein-calorie malnutrition because their parents fed them no animal food other than breast milk. At least one child died as a result.

Studies of vegan infants and young children are alarming. A Seattle home economist studied 8 children on vegan diets, 7 others on ovolacto- or lactovegetarian diets, and 12 children on ordinary diets. They ranged in age from one to five years and were from comparable income groups. All of the vegan children, whom the researcher described as appearing "lethargic," were in the bottom half of the national statistics for weight, and one child was clearly malnourished. Six were receiving inadequate calories to support normal growth, and all the vegan children consumed much less calcium and riboflavin than the other children.

Although a few vegan communities are raising infants according to carefully spelled out vegan nutritional guidelines, in general this is unadvisable. Infant nutrition, even under the best of nutritional circumstances, is a risky affair. To assure proper growth and development, a baby's diet should contain some animal protein besides the breast milk of a vegan mother. By the time a child reaches school age, however, it is less difficult to supply adequate nutrients and calories on a vegan diet as long as sources of B_{12} and calcium are given to the child.

The situation is quite different if dairy products and/or eggs are included in a vegetarian child's diet. Dr. Mervyn G. Hardinge, dean of the Loma Linda University School of Health, points out that "if food is reasonably chosen, the nutritional adequacy of the lacto-ovo or lacto-vegetarian diet is above question for the feeding of all age groups, including infants. Our study of adolescents raised on this diet, some of them second- or third-generation subjects, showed them fully comparable in development and health to adolescents raised as nonvegetarians."

How to Eat and Cook Like a Vegetarian

The idea in a vegetarian diet is to move away from the highly processed, refined, sugar- and fat-laden foods in the typical American diet and to substitute fresh vegetables, dried peas and beans, whole grains, and naturally sweetened fruits wherever possible. While nuts are a fine source of vegetable protein, they are also quite high in fat (albeit unsaturated fat) and calories, so they should not be eaten to excess. Two to 4 tablespoons of nuts are quite enough in a meal for an adult. Nor should cheese—high in fat and cholesterol—become a steady standby for snacks and meals. A few ounces of hard cheese a day should be the outside limit for a vegetarian. (A 1-inch cube of cheese is approximately 1 ounce.)

Eggs, or more accurately, egg yolks, are another thing to eat in moderation. The yolk of one large egg contains 250 milligrams of cholesterol, and by itself nearly fulfills the recommended daily maximum intake of 300 milligrams of cholesterol for an adult. Thus, if you eat two eggs a day and several ounces of cheese, you'll be consuming as much cholesterol as the average meat eater.

The New York City Department of Health's Bureau of Nutrition has devised some sample menus for ovolacto- and lactovegetarians.* The menus are designed to provide adequate protein and the daily requirements of vitamins and minerals for teenagers and adults without overloading on saturated fats, cholesterol, and calories. If you require fewer than 2,400 calories daily, adjust portion sizes downward or cut

*"The Vegetarian Follows the Star Guide to Good Eating" can be obtained free from the Bureau of Nutrition, Department of Health, 93 Worth Street, Room 714, New York, New York 10013.

down on fats. Teenaged boys and menstruating women may need more iron in their diets than these menus provide, and pregnant and nursing women definitely require an iron supplement. Recipes follow for the starred items in the menus.

OVOLACTOVEGETARIAN MENUS

Sample Menu 1	*Sample Menu 2*

Breakfast

Cantaloupe, ½ medium	Grapefruit, ½
Shredded-wheat biscuits, 2	Sliced cheese, 1 ounce
Whole-grain or enriched toast, 1 slice	Whole-grain or enriched toast, 2 slices
Margarine, 1 pat (1 teaspoon)	Margarine, 1 pat
Skim milk, 1 cup	Skim milk, ½ cup

Lunch

Vegetable juice, 1 cup	Black beans and rice, 1 cup
Egg-salad sandwich:	Mixed green salad
2 slices whole-grain bread	Cottage cheese, ½ cup
1 medium egg	Salad dressing, 1 tablespoon
1 tablespoon diced celery	Whole-grain or enriched bread, 1 slice
1 teaspoon mayonnaise	Margarine, 1 pat
Pear	Cantaloupe, 1 slice

Snack

Dried apricot halves, 4	Yogurt, 1 cup
Almonds ¼ cup	Sunflower seeds, ¼ cup

Supper

Soy and brown-rice loaf*, 1 cup	Potato kugel*, 1 cup
Carrots, ½ cup	Baked acorn squash, ½
Broccoli, ½ cup	Coleslaw, ½ cup
Margarine, 1 pat	Mayonnaise, 1 teaspoon
Waldorf salad:	Whole-grain or enriched bread, 1 slice
½ cup diced apple	Margarine, 1 pat
1 tablespoon diced celery	Pear
1 tablespoon raisins	
1 tablespoon chopped walnuts	
1 tablespoon mayonnaise	
Vanilla pudding, ½ cup	

Snack

Buttermilk or yogurt, 1 cup	Milk, ½ cup
Graham crackers, 4	Bulgur wheat, ¾ cup
	Raisins, ¼ cup

Soy and Brown-Rice Loaf

2 cups cooked mashed soy beans
1 cup cooked brown rice
1 cup milk
½ cup enriched bread crumbs
1 tablespoon oil

1 tablespoon powdered vegetable broth
2 tablespoons minced onion
Salt, as desired (optional)

Mix all the ingredients well. Place in an oiled loaf pan. Bake in a 350-degree oven for 45 minutes. If desired, moisten the top of the loaf with tomato sauce. Yield: 4 servings.

Potato Kugel

6 medium raw potatoes
2–3 raw carrots
1 large onion
1 clove garlic, minced
2 eggs, beaten
3 tablespoons oil

2 teaspoons salt
¼ cup whole-grain or enriched bread crumbs
¾ cup dry skim-milk powder
Topping, if desired: 1 cup grated cheese

Grate the potatoes, carrots, and onion into a large bowl. Drain off the accumulated liquid. Stir in the remaining ingredients, adding the milk powder slowly to avoid lumps. Spread mixture in an oiled 7 × 7-inch pan and bake at 350-degrees for 45 minutes to 1 hour. The kugel is done when the edges are brown and a knife inserted in center of the kugel comes out dry. If desired, add the grated cheese on top of the kugel at this point and leave in the oven 5 minutes longer. Yield: 8 servings.

LACTOVEGETARIAN MENUS

Sample Menu 1	Sample Menu 2

Breakfast

Grapefruit juice, ½ cup	Orange, 1 medium
Oatmeal, 1 cup	Cottage cheese, ¼ cup
Whole-grain or enriched toast, 1 slice	Whole grain or enriched toast, 2 slices
Margarine, 1 pat	Margarine, 1 pat
Skim milk, ½ cup	Skim milk, ½ cup

Snack

Yogurt, ½ cup	Part-skimmed cheese, 1 slice
Sesame bread sticks, 4–6	Whole-grain or enriched crackers, 4–6

Menus continue on next page

Lactovegetarian Menus continued

Sample Menu 1	Sample Menu 2

Lunch

Grilled cheese sandwich: Split-pea soup, 1 cup
 2 slices whole-grain toast Sesame crackers*
 1 ounce cheese   Tomato and cucumber salad
 1 pat margarine   Salad dressing, 1 tablespoon
Tossed green salad   Baked apple
Salad dressing, 1 tablespoon Skim milk, ½ cup
Fresh fruit cup

Snack

Raisins, ¼ cup   Prunes, 2
Peanuts, ¼ cup   Roasted soy beans, ¼ cup

Supper

Tomato juice, ½ cup   Fresh fruit cup
Mixed bean salad,* 1 cup Baked macaroni and cheese, 1 cup
Pancake delight*   Collard greens, ½ cup
Apple   Whole-grain or enriched bread, 1 slice
          Margarine, 2 pats
          Junket, ½ cup

Snack

Whole-grain or enriched cereal, 1 cup Whole grain or enriched roll, 1
Milk, ½ cup   Buttermilk, ½ cup

Sesame Crackers

1½ cups whole-wheat flour ¾ teaspoon salt
¼ cup soy flour   ⅓ cup oil
¼ cup sesame seeds   ½ cup water (as needed)

  Stir the flours, seeds, and salt together. Add the oil and blend well. Add enough water so that the dough can be kneaded into a soft ball and can be rolled easily to a thickness of ⅛ inch. Cut the dough into cracker shapes and place on an ungreased sheet. Bake at 350 degrees for about 15 to 20 minutes or until the crackers are crisp and golden. Yield: 3 to 4 dozen crackers.

Mixed Bean Salad

1 cup cooked garbanzos (chick-
peas) (½ cup dry)
1 cup cooked kidney beans (½
cup dry)
1 cup cooked black beans (½ cup
dry)
1 cup cooked string beans

¼ cup diced pimiento
¼ cup diced onion
2 tablespoons oil
1 tablespoon lemon juice
¼ teaspoon salt
¼ teaspoon dried basil
Dark leafy greens

Cook the garbanzos, kidney beans, and black beans separately until they are tender but still firm. Drain well. Combine the beans with the rest of the ingredients except the greens. Toss well and refrigerate. Serve on bed of leafy greens. Yield: 4 to 6 servings.

Pancake Delight

1 cup buckwheat flour
1 cup whole-wheat flour
2 teaspoons baking powder
½ teaspoon baking soda
¼ teaspoon salt (optional)
¼ teaspoon caraway seeds

¼ teaspoons turmeric
¼ teaspoon curry
¼ teaspoon powdered allspice
⅛ teaspoon celery seeds
¼ teaspoon onion salt
2 cups buttermilk

Place the flours, baking powder, baking soda, salt, spices, and onion salt in a large bowl. Add the buttermilk, stirring lightly until the mixture is well blended. Pour some of the mixture onto a lightly greased griddle or frying pan. Cook until pancakes are golden brown underneath. Turn once. Yield: 16 pancakes.

Menu planning for a strict vegetarian is much trickier than for an ovolactovegetarian. The following two sample menus were devised by the Department of Nutrition of the School of Health at Loma Linda University.* They provide 2,800 to 2,900 calories a day and about 80 grams of protein each, so if you need fewer calories, smaller portions may be consumed without stinting on needed protein. However, a better approach would be to eat less fat. Recipes follow for starred items.

*Complete seven-day menu plans for strict vegetarians and for ovolactovegetarians plus recipes can be obtained from the Educational Materials Center, School of Health, Loma Linda University, Loma Linda, California 92350.

VEGAN MENUS

Sample Menu 1	*Sample Menu 2*

Breakfast

Orange, 1	Orange, 1
Oatmeal (⅔ cup dry) with	Whole-wheat cooked cereal,1 cup with
1 tablespoon molasses	1 tablespoon molasses
¼ cup raisins	¼ cup raisins
⅔ cup nondairy creamer or	⅓ cup nondairy creamer or
powdered soy milk	powdered soy milk
Whole-wheat toast, 2 slices	Banana, 1
Margarine, 2 pats	Whole-wheat toast, 2 slices
Peanut butter, 1 tablespoon	Margarine, 2 teaspoons
	Peanut butter, 2 tablespoons

Lunch

Savory patties,* 2 servings	Black beans on rice,* 2 servings
Baked potato, 1	Diced carrots, ½ cup, cooked, or
Margarine, 1 tablespoon	summer squash, 1 cup, diced
Cooked turnip greens, 1 cup	Coleslaw, ⅔ cup
Large tomato, sliced, 1	Date bread, 2 slices
Whole-wheat bread, 1 slice	
Margarine, 1 teaspoon	

Supper

Wheat tortillas with filling*, 2 servings	Thick vegetable soup*, 2 servings
Apple, 1 medium	Kale (no stems), ¾ cup cooked
Figs, 5 large dried	Whole-wheat bread, 1 slice
Raw almonds, 15	Margarine, 1 pat

Savory Patties

⅔ cup dry soybeans	1 teaspoon Italian seasoning
3 cups water	2 tablespoons soy sauce
1¼ cups water	½ teaspoon salt
1 teaspoon onion powder	1⅓ cups rolled oats
or 1 chopped onion	2 tablespoons oil

Soak the soybeans overnight in 3 cups water, then drain (yields 2 cups soaked beans). Grind the soybeans or blend in 1¼ cups water until the texture becomes quite fine. Add the seasonings and the rolled oats. Allow the mixture to stand 10 minutes until oats absorb the liquid. Stir again and drop by rounded tablespoon into a lightly oiled skillet over moderate heat (350-degrees in an electric skillet). Cover and cook the patties for about 10 minutes or until brown. Turn, cover, and cook until browned. Reduce the heat and allow the patties to cook 10 minutes longer. Serve with tomato sauce (see the recipe below). Yield: 16 patties (2 per serving).

Tomato Sauce

1 large onion, finely chopped
1 tablespoon oil

2 cans condensed tomato soup (undiluted)
½ teaspoon orégano or basil

Sauté the onion in the oil over a very low heat; do not brown. Add the tomato soup and orégano or basil. Heat the sauce until bubbly and serve on warm Savory Patties.

Black Beans on Rice

1 pound dry black beans
6 cups boiling water
2 green peppers, chopped
6–8 green onions (scallions) with tops, chopped

1 clove garlic, minced
⅓ cup oil
2 teaspoons salt
Seasonings (optional)
1 pound brown rice, cooked

Cover the beans with the boiling water and cook for 1 hour. Sauté the green peppers, green onions (reserve 1 to 2 tablespoons), and garlic in oil. Combine the vegetables with the beans, add the salt and other seasonings (as desired), and cook until the beans are tender and the liquid is thick. Serve over brown rice. Garnish with the reserved chopped green onions. Yield: 16 servings, ¾ cup each.

Wheat Tortillas with Filling

1 cup dry pinto beans
1 can tomato soup
1 teaspoon onion salt
3 cups whole-wheat flour
1 teaspoon salt
⅓ cup oil

1 cup water
6–8 tablespoons chopped parsley
6–8 leaves salad greens (e.g., cabbage, lettuce), shredded
5–6 green onions (scallions) with tops, sliced

To make the filling: Soak the pinto beans overnight in water to cover. Drain. Cook the beans in fresh water until they are tender. Drain again. Add the tomato soup and onion salt to the beans and cook the mixture while preparing the tortillas.

To make tortillas: Mix the flour with the salt. In a separate bowl, combine the oil and water and beat together with a fork. Stir the oil-water mixture into the flour, wetting the flour as evenly as possible. Mix. Divide the dough into 12 parts. Roll or pat each piece of dough into a thin circle of about 5 inches in diameter. Cook the tortillas on an ungreased skillet or on a grill.

Turn when bubbles form and the bottom is browned slightly. Cook about 10 minutes longer. The tortillas should be pliable and easy to roll.

Fill the tortillas with the bean-tomato mixture. Top with parsley, salad greens, and green onions. Yield: 12 tortillas (2 per serving).

Thick Vegetable Soup (for 30 persons)

1 pound dry pinto beans
1 pound dry lentils
10 potatoes, diced
2½ cups carrots, chopped
1 pound dry barley
1 bunch parsley, chopped (8 tablespoons)

5 medium onions
½ cup oil
2 tablespoons soy sauce
10 small tomatoes (canned if not in season)
1 gallon can green beans
Seasonings (to taste)

Soak the pinto beans and lentils overnight in water to cover. Drain. Cook the beans and lentils in fresh water until they are almost done. Add the potatoes, carrots, barley, parsley, and onions and cook until vegetables are tender. Add other ingredients at the end of cooking. Simmer to blend flavor. Add other seasonings to taste (e.g., Kitchen Bouquet, pepper, garlic, Royal soup flavoring). Yield: 30 servings, 1¼ cups each.

The above menus and recipes are merely guidelines for sensible vegetarian diets. If you are serious about being a vegetarian (or remaining a meat eater but reducing your dependence on animal foods), you would be wise to consult one or more cookbooks devoted to vegetarian diets. Reliable sources include:

Frances Moore Lappé, *Diet for a Small Planet,* rev. ed. (New York: Ballantine, 1975).

Ellen Buchman Ewald, *Recipes for a Small Planet* (New York: Ballantine, 1975).

Julie Jordan, *The Wings of Life* (Trumansburg, N.Y.: The Crossing Press, 1976).

Laurel Robertson, Carol Flinders, and Bronwen Godfrey, *Laurel's Kitchen* (Petaluma, Calif.: Nilgiri Press, 1978).

Anna Thomas, *The Vegetarian Epicure* (New York: Vintage, 1972).

Anna Thomas, *The Vegetarian Epicure, Book 2* (New York: Knopf, 1978).

Lindsay Miller, *The Apartment Vegetarian Cookbook* (Culver City, Calif.: Peace Press, 1978).

Florence Lin, *Florence Lin's Chinese Vegetarian Cookbook* (New York: Hawthorn, 1977).

Mollie Katzen, *Moosewood Cookbook* (Berkeley, Calif.: Ten Speed Press, 1977).

Mollie Katzen, *The Enchanted Broccoli Forest* (Berkeley, Calif.: Ten Speed Press, 1982).

Though not a cookbook, *The Vegetarian Alternative,* by Vic S. Sussman (Emmaus, Pa.: Rodale, 1978), is a good overall guide to vegetarian diets and meal preparation.

How to Use the Meat Analogues

If you would like to switch partly or completely to a vegetarian diet but are not quite ready to give up meat, the soybean may be your answer. For centuries, Asians have used this high-protein legume as a major protein source, primarily as bean curd, sprouts, and paste. Since the early 1800s, Americans have grown soybeans mostly to feed cattle and, in the last sixty-five years, as a source of vegetable oil. But only since the 1950s has this most nutritious of vegetable proteins been technologically transformed into forms that might suit the wide range of tastes and dietary habits of Westerners.

Today, vegetarians and nonvegetarians alike can sit down to a meal of sausages, burgers, bacon, chicken, chili con carne, ham, or scallops that contains not a speck of meat, fish, or poultry. It's all made with soybeans, molded into "analogues" by a process similar to the one used for producing rayon. You've probably seen it in your market as *textured vegetable protein (TVP),* boxed or premixed with ground beef or as imitation bacon bits. TVP is a popular, inexpensive, and highly nourishing meat extender among nonvegetarians in many parts of the nation.

To make the ersatz "meat," first the oil is pressed out of the soybeans and then the carbohydrates are removed, leaving a honeylike slurry of pure protein. This is pumped through a "spinnerette"—a showerheadlike device with microscopic holes—and as the protein emerges from the holes, it hits an acid bath that converts it into fibers. After being neutralized and washed, the tasteless, odorless, off-white fibers are mixed with flavorings, colorings, fat, water, and sometimes egg white as a binder. By varying the stretch on the fibers as they go through the spinnerette, they can be spun into a variety of meatlike textures.

A second process for making vegetable meat analogues uses soybean flour or defatted soybean concentrate instead of isolated protein. This is mixed with water and flavorings, subjected to heat and pressure;

and then forced through small holes of various sizes and shapes. The resulting product is then cooked and ready to eat. Or it may be frozen, canned, or dried. The spun protein can be sliced, cubed, cut into chunks, ground into bits or molded into rolls. In addition to soybeans, textured vegetable protein can be made from peanut, cottonseed, sunflower, safflower, and other oil seeds.

Because their nutritive content can be precisely controlled, meat analogues can be prepared with the identical food value of the foods they imitate. In fact, they may be healthier than the "real thing" because they can be made with little or no animal fats and cholesterol and sometimes fewer calories. The analogues are also easy to store and to prepare, and they contain no waste—you get to eat everything you've paid for. Their main nutritional drawback is their usual high salt content.

Some people who have become vegetarians because they want a "natural" diet object to the extensive processing and large numbers of additives and salt used in making meat analogues. But for others, the meat imitations make it easy to give up the foods they grew up on and instead stick to a vegetarian diet. Even if you're not a vegetarian, you may find some of the analogues to be attractive, economical, and healthy alternatives to meat. TVP can go a long way to stretch your food dollar when you use it in ground-meat dishes to make them go further.

The following is a list of manufacturers of meat analogues and of stores that are likely to carry their products. If you have difficulty finding the products in your area, write to the company's marketing or customer service department. These departments will also send recipe booklets upon request.

Worthington Foods, a division of Miles Laboratories Inc., 900 Proprietors Road, Worthington, Ohio 43085. Products found in most health-food stores.

Loma Linda Foods, 11503 Pierce Street, Riverside, California 92515. Products found in many supermarket chains and in some health-food stores.

Morningstar Farms, a division of Miles Laboratories Inc., 7123 West 65th Street, Chicago, Illinois 60638. Nationally distributed in supermarkets and grocery stores.

A Postscript for Meat Eaters

You don't have to become a total vegetarian to derive many of the benefits of the vegetarian diet. Even if you have no interest in vegetarianism, *there's no reason why you should have animal protein at every meal or even every day.* By including vegetarian dishes in your daily menu and adapting the vegetarian approach to menu planning, you can greatly reduce your dependence on animal protein and especially on high-fat, high-calorie meats.

If, for example, you prepare a soup or vegetable casserole containing a substantial percentage of balanced vegetable protein, you need not eat three or more ounces of meat, poultry or fish to complete your meal. An ounce of animal protein will be more than enough.

Or, instead of eggs and bacon for breakfast, how about a bowl of oatmeal cooked in half water, half skim milk? Far less fat and cholesterol (and less expensive). For the adventurous, an especially delicious and nutritious breakfast is fried rice with scraps of leftover meat or chicken and vegetables.

We would all be better off if we stopped thinking of vegetables and grains as merely side dishes to embellish a chunk of animal protein and to provide vitamins, minerals, and roughage. *Vegetables can be an important source of protein for everyone.*

PART SIX

What's in Your Food

25 ✎ ADDITIVES: FEASTING ON FOOD OR CHEMICALS?

IT'S SATURDAY. You're in the supermarket procuring the family food supply for the coming week. You pick up an item and read the label: *"Contents: water; triglycerides of stearic, palmitic, oleic, and linoleic acids; myosin and actin; glycogen; collagen; lecithin, cholesterol; dipotassium phosphate; myoglobin, and urea. (Warning: May also contain steroid hormones of natural origin.)"*

Dropping this chemical concoction like a hot potato, you move down the aisle and reach for something else. This label reads: *"Water, starches, cellulose, pectin, fructose, sucrose, glucose, malic acid, citric acid, succinic acid, anisyl propionate, amyl acetate, ascorbic acid (vitamin C), beta carotene (vitamin A), riboflavin, thiamin, niacin, phosphorus, and potassium."* Again, with a shudder of disgust, you put the product back and move on.

The next item has a shorter list but even stranger sounding ingredients: *"Caffeine, tannin, butanol, isoamyl alcohol, hexanol, phenyl ethyl alcohol, benzyl alcohol, geraniol, quercetin, 3-galloyl epicatechin, and 3-galloyl epigallocatechin."* Back on the shelf it goes.

And so on down all eight aisles of the market. *Everything* was full of chemicals, and there was nothing you felt comfortable about buying.

You're right. Everything *is* full of chemicals. But you're also wrong. Because the items you passed up were not concocted in a chemist's laboratory to undermine your family's health. Rather, they were *100-percent natural, unadulterated foods from farm and field.* The first was beefsteak, the second cantaloupe, and the third tea. Milk, as it comes from the cow, is a combination of 95 chemicals, including 12 fats, 6 proteins, lactose, 9 salts, 7 acids, 3 pigments, 7 enzymes, 18 vitamins, 6 miscellaneous compounds, and 3 gases. And the potato, just as it's dug up from untreated soil, contains 150 different chemical ingredients, including one—solanine—that's a poison.

All this is not meant to win converts for the food-chemical industry but to make a point crucial to understanding the nation's food supply: food *is* chemicals, and all creatures that eat are chemicals, too.

If we refused to eat foods containing chemicals, we'd starve to death very quickly. Not all chemicals are bad, whether they're natural or added in a factory. Neither are all chemicals good, including many natural chemicals. In fact, some of the most poisonous chemicals known to humankind are perfectly natural. And some of the most beneficial chemicals in our foods are wholly synthetic. Your body can't tell the difference between a natural poison and an artificial one. Both can cause harm. Nor can your body distinguish between a natural beneficial chemical and one devised in a test tube. It's grateful for any chemical that helps it to function.

The American aversion to chemicals is hardly a new phenomenon. Many years ago, the food industry—knowing the public wariness of anything "chemical"—adopted the word "additives" to describe chemicals used in processing foods. The industry won the right to list several additives by their initials instead of their more forbidding chemical names. Thus, BHT on the label stands for butylated hydroxytoluene, and CMC is really sodium carboxymethylcellulose. And in some products covered by federal food standards (lists of mandatory and optional ingredients), certain food additives don't have to be listed on the label at all.

Why Chemicals Are Added to Food

Following the Civil War, the American pattern of food production and consumption changed dramatically as industrial development brought rural residents to cities, which depended on food from distant sources. As American industry and cities grew, more and more people relied upon the foods produced and preserved by fewer and fewer people. Instead of growing it in their back yards, urban folk got their food from stores. Fewer women spent their days preparing meals "from scratch." Instead, they got jobs and became increasingly dependent on canned and packaged convenience foods from the local market. Today, 92 percent of Americans rely on foods grown and processed by others. Even the remaining 8 percent who are still "down on the farm" don't really feed themselves. They get most of their food from farms and factories hundreds or thousands of miles away. Instead of making a daily trip to the local general store and greengrocer, most Americans shop for food once a week. The food they buy may have left the factory weeks or months earlier, the farm even longer ago than that. Something has to keep it looking and tasting good and free from insects or disease-causing microorganisms. That something is food additives.

However, additives today serve a wide variety of purposes, not all laudatory. They make possible many nutritious convenience foods, such as packaged breads, canned fruits and vegetables, canned and packaged soups, margarine, and ready-to-eat cereals. But additives also permit the concoction of junk foods, trumped-up "imitations," nutritionally deficient replacements for nourishing natural foods, and entirely new "foods" for which there is no demand until one is artificially created by the manufacturer. The explosive growth of the food-processing industry in recent decades has led to more than a 50-percent increase in the use of additives since 1960.

The most serious problem with additives is less the safety of the chemicals themselves (although for some this is certainly a legitimate concern) than the kinds of foods that are most heavily laden with them: foods processed to a fare-thee-well with lots of sodium, sugar, and/or fat, adding little of real nutritive value to the American diet. We don't need all those presweetened, heavily fortified cereals; fatty and salty processed meats, chips, and dips; sugary soft drinks; and the endless stream of heat-and-serve, mix-and-match, and eat-and-run products the American food industry foists on the public.

But to revert to a wholly unprocessed, additive-free food supply just isn't practical for many reasons.

Many foods could only be purchased in small quantities because they would spoil quickly without preservatives. And few of us have the time or inclination for the frequent shopping and lengthy food preparation that unprocessed foods require.

If everyone insisted on only fresh carrots, peas, green beans, broccoli, tomatoes, and the like, during much of the year there wouldn't be enough of them to go around. Nor would it be possible to get fresh supplies to all parts of the country often enough.

The limited shelf life of most fresh foods would lead to a great deal of waste, further diminishing the available food supply.

The food left might cost more. Distribution of conveniently packaged and processed foods is already extremely expensive, and likely to get more so as energy supplies dwindle. Transporting fresh foods, which are less compact and far more perishable, could cost many times more.

So, like it or not, we are stuck with a food-processing industry and the chemical additives it uses to keep food in good condition until it reaches the consumer's table. What's more, we have come to expect a quality product when we buy food, whether it comes from farm or factory. We want to be sure that every time we buy a loaf of Pepperidge Farm 100% Whole Wheat bread, it's going to be like the last loaf we had. We don't want ice crystals in our ice cream, bugs in our flour, rancid crackers, crumbly cakes, or mushy vegetables. High standards of uniformity and safety from food spoilage are the hallmarks of the modern American food industry. And when food processors occasionally fall down on the job, consumers complain loudly and clearly.

What Are Food Additives?

Additives are substances purposely added to foods to prevent spoilage, improve appearance, texture, or taste, or enhance nutritive value. For example, calcium propionate might be added to bread to prevent mold growth, green coloring to mint ice cream to give the ice cream a "minty" look, or iron to cereal to make the cereal more nutritious. Other chemicals accidentally get into foods during production, processing, or packaging. Molecules from plastic wrap that get into packaged foods and the lead in tuna and evaporated milk that comes from the solder used to seal the cans are examples of such *unintentional additives.*

The actual chemicals used as food additives come from a variety of sources. Many are *natural substances* extracted from foods or other living creatures: carrageenan and agar from seaweed; lecithin from soybeans; gelatin from bones; monosodium glutamate (MSG) from corn; sodium caseinate from milk protein; glycerol from fats; gum tragacanth and guar gum from trees; sorbic acid from berries; and sugar from sugar cane.

Some additives are *synthetic copies of natural substances,* such as vanillin from the vanilla bean; ascorbic acid, which is vitamin C; beta carotene, the orange coloring in carrots; or calcium propionate, a preservative found naturally in Swiss cheese. A laboratory-made carbon copy of a natural chemical means greater availability at lower cost; when two chemicals have identical structures, the body cannot tell whether these chemicals come from a laboratory or a living thing.

Still other additives are *wholly synthetic chemicals* that have no natural counterpart. They include saccharin (which millions of consumers fought to keep when it faced a threatened ban), sorbitan monostearate, sodium bisulfite, butylated hydroxyanisole (BHA), calcium stearoyl lactylate, and ethylenediamine tetraacetic acid (EDTA). Consumers are most fearful of synthetic chemicals. But just because a substance is not found in nature doesn't make it necessarily bad. EDTA, for example, is a safe synthetic used in many processed foods

Chart 15 • HOW MANY ADDITIVES WE EAT

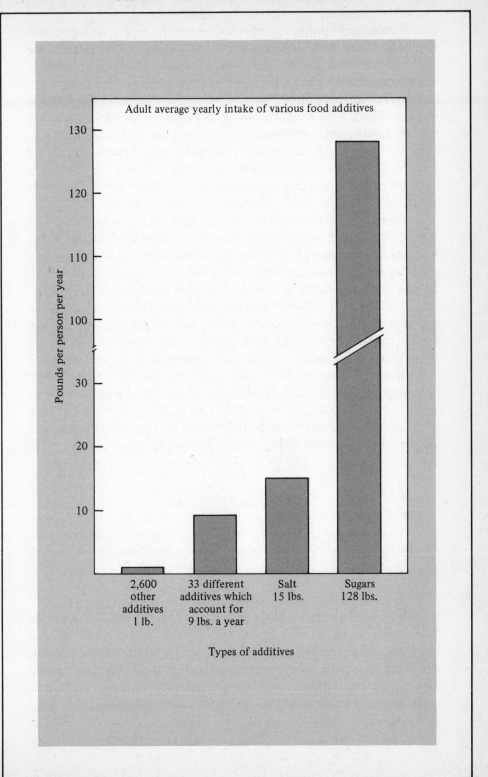

to trap metallic impurities that would otherwise cause the food to turn rancid and lose its natural color. And synthetic vitamins—also perfectly safe in recommended amounts—are added to bread and milk to make them more nutritious.

In fact, no matter how "natural" your diet is, *if you use substances like sugar, salt, pepper, spices, baking soda, lemon juice (ascorbic acid), vinegar (acetic acid), or cornstarch, you're using food additives.* The additives consumed by Americans in largest amounts (see Chart 15) are natural substances, including sugar (sucrose), 95 pounds per person a year; other sweeteners (corn syrup, dextrose, fructose, etc.), 33 pounds per person a year; and salt, 15 pounds per person a year. The 33 next most commonly used additives include both natural and synthetic substances that total 9 pounds per person a year. Among them are MSG, mustard, black pepper, hydrolyzed vegetable protein, sodium caseinate, modified starch, yeasts, bicarbonate of soda, acetic acid, lecithin, carbon dioxide, and caramel. Finally, there are another 2,600 additives, half of which are consumed in amounts of less than ½ milligram per person a year. They include most colors and flavors and together add up to 1 pound per person a year.

To put this chemical "feast" into perspective, the average adult American consumes approximately 1,500 pounds of food each year, including about 150 pounds of additives, 93 percent of which are sweeteners and salt. In other words, additives make up 10 percent of our total food consumption, and more than 90 percent of them are the sugars and salt we add to our food. Other chemicals make up only 1 percent of the total.

What Do They Do?

The thousands of chemicals used as food additives serve more than forty different functions, many of which we've come to take for granted. Some are more important to our nutritional health than others.

Flavors. Flavorings comprise the largest category of food additives. Many are natural and safe, including citrus oils, amyl acetate (the flavoring in bananas), cinnamon, and cloves. Some are natural and dangerous. Nutmeg, for example, can cause hallucinations in amounts not much larger than those commonly used in food. And one natural flavor, safrole (the natural root-beer flavor from sassafras), was banned when it was found to cause cancer in test animals. Finally, a synthetic flavoring agent, cinnamyl anthranilate, widely used since the 1940s as an imitation grape or cherry flavor in beverages, ice cream, candy, baked goods, gelatins, puddings, and chewing gums, was banned in December, 1985, after it was found to produce cancer when fed to rats and mice.

Many synthetic flavors—for example, vanillin, limonene, and l-malic acid—are chemically identical to naturally occurring flavors in foods and spices we regularly consume. So just because a label says "artificial flavoring added" doesn't mean the product contains a chemical that was made up by a scientist. Some flavoring agents enhance the flavor of other substances rather than impart one of their own—for example, MSG and maltol.

Colors. These chemicals are put into foods mainly to give them an appetizing appearance. Many consumers refer to them as "window dressing," an unnecessary source of chemical contamination in our diet primarily used to disguise overprocessing and poor quality. Food processors retort that consumers are reluctant to buy mint ice cream that's white instead of green, gray hot dogs, green oranges, pale-yellow cheese, or white butter and margarine. To which the consumer is likely to reply, "You have conditioned us to expect foods to have such bright, artificial colors. If all hot dogs were gray, we'd eat gray hot dogs."

When food colors are used to mask poor quality, or to hide the absence of a desirable ingredient, or to entice people to eat nutritionally deficient foods, they're bad even if they're perfectly safe. When they enhance the appeal of nutritionally valuable foods—say, by compensating for natural color variations that might otherwise turn people off—they're okay. But when they're of questionable safety, they're bad, no matter what other good they might do. (See page 477 for further discussion of the safety of food colors.)

Some food colors are natural chemicals—chlorophyll, beta carotene, annatto, anthocyanins, caramel, and cochineal, among others. But more than 90 percent of the colors used today are synthetic dyes, highly purified chemicals tiny amounts of which are needed to produce the desired effect. However, if any coloring is added to food—natural or not—the label must state "artificial coloring added."

Preservatives. These are the most important class of food additives because they help to assure us of a year-round, unspoiled, palatable food supply. One group are *antioxidants* that prevent fats and oils from turning rancid and stop the enzyme action that causes certain fruits and vegetables (for example, apples, pears, and potatoes) to turn brown after they are sliced.

Among the most widely used antioxidants are BHT, BHA, ascorbic acid (vitamin C), alpha tocopherol (vitamin E), propyl gallate, lecithin, citric acid, stearyl citrate, isopropyl citrate, and stannous chloride. Although the safety of BHA and BHT has been challenged, they have also been shown to block the action of a large group of chemicals that cause cancer. Some scientists, in fact, think they are partly responsible for the decline in stomach cancer among Americans. BHT can also inactivate certain viruses, protect against poisoning by carbon tetrachloride, and—in mice at least—delay aging.

The second group of preservatives are *antimicrobial agents,* which stop the growth of molds, bacteria, and yeasts that can render food inedible and sometimes poisonous. Some molds and bacteria—salmonella and Clostridium botulinum for example—produce toxins that can cause serious illness or death.

Sanitary food-processing techniques, the use of chemical preservatives, and refrigeration have helped to reduce the incidents of food poisoning from processed foods. Among the commonly used preservatives are sugar, salt, vinegar, calcium and sodium propionate (which inhibit mold growth in bread), sodium benzoate, benzoic acid, sorbic acid, calcium, sodium and potassium sorbate (used in cheeses), sulfur dioxide, sodium bisulfite, methyl paraben, sodium nitrate, and sodium nitrite (used to prevent the growth of botulism bacteria in cured and processed meats and smoked fish). (See page 480 for further discussion of nitrates and nitrites.)

Sometimes perservatives help to make foods more nutritious. Sulfites increase the stability of vitamin C; sulfur dioxide preserves vitamin C and beta carotene, the precursor of vitamin A; ascorbic acid prevents iron and copper from damaging vitamins A, E, thiamin, and folacin; and BHA, BHT, and alpha tocopherol protect vitamins A and D from chemical breakdown.

It's an irony typical of our times that many bread producers, wanting to cash in on the market for "natural" foods, have stopped adding calcium propionate to their products. The label can now read "no preservatives." But instead of benefiting, the consumer suffers: not only does the bread get moldy in a few days in warm weather, it also now lacks a perfectly safe chemical that was a source of an essential nutrient, calcium.

In an effort to avoid or reduce the risks of chemical preservatives and residues of pesticides that counter spoilage, the Food and Drug Administration has begun to phase in irradiation as a preservative. Approvals have already been granted for spices, pork, and fresh fruits and vegetables. Some consumer and health organizations have opposed food irradiation as ineffective, potentially hazardous, and inadequately tested, since the long-term consequences of eating irradiated food have not been assessed. It does not render the food radioactive, and no workers are exposed to the radiation.

Texture agents. *Emulsifiers* assure a more uniform product by keeping in suspension substances that would ordinarily separate (for instance, oil and water). They are important in the production of ice cream, salad dressings, breads (where they improve the consistency of batter and dough), and beverages made with oils and flavors that don't mix with water. Among widely used emulsifiers are phosphoric acid and phosphates; polysorbate 60, 65, and 80; sorbitan monostearate, and lecithin.

Stabilizers and *thickeners* are also used to give processed foods a uniform texture. Stabilizers keep bits of chocolate from separating in chocolate milk, prevent ice crystals from forming in ice cream, and keep flavoring oils stable in cake and pudding mixes. Stabilizers are usually also thickeners, and most are derived from natural sources: agar, alginates, and carrageenan from seaweed; gelatin from animal bones; sorbitol and pectin from fruits and berries; a long list of gums derived from various plants (locust bean, guar, furcelleran, arabic, karaya, tragacanth, and ghatti); and sodium carboxymethylcellulose (CMC), a combination of cellulose and vinegar. Another widely used thickening agent is starch or modified (chemically treated) starch derived from flour, potatoes, and corn. Its main disadvantage is that it makes foods look thicker and richer than they really are, and thus may prompt the consumer to buy a nutritionally inferior product.

Acid controllers. Various acids, alkalies, buffers, and neutralizing agents are added to processed foods to maintain a desired degree of acidity or alkalinity, thereby affecting flavor, texture, and cooking characteristics. They are widely used in dairy products and also to flavor soft drinks, prevent discoloration in canned vegetables, and to peel fruits and vegetables before canning. They include phosphoric acid, citric acid, lactic acid, and acetic acid (vinegar).

Leavenings. Yeast, baking powder, and baking soda are used in breads, cakes, pancakes, biscuits, and other baked goods to make dough rise. They work by releasing a harmless gas (carbon dioxide) into the batter or dough. Baking soda is sodium bicarbonate; double-acting baking powder is a combination of leavening agents—baking soda, sodium aluminum sulfate, and calcium phosphate.

Nutrients. Vitamins and minerals may be added to certain foods either to improve on nature or to replace micronutrients lost in food processing. The most notable examples are breads enriched with B vitamins (although not all the vitamins lost in refining grain are replaced), milk fortified with vitamins A and D, cereals enriched with iron, salt supplemented with iodine (to prevent goiter), and soft drinks with vitamin C (see page 526 for a discussion of fortification).

Sometimes other additives must be used to make this enrichment possible. For example, the stabilizers polysorbate 80 and propylene glycol help in adding water-soluble vitamins and vitamin A to foods. And mono- and diglycerides are used to coat thiamin, riboflavin, and niacin to prevent them from breaking down and producing off-odors and a bitter taste in enriched foods.

Other additives. *Bleaching and maturing agents,* such as acetone peroxide and azodicarbonamide, make flour whiter and improve its baking characteristics. *Sequestrants,* such as EDTA and citric acid, are used in shortenings and elsewhere to prevent metal contaminants from causing rancidity. *Humectants*—glycerol, propylene glycol, and sorbitol—absorb and hold water, thereby minimizing the effect of atmospheric changes on foods such as candy and shredded coconut. *Anticaking agents*—various silicates and yellow prussiate of soda—keep salts and powders flowing freely. *Firming agents*—various calcium salts—prevent canned fruits and vegetables from becoming too soft. There are also *foaming agents* that keep whipped toppings whipped and *foam inhibitors* that keep down foam where it's not wanted; *clarifying agents* that keep liquids from clouding up; *solvents* that carry flavors, colors, and other additives into some foods and remove chemicals (for example, caffeine) from others; *glazing agents* that make food surfaces shiny and help prevent spoilage; and *releasing agents* that help separate food from its surrounding surfaces during processing and transport.

Are They Safe?

If you're asking for absolute safety, the answer is "no." Absolutes in scientific research do not exist. Many things, natural and synthetic, consumed in excessive amounts are harmful, and it is possible to design an animal test that would demonstrate the toxicity of most "harmless" substances (that is, harmless in the manner in which it's usually consumed). For the most part, however, food additives have been far better tested than the natural chemicals in foods.

Certainly, additives are safer and more closely scrutinized today than in the "good old days" at the turn of the century, when America's burgeoning food industry was not above using copper sulphate, a powerful emetic, to give canned vegetables a fresh look. Other potential poisons, such as salicylic acid, borax, and formaldehyde, were used in generous amounts. The industry goal was not food purity or safety, but simply to keep the food—even spoiled food—looking and smelling good until it reached the consumer.

In 1906 Congress passed the nation's first Food and Drugs Act to prohibit the adulteration of processed foods with toxic ingredients. It succeeded in keeping many harmful additives out of foods, but did nothing to counter contamination by pesticides. The law also had weak enforcement provisions. It was up to the government to prove a substance hazardous; inspectors could enter plants only with management permission and the penalties they could impose were light. So in 1938 a new law was passed—the Food, Drug and Cosmetic Act—still in effect, in amended form, today. This act prohibited the use of poisonous or harmful substances in food, but it exempted certain substances and mandated "safe" tolerance levels for others that were either unavoidable contaminants or necessary for production. But it was still up to the government to prove a substance hazardous *after* it was in the food supply.

In 1958 the law was amended by the passage of the *Food Additives Amendment,* which required that new food chemicals (both intentional and incidental additives) be shown to be safe *before* they could be added to foods. But it exempted from premarket testing requirements 670 substances "Generally Recognized as Safe"—or *"GRAS"* substances— on the basis of available scientific data or previous experience of their safe use in foods. Other substances were awarded *"prior sanctioned"* status since their use in foods had already received official approval; they, too, were exempt from further testing requirements.

The GRAS list contains some of our most prominent food additives: sugar, salt, ascorbic acid, nitrates (nitrites were prior sanctioned), cornstarch, MSG, lecithin, a host of food colors both natural and synthetic, vitamins and minerals, leavening agents, sorbitol, the fumigants methyl bromide and ethylene oxide, propellants, solvents like alcohol and glycerine, gums, waxes, and the preservatives sodium benzoate and calcium propionate. Until 1972, when evidence of its cancer-causing potential became impossible to ignore, saccharin had also been a GRAS substance.

In 1980 a national group of independent scientists, who report back to the Food and Drug Administration, completed a review of 415 substances on the GRAS list. Of the chemicals examined, 305 (73 percent) were declared safe, including sodium benzoate, sorbitol, cellulose, mustard, and many phosphates. Another 68 (16 percent) were said to be all right but more information was needed; in the interim the amounts permitted in food might be restricted. These include natural gums, agar, sulfur dioxide, licorice, sucrose (table sugar), and corn sugar. Nineteen (5 percent) of the chemicals fell into a third category —"uncertainties exist requiring that additional studies be conducted" —among them BHT, caffeine, carrageenan, and nutmeg. Another 5 additives (1 percent) were said to warrant restrictions as currently used. These include salt and four modified starches, as well as the use in baby foods of MSG and hydrolyzed vegetable protein. And 18 additives (4 percent) fell into a final category for which there were inadequate data to make a judgment, including waxes used on fruits, vegetables, and food packages.

The remaining 100 GRAS substances include spices and natural flavors that will be evaluated by another group of experts as part of a review of 1,350 flavorings. In addition, all 31 approved color additives and 11 provisionally accepted colors are being examined. A total of 1,571 food additives are now being looked at to determine if any regulatory changes are necessary.

Additives not prior sanctioned or on the GRAS list, new ones introduced since 1958, and old additives to be used in new ways must undergo a series of safety tests that include the following:

An "acute toxicity" test, in which a large single dose is given to laboratory animals to determine a chemical's possible poisonous effects.

Subchronic toxicity tests, in which various concentrations of a chemical are fed to groups of animals for ninety days to determine effects on growth, behavior, appearance, body organs, disease, and death rates.

Long-term toxicity tests in laboratory animals—lasting at least two years and usually more—to determine the effects of lifelong exposure to a chemical. In some cases, effects on reproduction and lactation are evaluated by giving the chemical for more than one generation.

Many of the controversies about additive safety surround the adequacies of these tests, which are done under the manufacturer's auspices and submitted to the FDA for evaluation. It is economically and logistically impossible to test additives in the manner and amounts to which humans are exposed to them. Large doses of a chemical are required to get results in a relatively small number of animals within their brief life span. Thus, the daily dose given to an animal could equal several years' worth of human exposure. Some scientists believe that the large doses used in animal testing make a chemical seem a lot worse than it would be under ordinary conditions of human use. The error —if there is one—is thus presumably on the side of safety.

Questions have also been raised about applying test results obtained in short-lived laboratory rodents, exposed to only one chemical at a time, to long-lived humans who are bombarded with hundreds of different chemicals at once. But no one has yet come up with a better testing scheme that is still practical.

If a chemical is approved, the FDA usually sets a limit—the least amount needed to do the job—on how much can be used in various foods. In most cases the maximum allowed is a hundredth the level that caused toxic effects in test animals. In other words, the toxic dose is at least one hundred times greater than the amount allowed in foods. Several natural beneficial additives, including vitamins A and D, fall short of this built-in margin of safety (their safety margins are a twenty-fifth and a fortieth, respectively) and other synthetic additives go far beyond it. The levels typically permitted are in the range of parts per million. For example, the FDA permits 50 parts per million of BHT in dry cereal (1.6 ounces in each ton of cereal).

The 1958 Food Additive Amendment included a clause that was both highly praised for helping to maintain safety in processed foods and widely blamed for creating public hysteria about additives. This is the so-called *Delaney Clause* which states that *no additive can be used if it causes cancer when fed to animals or people or if it causes cancer in human or animal tests "appropriate for the evaluation of the safety of food additives."*

Substances on the GRAS list are exempt from the clause, although at any time the FDA could remove the GRAS designation from a suspect chemical (as it did with saccharin) and bring it within Delaney jurisdiction. The clause was responsible for the banning of the colors Red Dye No. 4, Violet No. 1, and carbon black; a vermouth flavoring, and the root-beer flavor safrole. It was also invoked to disallow the use of the growth hormone DES in cattle; but the FDA ruling was overturned in the courts on technical grounds, and this substance—which has caused cancer in the daughters of women who received it during pregnancy—remained a possible incidental additive in the American food supply for five years longer (see further discussion on page 478).

One problem with the Delaney Clause is that while it theoretically allows discretion on the part of the FDA to decide what are "appropriate" tests for food additives, in fact—because of political pressure—most feeding tests that have resulted in cancers in test animals have been considered appropriate.

Another dilemma is that the Delaney Clause permits consideration only of an additive's risks, not its possible benefits. Thus the finding that saccharin caused cancer when fed to test animals compelled an FDA ban despite its presumed (though unproven) benefits to people with diabetes and weight problems. It took an act of Congress to stay the agency's hand—at least temporarily. (See pages 483–486 for further discussion of the safety of artificial sweeteners.)

There are still other unknowns about the safety of food additives. In most cases, each additive is tested by itself. Little is known about possible interactions with other substances that might be used in the same product or in products that are eaten together. Interactions might also occur with chemicals naturally present in foods or that get into foods as environmental contaminants. For example, the preservative sorbic acid and its salts (sorbates) can combine with nitrites, which are present in digestive juices and used as food additives, to form potent compounds that can damage the genes. Such damage, called mutation, might result in birth defects or cancerous changes in cells. In another example, the pesticide atrazine, which contaminates some drinking-water supplies, can also react with nitrites to form a possible cancer-causing substance, N-nitrosoatrazine. No one yet knows what hazard such interactions may present to human consumers. And while it is assumed that the toxic effects of different food chemicals are not cumulative, it is not a certainty in all cases. In some situations, one chemical can wipe out the toxic effects of another. Could they enhance one another under other circumstances?

A Few Bad Apples

Public doubts about the safety of food additives have been nurtured by disclosures that certain long-assumed-to-be-safe chemicals are, in fact, hazardous to health and some are too dangerous to be used at all. These few "bad apples" have prompted some consumers to discard the whole barrel, barring forever from their pantry and palate any and all chemicals that "contaminate" foods.

To be sure, disclosures of real and potential dangers from various food additives have been frequent enough to stir the complacency of the most trusting consumer. Among the more notable additive scares are these.

MSG

Glutamate has been used as a flavor enhancer in Oriental cooking for thousands of years. At the beginning of this century, a Japanese chemist isolated monosodium glutamate from a seaweed that was often used in Japanese cooking to improve flavor. It wasn't long before MSG found its way into Western cooking as well. (Remember "Pour on the Ac'cent and bring the flavor out"?) By 1967 Americans were using about 45 million pounds of MSG a year, which is also marketed under the brand name Ajinomoto, as plain MSG, or mixed with other spices.

Then, in 1968, an American physician of Chinese extraction described a series of strange symptoms he experienced within half an hour of starting a meal in a Chinese restaurant: a burning sensation in the back of his neck and forearms, a tight feeling in his chest, and a headache. He dubbed it *"Chinese Restaurant Syndrome."* Upon reading this description, fellow sufferers emerged like so many dishes at a Chinese banquet. A team of New York physicians traced the syndrome to the soup he had eaten, specifically to the MSG that is commonly added in large quantities to Chinese soups.

Chinese Restaurant Syndrome is a temporary discomfort of no known lasting significance (and usually avoidable by skipping the soup course). Soon after its discovery, however, more serious questions were raised about MSG. Dr. John W. Olney of the Washington University School of Medicine in St. Louis found, in 1969, that feeding MSG to infant mice destroyed nerve cells in the part of the brain that controls appetite, body temperature, and other important functions. MSG was subsequently removed voluntarily from baby foods; many Chinese restaurants reduced their dependence on the chemical or offered to omit it upon a diner's request. But MSG has remained on the GRAS list, and no regulatory action has been taken to ban its use in baby foods. A scientific review panel for the FDA concluded in 1980 that MSG was not hazardous to adults as it is presently used, but recommended that manufacturers use restraint in how much they add to foods.

FOOD COLORS

These are certainly the most controversial of additives. Since their purpose is purely cosmetic, even the slightest risk associated with their use is too great. The controversy has focused on a relatively small group of artificial colors that were originally derived from coal tars and now are synthesized in pure form. Nothing like them is found in nature. They are far and away the most widely used coloring agents in the American food supply.

In the past half century, *more than a dozen coal-tar food colors have been banned because they were found to damage internal organs or cause cancer in laboratory animals.* In fact, a number of industrial (nonfood) dyes derived from coal tars have also been shown to cause cancer, in people as well as test animals. Among the banned food colors have been FDC Orange No. 1 and No. 2; Yellow Nos. 1, 2, 3, and 4; Violet No. 1; Red Nos. 2 and 4; and carbon black. Citrus Red No. 2 can only be used to dye the outer skin of oranges; in animals it can cause internal organ damage and cancer.

All but one of the six remaining coal-tar dyes are suspect, especially Red No. 40, which replaced the banished reds and is now the most widely used food color. It promotes the growth of cancers in mice. Red No. 3, another widely used food color, has been shown to partially block the uptake by rat brain cells of a crucial neurotransmitter called dopamine, which carries messages between brain cells and, in people, has a pronounced effect on moods and behavior. Red No. 3 is also suspected of causing cancer.

Other colors among the 16 synthetic food dyes now approved by the FDA are as yet very poorly tested, so little is known about their safety or potential hazards. Some nations are far less liberal than ours about synthetic food colors. Norway and Greece forbid them entirely, and Canada permits the use of only 9. The World Health Organization evaluated 29 colors, and found for only 6 sufficient evidence to establish acceptable levels for daily consumption. Another 9 were given provisional acceptable intake levels pending additional data.

More than 10 percent of the foods Americans eat are artificially colored. *If there is a battle to be fought against food additives, it's best directed at these synthetic food colors, which have little or nothing to do with good nutrition or the availability of an adequate and healthful food supply.* Meanwhile, you can avoid a lot of them by not eating factory-concocted junk foods.

DES

In full chemical regalia, this substance is known as diethylstilbestrol. It is a synthetic hormone that acts like the female sex hormone estrogen and is used as a growth stimulant for cattle. It helps the animal put on lean meat more quickly, thus reducing the amount of grain needed as feed and the resulting cost of beef to the consumer. Residues of DES occasionally appear in meat, especially liver, from DES-treated animals.

DES also causes cancer in people. Cancers of the vagina and cervix have developed in young women whose mothers were treated with large doses of DES during pregnancy. While nothing like these doses could ever result from eating DES-contaminated meat, DES is a carcinogen when consumed and such carcinogens cannot be added, intentionally or accidentally, to human foods.

The FDA tried at first to prevent DES contamination of retail meats by requiring a preslaughter grace period of seven days during which DES could not be used. But it didn't work; even with the week-long restriction DES residues could still be found in 2 percent of cattle livers tested. So the FDA banned the use of the hormone entirely. The manufacturers of DES took the matter to court in 1974 and won the case on a technicality. The FDA issued a new ban, however, which finally took effect on November 1, 1979. Still, some producers illegally sold DES, and it continued to be used in livestock into 1980.

Sulfites

An estimated one million Americans are sensitive to sulfites, although the actual number could be much higher. Sulfite preservatives are commonly used on shrimp (especially those that go to the fresh market), frozen vegetables like potatoes that darken upon exposure to air, the ingredients in many salad bars and buffets, fresh mushrooms sold in packages, and dried fruits. In addition, nearly all wine is made with sulfites.

While not everyone is unlucky enough to suffer adverse reactions to these widely used preservatives, when reactions occur, they can be —and in a few cases have been—fatal. Most likely to be affected are people with asthma, but serious reactions, including death, have occurred in people with no history of asthma or serious allergies. Reactions to sulfites have included shortness of breath, weakness, tight feeling in the chest and/or throat, hives, severe wheezing, swelling of the tongue, and loss of consciousness.

Consumer advocates have been clamoring for labeling of all sulfite-treated foods, in addition to finding safer alternatives and banning their use in restaurants. Some salad bars now advertise their wares as free of sulfites. However, the restaurant diner can truly be in jeopardy, especially when the sulfites are added to bulk shipments at a processing plant (or, in the case of shrimp, on the boat) and the ingredients used by the chef have been transferred to unlabeled containers. Also potentially hazardous to the sulfite-sensitive are dishes prepared with wine or champagne.

Nitrates and Nitrites

An Iowa firm that makes a nitrite-free bacon ran the following advertisement:

HERE IS A SPECIAL HEALTH

MESSAGE

RED

MAY MEAN

DEAD

FOR . . . . YOU

OR YOUR LOVED ONES

Most all sliced bacon contains a color additive listed on the package as nitrate or nitrite. This chemical causes the red meat portion of the bacon to assume a brighter than normal, red color that seems attractive to the purchaser.

Nitrite combined with the secondary amines found in the muscle fat of this same bacon creates cancer-producing Nitrosamines when fried in your frying pan at home at 370° Fahrenheit or higher; Nitrosamines that you eat when you eat panfried traditional bacon.

These Nitrosamines have entered the blood stream to produce cancerous tumors of the lung, liver, stomach and other areas of the bodies of thousands of test animals that have similar biological characteristics of the human being.

Whatever you might say about the taste of this sales tactic, the ad copy is scientifically accurate. And it went only as far as the evidence available at the time (1975). Since then, further evidence has strengthened the indictment of nitrates and nitrites (which, incidentally, are exempt from the Delaney Clause) that are used in nearly all frankfurters, ham, luncheon meats, bacon, knockwurst, and other processed meats, and in smoked fish (not, however, in bratwurst, sliced whitemeat chicken roll, or turkey roll).

Nitrates and nitrites have been used as curing agents for meat for more than 2,000 years. Although they both have the ability to retard the growth of microorganisms, notably the potentially lethal botulism bacteria, they are primarily used for coloring and flavoring. They give hot dogs, cold cuts, and ham their characteristic pink color. Without these additives, these meats would have a brownish hue—like bratwurst. They may also have a slightly different flavor, although meat products free of nitrates and nitrites have been produced that taste nearly the same as their chemically treated counterparts.

Government scientists have shown that nitrosamines can form in the normal process of cooking nitrite-treated bacon, that nitrosamines could be found in 6 percent of the samples of processed meats and cooked sausage products on the retail market, and that 1.6 percent of cured hams also had detectable amounts of these cancer-causing chemicals. And the discovery of highly potent nitrosamines in most of the tested brands of beer and Scotch is apparently due to the barley malting process from which these beverages are made. Alternative manufacturing methods that would eliminate the potential hazard from beer and Scotch were already under study when news of the contamination reached the public in mid-1979. The switchover to new methods was industry-wide by January, 1980, and now any malt beverages that contain nitrosamines at levels that can reliably be detected—above 5 parts per billion—are subject to regulatory action. However, trace amounts of nitrosamines below that level may still be present in beer and Scotch.

The safety of nitrates and nitrites is a complex, confusing, and unsettled issue. It centers around the fact that nitrates can be changed by digestive juices into nitrites, and nitrites can combine with other food substances called amines (prominent in meat and fish) to form nitrosamines. Nitrosamines can form in nitrite-treated foods before cooking and as a result of cooking at high temperatures. They also form in the acid stomach of laboratory animals and probably in human beings as well. They are among the most potent cancer-causing substances yet discovered, and readily induce several different types of cancers in virtually all species of laboratory animals. Further, a study conducted in 1979 at the Massachusetts Institute of Technology suggested that nitrite itself might cause cancer of the lymph system in laboratory rats, though this finding was considered "inconclusive" by a team of independent experts. No human case of cancer has ever been traced to nitrosamines in foods, and the FDA decided in August, 1980, that existing scientific evidence did not warrant banning sodium nitrate as a cancer-causing agent.

The nitrates and nitrites question is complicated by the fact that most of our exposure to these chemicals is totally natural, not artificially introduced. Nearly four times as much nitrite is produced in your own saliva each day as you would get from an average serving of cured meats. A much smaller amount would be derived from the consumption of vegetables that naturally contain very large amounts of nitrates, including spinach, beets, radishes, celery, eggplant, carrots, lettuce, potatoes, and collard and turnip greens. Following consumption, some of the nitrates in these vegetables are changed to nitrites by digestive juices. Nitrate may also come from drinking water contaminated by fertilizer from farmlands. All told, an estimated 20 percent of our daily exposure to nitrite comes from the use of food additives; most of the rest is natural.

Still, many researchers concerned about the healthfulness of our food supply say there is no point in adding to the already substantial number of potentially hazardous chemicals we are exposed to. A 20-percent cutback in potential exposure to a carcinogen can be significant, especially since, unlike vegetables rich in nitrate, the chemically treated meats and fish deliver a concentrated dose of the basic ingredients needed for forming nitrosamines—nitrites and amines (from protein).

The U.S. Department of Agriculture has mandated a reduction in the amounts of nitrates and nitrites allowed in certain products and has eliminated the use of nitrites entirely in others. The department specified that the reduced amount of nitrite now permitted in bacon must be used along with sodium ascorbate (a form of vitamin C) to block the formation of nitrosamines. The USDA is also periodically testing fried bacon from commercial sources, as well as other nitrite-cured meats, to be sure the levels of nitrosamines in them are at or below the lowest reliably detectable amount—10 parts per billion. At the same time, alternative preservatives and coloring and flavoring agents are under study.

If you want to avoid needless exposure to nitrates and nitrites, start reading labels (if present, these chemicals must always be listed) and restrict your purchases to those products that are prepared without them. Check the frozen-food compartment, "deli" section, or local health-food stores for brands of frankfurters, bacon, and other meats that are specially prepared without nitrates or nitrites. (The frankfurters may be labeled "uncured cooked sausage" or "uncured franks"; the bacon may be called "pork bellies" or "pork strips" or "uncured bacon.")

Don't keep uncured meats in an unfrozen state for more than four to seven days, and don't let them sit unrefrigerated for more than a few minutes. If you're worried about botulism, stick to products that have to be cooked after purchase since heat destroys the botulinum toxin.

But the best solution is to greatly reduce or eliminate from your diet bacon, frankfurters, and cold cuts which have other more serious nutritional shortcomings. They are very high in fat (mostly saturated animal fat), cholesterol, and sodium, and are thus a nutritionally poor source of protein.

Sweeteners

Our schizophrenic attitude toward the safety and healthfulness of our food supply was probably never more clearly demonstrated than in 1977, when *saccharin* was threatened with extinction because it caused cancer in laboratory rats. The very public and its congressional representatives who criticized the FDA and the food industry for "poisoning" our food with harmful additives this time clamored for keeping a cancer-causing additive on the open market.

Saccharin, after all, was special. Then the only noncaloric artificial sweetener permitted in foods, it was beloved by millions who wanted something—a sweet taste—for nothing. The obese said saccharin was their life line to slimdom, and diabetics claimed it was essential to controlling their blood sugar. Who cared if some rats got cancer? The public outcry over the threatened saccharin ban led to a congressionally voted eighteen-month moratorium on the ban, which has subsequently been indefinitely extended.

Although saccharin has been around since 1900, it really didn't come into widespread use until after 1969, when its noncaloric companion, *cyclamate,* was banned as a potential carcinogen. By 1980 some 50 to 70 million Americans—including one-third of children under 10—used saccharin regularly, and three-fourths of the 7 million pounds consumed each year was as a sweetener in diet soft drinks.

The test that spelled cyclamate's doom used a 10-to-1 combination of cyclamate and saccharin, but only cyclamate was banned. Although numerous subsequent tests showed no cancer-causing effect of cyclamate alone, attempts to get it back on the market have been spurned. Actually, no matter how unjustly a food chemical may have been treated, in the current cancerophobic climate the chances are slim that a once-suspected and banned substance will be returned to the marketplace.

Ironically, though, saccharin is far more likely to be the villain of the piece. The first hints of hazard date back to the 1950s when three animal experiments showed that feeding high doses of saccharin or implanting saccharin pellets in the bladder increased the incidence of bladder tumors. But these findings were virtually ignored until 1972, when another test of implanted saccharin pellets again produced bladder cancers. Based on this test, the FDA removed saccharin from the GRAS list and ordered that all products containing it must state that it is a *"nonnutritive sweetener for persons who must restrict their intake*

of ordinary sweets." However, the National Academy of Sciences in
1974 deemed the evidence for saccharin's cancer-causing potential to
be inconclusive, and its popularity continued to zoom.

Finally, in March, 1977, a Canadian study showed that feeding
large doses of saccharin to pregnant rats and their weanlings produced
bladder cancers in the male offspring. The Canadians immediately
banned saccharin, and the FDA announced its intention to follow suit.
Shortly thereafter, Congress enacted the Saccharin Study and Labeling
Act, which stayed the FDA's hand temporarily and ordered a stronger
warning on all saccharin products:

Use of this product may be hazardous to your health. This product contains
saccharin which has been determined to cause cancer in laboratory animals.

The warning had less of an effect than the one on cigarette packs,
judging from how Americans continued to guzzle saccharin-sweetened
drinks.

Again in 1978, the National Academy of Sciences reviewed the
saccharin evidence and this time concluded that the sweetener was a
weak carcinogen in animals and probably also capable of causing cancer
in people. The academy scientists suggested that saccharin might act
primarily as a *co-carcinogen,* or promoter of other cancer-causing
agents.

While the tests of saccharin's cancer-causing ability in people have
been equivocal, experts point out that none has been designed well
enough to detect a generalized cancer-promoting role. But the issue has
become somewhat moot now that another artificial sweetener without
known carcinogenic properties has come on the scene. In 1981, after
years of waffling over controversial safety tests, the FDA finally approved aspartame, a substance 200 times sweeter than sugar (1/10
calorie's worth of aspartame is equivalent in sweetening power to 1
teaspoon of sugar containing about 16 calories.) Aspartame, a chemical
combination of two amino acids (aspartic acid and phenylalanine) that
are ordinarily found in protein foods, was introduced by G. D. Searle
as a table top sweetener called Equal and as a food additive called
Nutrasweet.

Ironically, manufacturers of diet drinks were not too delighted
with aspartame's arrival because it cut seriously into their profits. For
decades they'd been selling diet sodas at the same price as regular
sugar-sweetened ones, but the saccharin cost only a tiny fraction of
what they spent on sugar. Now, here was an artificial sweetener almost
as expensive as the real thing! But the manufacturers had no choice: the

public demanded aspartame, which has a flavor much closer to sugar's and which lacks the bitter aftertaste so common to saccharin. It wasn't long before soft drink manufacturers clamored to shed the saccharin taint and replace it with the "hot" new substitute. Sales of aspartame and diet drinks soared and, for the moment at least, both the manufacturers and the public were thrilled.

But with millions now downing aspartame, complaints started trickling in and researchers began to look at it more critically. While aspartame has thus far been spared any link to cancer, it has hardly escaped without charges of health hazard. It was known from the outset that aspartame could not be used safely by people—about one in 15,000 —who suffer from an inherited metabolic disorder called phenylketonuria (PKU), who lack an enzyme needed to process phenylalanine. If this amino acid is allowed to build up in the blood, it damages the brain and causes mental retardation. But what wasn't recognized until millions started consuming aspartame is that certain people—the percentage is not yet known—who are free of PKU nonetheless seem to have some peculiar reactions to aspartame. Complaints have included depression, severe headache, behavioral abnormalities, and seizures, in addition to more pedestrian problems like hives and stomach upset. The national Centers for Disease Control evaluated some 600 of such complaints and, while failing to find a clearcut pattern, also felt unable to give aspartame a clean bill of health. Rather, continued monitoring of complaints and further well-designed studies of people using aspartame were recommended. Such studies are now underway under Searle's sponsorship. Meanwhile, the Council on Scientific Affairs of the American Medical Association, an organization not noted for aggressive action to protect the public health, has concluded that "available evidence suggests that consumption of aspartame by normal humans is safe and is not associated with serious adverse health effects."

Ironically, through all this tumult about artificial sweeteners, none have ever been shown to be of any particular benefit to anyone. Not one study has ever demonstrated that artificial sweeteners actually help diabetics control their blood sugar or that they help dieters shed excess pounds. If anything, while the popularity of artificially sweetened foods and drinks soared, Americans got heavier! At best, artificial sweeteners simply perpetuate your sweet tooth and make it more likely that you'll succumb to a highly sugar-sweetened food when tempted.

Your best bet, then, is to try to break your sweet addiction. Start by cutting out diet drinks, which have nothing to offer nutritionally in any case. Try substituting fruit juices mixed half-and-half with unsweetened beverages like seltzer, club soda, mineral water, or just plain water. Or leave out the fruit juice altogether. After a few weeks, you just may find that diet pop tastes sickeningly sweet (see Chapter 6 for other sweet suggestions).

Additives and the Hyperactive Child

An estimated 5 to 10 percent of school-age children are said to be hyperactive, far more boys than girls. Their restlessness, short attention span, and disruptive behavior interfere with learning and disturb others around them. Many factors have been suspected as causes—including prenatal brain damage, inherited abnormalities, birth injuries, low-level lead poisoning, excessive sugar consumption, and vitamin deficiencies. In all likelihood, there are many causes which in different children produce a similar set of symptoms.

But in 1973 Dr. Ben F. Feingold, a pediatric allergist at the Kaiser-Permanente Medical Center in San Francisco, proposed that half of children described as being hyperactive can benefit from a diet that excludes all artificial colors and flavors and various foods that naturally contain chemicals called salicylates (relatives of aspirin). Younger children were said to respond best to the modified diet.

The Feingold diet virtually eliminates all factory-made soft drinks, candies, cakes, puddings, ice cream, luncheon meats, margarine, many processed cheeses, plus a host of other processed foods. In addition, the restriction on salicylates means no grapes, raisins, cucumbers, cherries, apples, apricots, oranges, nectarines, peaches, plums, prunes, tomatoes, strawberries, or raspberries; nothing flavored with natural mint or wintergreen; no aspirin-containing medications; and no tea. However, a return to the salicylate-containing items is permitted after four to six weeks of a favorable response.

Dr. Feingold's theory, supported by clinical observations and anecdotal reports of dramatic improvement among children who followed the restricted regimen, was naturally attractive to parents struggling to care for their frenetic offspring. Many were disillusioned with other treatments, especially with the use of powerful drugs that could impair a child's physical development while controlling his or her hyperactivity.

The "good word" spread quickly after publication in 1974 of Dr. Feingold's book *Why Your Child Is Hyperactive,* describing his behavior-changing diet and the remarkable effects it supposedly had on half the affected children. "Feingold Associations"—clubs of enthusiastic parents—were formed throughout the nation while scientists tried to verify Feingold's claims. Unlike Dr. Feingold, they performed controlled, double-blind tests in which neither the child nor the observers (parents, teachers, testers, and independent evaluators) knew which child was on which diet at which time. In the typical study, half the children were placed on the Feingold diet and the other half on a similarly constituted diet that contained the prohibited substances. Then after a time (several weeks to a month), the diets were switched. The results of such trials have been inconsistent. Some showed no benefit; others showed some improvement in a small group of young children; still others showed benefit only on the basis of the parents' observations but not as assessed by teachers, testers, and independent observers. In no study was the extensive improvement reported by Dr. Feingold seen.

In a second series of studies—eight to date—some hyperactive children were fed artificial colors hidden in special foods, and others were given the same foods without the colors. After a time, the groups were switched. Again, no dramatic results were observed, but two studies showed a small but significant increase in hyperactivity after the additives were eaten. In a third study, 1 of 22 children—a 3-year-old girl—responded with a dramatic worsening of her behavior problems after eating disguised doses of artificial colors.

Yet another study in Toronto examined the effects of a much larger dose of artificial colors on a group of 40 children, 20 of whom had been diagnosed as hyperactive. The amount of dye used was said to be twice the average daily intake for young children. Rather than behavior observed by parents or teachers, the Toronto researchers measured the children's performance on a learning test. The hyperactive children—but not the others—made many more errors on the test after consuming the food-dye mixture. The scientists concluded that the dyes can act like toxic drugs in hyperactive children and interfere with learning by decreasing the children's ability to pay attention. The Toronto researchers criticized previous studies for using dye doses far too small to be meaningful.

In other studies on isolated nerve cells, Red No. 3 was shown to disrupt substances that transmit nerve messages. Although it is not known if the dye can get into the brain under normal conditions, when fed to rats it causes behavioral disturbances.

How can these confusing results be interpreted? First, they show nothing like the spectacular changes in behavior that Dr. Feingold claimed for his diet. Second, they indicate that *while some young hyper-active children might be affected by certain additives, the vast majority probably are not.* In fact, the observed effects of the Feingold regimen may have less to do with additives per se than with an overall improvement in the child's nutritional status when all junk foods and most heavily processed foods are eliminated from the diet. Another factor may be the enormous amount of family cooperation and attention to the child that the Feingold diet demands.

Nonetheless, the studies do suggest that food dyes can affect behavior and learning in some children. And they point to a deficiency in the safety testing of food additives—the lack of any systematic screening of these chemicals for toxic effects on behavior.

AN EATER'S GUIDE TO ADDITIVE SAFETY

The following list is based on scientific evidence available in mid-1980 about the risks of various popular food additives. It is derived largely from "Chemical Cuisine," a poster prepared by the Center for Science in the Public Interest, but has been updated according to recent information available to this author. For some items in the "Avoid" column, there is no known clear-cut risk, but the chemicals have been poorly tested and serve no essential role. For some additives listed under "Caution," testing has been inadequate or has raised suspicions of a possible hazard and safer substitutes are available.

Avoid

Artificial colorings: Blue No. 1, Blue No. 2, Citrus Red No. 2, Green No. 3, Red Nos. 3 and 40, Yellow No. 5
Brominated vegetable oil (BVO)
Caffeine (for children and pregnant women)
Monosodium glutamate (MSG) (for children)
Quinine
Saccharin
Sodium nitrate
Sodium nitrite

Caution

Artificial coloring Yellow No. 6
Artificial flavorings
Butylated hydroxyanisole (BHA)
Butylated hydroxytoluene (BHT)
Caffeine (for nonpregnant adults)
Carrageenan
Heptyl paraben
Mono- and diglycerides
Monosodium glutamate (MSG) (for adults)
Phosphoric acid and phosphates
Propyl gallate
Sodium bisulfite
Sulfur dioxide

Safe

Alginate and propylene and glycol alginate
Alpha tocopherol
Ascorbic acid
Beta carotene
Calcium (or sodium) stearoyl lactylate
Carboxymethylcellulose (CMC)
Casein and sodium caseinate

Guide continues on next page

An Eater's Guide continued

Citric acid and sodium citrate
EDTA
Erythorbic acid
Ferrous gluconate
Fumaric acid
Gelatin
Glycerin (glycerol)
Gums: arabic, furcelleran, ghatti,
  guar, karaya, locust bean,
  tragacanth
Hydrolyzed vegetable protein (HVP)

Lactic acid
Lactose
Lecithin
Mannitol
Polysorbate 60, 65, and 80
Sodium benzoate
Sorbic acid and potassium sorbate
Sorbitan monostearate
Sorbitol
Starch and modified starch
Vanillin and ethyl vanillin

And don't forget those most popular food additives, sugars and salt, which should always be consumed with discretion (see Chapters 6 and 10).

A Rational Approach to Additives

Additives—especially those of questionable safety—are most abundant in foods that we would all be better off without. Candy, cold cuts, sausages, artificial beverages, packaged cakes, snack foods, and various ersatz products are additive-laden foods that offer little nutritional benefit or that contain too much fat or sugar to be worth the calories. Here are some tips to help you reduce your exposure to needless additives and minimize any possible adverse effects from the rest. Several of the recommendations come to you compliments of *Environmental Nutrition,* a bimonthly newsletter for consumers.

• Eat a wide variety of foods. This will help to dilute the concentration of additives in any one food and thus minimize the chances that it will reach hazardous levels in your body. Don't have a salami sandwich for lunch every day or guzzle two or more cans of diet pop. Foods that are primarily additives or are heavily dosed with them should be, at most, a sometime thing in your diet.

• Use fresh or minimally processed foods. Those that are boxed or canned have more additives than those that are frozen. Fresh foods have the least amount of additives (usually none). The further removed a food is from its natural form, the more additives it's likely to contain.

• Use "real foods," not their artificial equivalents. Drink *real* fruit juice (freshly made or frozen), not powdered imitations or fruit drinks that are artificially flavored, colored, sweetened, and stoked with vitamins and/or minerals.

• Make reading labels a regular habit before you toss foods into your shopping cart (see Chapter 27). Though not all additives must be listed, most are in the ingredients list on the package. If your eyesight is poor, take a hand magnifying lens with you when you shop. Compare brands of similar items, and choose those that are prepared with the fewest additives or that leave out additives that are suspect.

• Don't be fooled by the word "natural" on the package. *All-natural* does not mean additive-free, since many additives *are* natural substances (see Chapter 26). In fact, it's possible to make an entirely synthetic food from completely natural chemicals. This, of course, does not mean that the product is hazardous or undesirable, but you should know that what you're paying for is not what naturally sprang from the earth in that form.

• In reducing your consumption of additives, don't forget the two leading ones: *sugar and salt.* In many ways, these two chemicals are the most hazardous ones on the American market today. And both are on the GRAS list! Remember what that means: "Generally Recognized as Safe." Don't you believe it.

In summary, food additives are neither inherently good nor inherently bad. When harmless chemicals are added to nutritious foods to enhance their palatability and make them available to more Americans than they otherwise could be, they are clearly the good guys in the nutritional war. But when they're used to concoct calorie-guzzling, nutritionally deficient "foods" that distract people from useful ones, they can appropriately be called a "poison" even though they themselves may be perfectly safe.

FOR FURTHER READING

Greta Bunin and Michael Jacobson, Ph.D., *"Does Everything Cause Cancer? A Food Safety Primer"* (Center for Science in the Public Interest, 1755 S Street N.W., Washington, D.C. 20009).

Marian Burros, *Pure and Simple* (New York: Berkley, 1978). An additive-free cookbook.

Michael E. Jacobson, Ph.D., *The Complete Eater's Digest and Nutrition Scoreboard: The Consumer's Factbook of Food Additives and Healthful Eating* (New York: Anchor/Doubleday, 1985).

Elizabeth M. Whelan, Sc.D., and Frederick J. Stare, M.D., *Panic in the Pantry* (New York: Atheneum, 1975).

26 ❧ HEALTH FOODS: ARE THEY HEALTHIER?

FRIGHTENED BY reports of "poisons" all around us and sacrifices of safety for the sake of profit, in the 1970s thousands of shoppers abandoned supermarkets for "health food" stores and "nutrition centers," where shelves were stocked with "natural" and "organic" foods. These terms inspired confidence in consumers, who had lost faith in traditional foods, a confidence readily bolstered by health-food literature that promised miraculous cures and preventives from eating chemical-free foods and taking nutritional supplements.

"Organically grown," "all natural," "no preservatives," "no additives," "nothing artificial" became the catchwords of this new movement. Many producers of ordinary foods jumped on the bandwagon and began selling "natural foods," too, proclaiming their products to be free of preservatives or additives or artificial ingredients. This did not slow the growth of the health-food industry, however, which in five years exploded from 245 manufacturers doing $500 million worth of business a year (mostly in California) to a nationwide industry of 1,100 manufacturers that today takes in several billion consumer dollars. At the same time, the health-food industry's emphasis shifted from an almost exclusive focus on vitamins, minerals, and other nutritional supplements to "whole" foods—cereals, flours, rice, grains, dried fruit, nuts, herbal teas, yogurt, fertile eggs, and unfertilized produce.

The health-food promise of better health through better eating is as yet unsubstantiated by scientific evidence. In fact, the Federal Trade Commission has proposed a ban on calling anything a "health food." Yes, some kinds of foods emphasized in health-food stores *are* more nutritious than typical supermarket fare. Yes, there *are* remains of some pesticides on ordinary foods. Yes, chemicals *are* added to most processed foods. Yes, some nutrients *are* lost in highly processed foods. And yes, pesticides and some additives *are* harmful to laboratory animals exposed to large doses. But no, *there is no evidence that foods called "natural" or "organic" are safer or more healthful than other foods.* Nor is there any guarantee that foods so labeled are free of the additives and pesticides that the health-foods consumer seeks to avoid.

In fact, there's evidence of consumer fraud in the health-food industry—of foods sold as "organic" that harbor residues of pesticides, of foods labeled one thing that are really another, and of foods called "natural" that are highly processed and filled with additives. Some manufacturers in the industry readily concede that when packaged health began to pay off, so did profiteering. In an interview in 1979 with *East West Journal,* Jeff Flasher, president of Erehwon, Inc., producer of more than 3,000 "health food" products, said, "The adulteration of quality has been dramatic compared to the last year, and much more dramatic compared to the year before. The number of products that I would consider to be 'questionable' in terms of ingredients, quality or raw materials, information on the label, or even mislabeling—that number has increased enormously, doubled from the year before." For example, Mr. Flasher said, while his company and a few other distributors of natural foods run periodic checks on the foods they call organic, most of the industry doesn't.

Ironically, the biggest boom in the health-food industry has been in the very same processed snacks and canned and ready-to-eat foods that health-food consumers initially rejected as unwholesome! Furthermore, many of the foods most popular among health-food enthusiasts are not particularly good for you—"natural" or not—because they're high in fat, saturated fat, cholesterol, sugar, or salt. According to Patricia Hausman, nutritionist with the Center for Science in the Public Interest, these include avocados (by weight avocados are 44 percent fat, one-fifth of it saturated), butter, coconut and coconut oil, nuts, cream cheese, egg yolks, granolas, cheese, honey, sea salt, miso, tamari, and soy sauce. In terms of fat, salt, calories, and cholesterol, a slice of "health food" quiche made with cheese, eggs, and cream, is no better nutritionally than a hot dog on a bun.

Yet, many people are willing to pay a premium price for health foods—often two to three times the price of comparable foods sold in supermarkets (see Table 26.1). A few items, such as rolled oats, unprocessed bran, dried fruits and nuts, that are sold in bulk form or packaged by the store may cost less at health-food stores. In some areas of the country, such stores are the only convenient source of certain desirable food products, such as unadulterated peanut butter, buckwheat flour, and bulgur. Grain products at health-food stores are generally of high quality and competitively priced. But other products, such as butter, fresh fruits and vegetables, eggs, meats, and poultry, may cost several times as much as the comparable items at the supermarket and yet be of inferior quality. Small and shriveled produce, rancid butter, and flavorless cheese are among typical costly health-food-store offerings.

Unless you buy at a store that is exceptionally clean and has a high product turnover, you may find an unexpected "bonus" in some health-food products—insects, especially in grains, dried fruits, and nuts that are free of preservatives and sold in bulk.

THE HIGH COST OF "ORGANIC" FOODS

The cost of selected foods labeled "organic" and sold at two stores in Washington, D.C., in February, 1976, was compared with the cost of regular foods sold at a Washington supermarket. Store No. 1 is a large natural-food store; Store No. 2 is a natural-food cooperative owned by the workers. The chart, compiled by Cynthia Cromwell of the U.S. Department of Agriculture, lists the cost of the organic products as a percent of the cost of comparable regular foods. Though a few organic products, like oats and wheat cereal, cost less than the regular version, most were considerably more expensive.

Table 26.1 • HOW MUCH DO "ORGANIC" FOODS COST?

Food	Amount	Dollar cost of regular food in supermarket	Cost of organic foods as percentage of regular foods Store No. 1	Store No. 2
Processed Foods				
Apple juice	1 quart	.45	198	182
Apple sauce	1 pound	.29	276	—
Cornmeal	1 pound	.26	154	115
Granola	1 pound	.69	—	132
Grits	1 pound	.37	214	116
Honey	1 pound	.94	120	115
Lentils	1 pound	.37	338	100
Oats, rolled	1 pound	.52	—	56
Peanut butter	1 pound	.79	—	170
Pickles	1 quart	1.00	150	150
Preserves, peach	1 pound	.87	151	—
Raisins	1 pound	.78	—	89
Tomatoes	1 pound	.23	326	296
Vinegar, cider	1 quart	.53	202	306
Wheat cereal	1 pound	.49	82	61
Whole-wheat bread	1 pound	.55	—	144
Whole-wheat flour	1 pound	.22	205	177

Table 26.1 continued

Food	Amount	Dollar cost of regular food in supermarket	Cost of organic foods as percentage of regular foods	
			Store No. 1	Store No. 2
Unprocessed Foods				
Apples	1 pound	.33	173	142
Beef, ground (regular)	1 pound	.75	313	—
Broccoli	1 pound	.55	125	129
Cabbage	1 pound	.10	550	430
Carrots	1 pound	.23	183	152
Chicken, whole fryer	1 pound	.65	254	—
Eggs	1 dozen	.79	165	—
Grapefruit	1 pound	.17	288	124
Green pepper	1 pound	.53	236	200
Lettuce, head	1 pound	.39	164	144
Onions	1 pound	.23	343	343
Potatoes, white	1 pound	.33	179	142
Spinach	1 pound	1.10	95	82
Tomatoes	1 pound	.52	208	138

Are Organic Foods Better?

The story of "organic" foods is not simple and straightforward. To start with, there isn't a legal definition of what *organic* means. Actually, *all food is organic.* Organic simply means made from compounds that contain carbon and were derived from plants or animals. The additive guar gum is organic, rice is organic, steak is organic, you are organic. But that's obviously not what most people mean when they think of so-called organic foods. They really mean foods that were grown without the use of chemical fertilizers, synthetic pesticides, antibiotics, and growth stimulants and that were processed without synthetic additives and preservatives. They mean foods that were grown in soil supplemented only with natural matter (manure or compost) and natural minerals, protected only by biological methods of pest control, and processed only with natural extracts and other organically grown foods.

But is this what you get when you buy "organic"? Often it's not. Since 1978, the Federal Trade Commission has been trying to introduce a legal definition of organically grown food and to prohibit the advertising as "organic" of any food that doesn't meet this definition. Currently, only a few states have laws that define *organic,* and even there, enforcement is questionable. In most of the nation, anyone can call anything organic, and it's up to the consumer to prove otherwise. Since people pay premium prices for organically grown foods, there's plenty of temptation to cheat, and consumer fraud in this area is rampant. Many purveyors of foods labeled "organically grown" have no idea where these foods come from and have never checked on the authenticity of the grower's claim.

In an analysis in 1972 by the New York State Food Laboratory, 30 percent of products labeled "organic" and purchased at health-food stores by government agents were found to contain residues of pesticides; among comparable foods lacking the "organic" claim, only 20 percent had such residues. Some proprietors of health-food stores have been seen to purchase ordinary food at nearby markets, remove the store package, jack up the price, and palm it off to customers as organically grown.

The truth is, there's more food being sold as "organically grown" than is actually grown organically. Furthermore, it can take years for residues of pesticides to disappear from the soil; even though a farmer may not add any synthetic pesticides, his first five to ten years of "organic" crops may still be contaminated with the unwanted chemicals. Crops may also become contaminated with pesticides used on nearby farms or along railroads or roadways.

Then there's the fact that it makes not a whit of difference to the nutrient content of the food if the food is grown with natural or chemical fertilizers. The nutrient content of a crop—the amount of protein, carbohydrates, fats, vitamins, and most minerals—is primarily determined by its genes, the weather, and the time at which it's harvested. A plant needs certain basic things in the soil to grow, and if those things are deficient, it will produce very poor yields, grow abnormally, or fail to grow at all. But if needed elements are there—supplied naturally or synthetically—the harvest will be a good one.

Only trace minerals in plants are influenced by how much of these minerals are present in the soil. Soils that are "organically fertilized" are even more likely than chemically fertilized soils to be deficient in essential trace minerals. If the soil in an area is lacking a particular mineral, say selenium, then the animals that eat plants grown on it also lack selenium and so will the manure these animals produce that's used as organic fertilizer on the same deficient soil. Chemical fertilizers, however, can supply the missing minerals in the required amounts.

No amount of fertilizer, organic or synthetic, will bring an apple up to the vitamin A content of a carrot or a carrot up to the vitamin C content of an orange. And no manipulation of the soil will raise the protein content of a green bean up to that of a soybean. At any given level of soil fertility, the content of the major nutrients in the plant is determined by its species, *not* by the organic constituents of the soil.

Three long-term studies—together totaling sixty-nine years of agricultural research—have shown no nutritional advantage to growing foods organically. No laboratory tests or animal-feeding studies have been able to distinguish between crops grown on organic versus chemically fertilized soil. Nor can consumers discern a difference in taste, according to studies conducted by the University of California at Davis and the University of Florida.

What's more, there's no evidence that organic fertilizer is a better way of providing plants with essential elements. Plants do not absorb nutrients in organic form. The elements that support plant growth must first be broken down into water-soluble inorganic ions before they can be taken up by the plant. In soils that are organically fertilized, this job is done by bacteria that live in the soil. When soluble chemical fertilizer is added to soil, bacterial breakdown is unnecessary.

It's true that plants grow better and produce higher yields per acre in soils that are rich in organic material. This fact is well known to farmers who use chemical fertilizers, and most of them routinely add organic material to their fields, usually by plowing in unharvested stalks, straw, or manure. Thus, in comparing organic with ordinary growing methods, you're seeing the results of two approaches to organic farming, one of which supplements nature with man-made fertilizer and the other which leaves nature to do the entire job. Organic fertilizer by itself is often unbalanced in nutrient content, and a good farmer will periodically analyze the soil and add to it inorganic chemicals in needed amounts. In addition, organic fertilizer, which is in short supply, is difficult and costly to distribute. About 1 pound of synthetic fertilizer supplies the nutrients in 20 pounds of manure, which is one reason why organically grown foods cost more.

Pesticide Residues and Other Contaminants

The use of pesticides, hormones, and antibiotics in producing ordinary foods is far more important to health than the way the soil is fertilized. There's no question that many foods sold to consumers contain *pesticide residues,* and no one would claim that the residues are good for you. The federal government determines the maximum amount of permitted pesticide contamination. Every two months the Food and Drug Administration does a "market basket" survey, analyzing pesticide residues in 117 kinds of foods in five regions of the country. The amounts allowed are extremely small—usually only a few parts per billion—and are based on toxicity tests in laboratory animals. In some foods, and for certain particularly hazardous chemicals, no detectable pesticide residues are permitted at all. The surveys have revealed some dramatic declines in residues of certain environmental contaminants, such as DDT and mercury, after their use was banned or curtailed.

Many researchers lament our current dependence on chemical pesticides because the pesticides cause serious environmental pollution, and because many pests have become resistant to the usual chemical killers, necessitating the use of larger amounts of more potent chemicals to keep them in check. Only belatedly has the agricultural establishment begun to take a serious look at alternative methods of pest control. Farmers, forced by the failure of chemicals, are coming to rely more on biological methods of pest control, such as the introduction of a beneficial insect species to eat the pest or a disease to attack it. The emphasis is now on "integrated pest management"—biological control techniques coupled with the judicious use of pesticides in small amounts for a limited time. The result should be more food available at lower cost and fewer potentially harmful chemicals reaching the consumer.

It would be great if we could abandon all use of pesticides right here and now, but the results would be disastrous. We already lose about a third of our crops to pests; without any pesticides, losses would soar to 50 percent or more and food costs would climb. The abandoning of pesticides would also mean the need to diversify crop production so that a single pest or disease could not wipe out an entire crop. But unless very carefully planned, such diversity may also mean lower yields and higher food prices.

Like it or not, American agriculture will be relying on synthetic pesticides for some time to come—perhaps forever. But the emphasis is finally beginning to shift, and the outlook is bright for diminished pesticide contamination of the food supply and the environment.

Organic food enthusiasts tend to forget another important form of food pollution—one, in fact, that has more direct effects on health than pesticide residues. That is the contamination of foods by disease-causing microorganisms. Unless properly sterilized, fertilizers from cattle and human wastes may contaminate foods with bacteria and parasites that cause serious gastrointestinal disease.

As for the use of *feed additives—antibiotics and stimulants* like the hormone DES—to promote the growth of farm animals, many scientists and government officials have long recommended an end to these practices. Nearly 40 percent of the antibiotics produced in this country are used in agriculture. They are routinely included in small amounts in animal feed to suppress infections that may limit growth. Unfortunately, this procedure promotes the development of resistant strains of infectious organisms that may contaminate the meat and poultry you buy. The hazard, if any, of this contamination is not known, but it is possible that some of the bacteria may infect people directly or may transfer their resistant genes to human pathogens.

Livestock producers claim that without feed additives it would cost more to produce meat and poultry because the animals would grow more slowly or succumb to infectious diseases. Their opponents say that feed additives are used to compensate for substandard maintenance and feed, and that animals raised under the best conditions show no added benefit from the additives.

The absence of feed additives in organically produced livestock, therefore, might be considered a plus for consumer health. But organically produced meat and poultry now sells for about three times the cost of comparable supermarket foods, and much of it must be frozen because it is transported long distances and turnover is slow.

Tips for the Organic Shopper

Remember the following if you choose to buy organically produced foods.

- Shop only at reputable stores.
- Find out on which days the store gets deliveries of produce, and shop on those days for peak quality.
- Keep in mind that the products in health-food stores are not all necessarily organically grown. Remember, there is no policing of the health-food industry.
- Ask to see affidavits or scientific tests by independent laboratories that attest to freedom from pesticides and additives.
- Ask the manager about the suppliers and whether they have

been personally visited to check on claims of organic production. Or visit the suppliers yourself. You should have more than someone's word to justify spending two to three times as much for food as you have to.

Another alternative, of course, is to grow your own produce. This can be done on a small scale in rural and suburban yards and even in city gardens—on rooftops, decks, and in street-level plots. If you grow more than you can eat fresh, freeze or can the rest for year-round consumption of organically grown fruits and vegetables.

But be especially careful about how you handle organically grown foods, or foods free of preservatives, to avoid harmful contamination with toxic microorganisms.

• All produce should be very carefully washed, preferably scrubbed, if not peeled before you eat it.

• Breads without preservatives should be kept in the refrigerator (unless eaten within two or three days) to prevent mold growth.

• Meats should not be eaten raw. Cured meats without nitrates or nitrites are best stored frozen.

• Cereals rich in nuts, seeds, and oils should not be kept for months; refrigerate or freeze them to prevent rancidity.

• All home-preserved foods should be canned according to instructions that come with the jars and lids or contained in an authoritative book on canning, such as "Home Canning of Fruits and Vegetables," a United States Department of Agriculture booklet that can be purchased from the Superintendent of Documents, U.S. Government Printing Office, Washington, D.C. 20402. Other government booklets on food preservation include "Home Freezing of Fruits and Vegetables," "Freezing Meat and Fish in the Home," "Freezing Combination Main Dishes," and "How to Make Jellies, Jams and Preserves at Home." An up-to-date, all-purpose canning and freezing guide is *The Ball Blue Book*, sold by the Ball Corp., Box 2005, Department PK 6A, Muncie, Indiana 47302.

"Natural"-ly Good?

If you think there's confusion about what's "organic," when it comes to "natural" there's total chaos. "Nature" sold big in the 1970s —bigger than "value," "convenience," "newness," "flavor," and "quality," according to the results of a consumer survey in 1977. More than two-fifths of those questioned by the Consumer Response Corporation, a New York survey organization, said they believed products labeled "natural" were safer and more healthful than other products. In another survey by the Federal Trade Commission, nearly half of those interviewed said they would pay more for food labeled "natural."

Clearly, the time was ripe for a Madison Avenue hype for Mother Nature. And predictably, the word "natural" began appearing on all sorts of products, including some highly processed foods. Consumers gobbled up natural cereals, natural beer, natural cheese, natural mineral water, natural bread, natural yogurt, natural flavors, natural colors, natural fiber, even natural candy and natural potato chips. And those products that couldn't be called natural in whole or part (because they were entirely artificial) were described as being "a natural"— "Coke is 'a natural,' " said one advertisement—with no one ever saying a natural what!

The irony behind this big vote of confidence for nature is that none of the truly "natural" foods people eat were created with human welfare in mind. Most, in fact, were present on earth long before our species evolved. The potato plant produces tubers to store starch, which in turn supports the growth of new sprouts. The chicken produces eggs to make more chickens. The broccoli plant makes a flowering head to seed itself. The cow produces milk to feed its calf. Agricultural research has resulted in better yields and growing characteristics and some improvements in nutrients, but it hasn't changed the basic chemistry of most foods. None of the natural foods we eat originated to promote the survival of Homo sapiens, who, after all, has only been on earth for a very short segment of evolutionary time. And just because human beings happen to be at the top of the food chain doesn't mean that every lower form of life is good for them to eat.

Early humans, like all animals before them, learned to distinguish edible from inedible by trial and error. Our prehistoric ancestors learned to avoid "foods" that caused illness or death. Those who consumed nourishing foods that enhanced short-term survival lived to tell their friends. But even evolution doesn't always make the best choices because it has no influence on events that take their toll beyond the peak reproductive years. Thus foods that may contribute to ill health and "premature" death decades later were not screened out by the forces of evolution and, as a result, we learned to eat many things that may compromise long-term survival.

Most of our popular foods, in fact, contain potent *natural poisons.* Other natural constitutents of foods can interfere with good nutrition. And many foods contain toxic metals, naturally acquired from soil and water as part of the chemistry of earth. For example, whole grains contain phytic acid that binds up some of the calcium and iron you eat and interferes with the body's ability to absorb these essential minerals. Estragole, an oil in the widely used herb tarragon, and safrole, the root-beer-flavored oil in sassafras (long used to make herb tea), both cause cancer in laboratory animals.

Among the 150 different chemicals in the common potato are such toxins as oxalic acid, arsenic, solanine, tannins, and nitrates, none of which does people any nutritional good and could in large doses do some harm. If it were possible for you to eat your year's quota of potatoes—120 pounds—all at once, you'd be killed outright by the 10,000 milligrams of solanine, a relative of the poison in deadly nightshade. Seafood naturally contains arsenic; broccoli has five different chemicals that disrupt the body's ability to use iodine (thus promoting goiter); eggs are rich in vitamins A and D, which are toxic in doses not much greater than those needed for good health; and lemons and oranges contain citral, which blocks the beneficial action of vitamin A. In addition, natural poisons can contaminate otherwise healthful foods, such as the cancer-causing aflatoxin produced by a mold that grows on peanuts, corn, and grain.

I think you get the point: "natural" doesn't necessarily mean "good." And, by the same token, just because something is toxic doesn't mean it's necessarily harmful as ordinarily consumed. It takes more than just the presence of a chemical to make a toxic substance a poison. It also requires a dose sufficiently large to have an effect. We are protected from the effects of natural poisons in most foods because they are present in only tiny amounts and are eaten along with a variety of other foods. *The greater the variety of foods you consume, the less the chance that you will accumulate a hazardous dose of a toxic chemical from any one food.*

Two of my friends discovered the hard way the importance of variety in the diet and of not depending too heavily on one food or type of food. One young woman, who became a fish-eating vegetarian to escape the antibiotics and hormones in meat and poultry, developed mercury poisoning because she ate two or more cans of tuna every day. And a 26-year-old man suffered a severe attack of gout from lunching daily on liverwurst sandwiches. His body simply couldn't handle the enormous amounts of uric acid he consumed in his daily diet of liver.

I had a similar experience during college when I ate two or more bowls of whole-grain cereal each day and regularly snacked on graham crackers. After a while I developed ugly, painful boils on my back, chest, and buttocks. Unfortunately, it took five years to discover that these horrid eruptions were the result of an allergic reaction to the enormous amount of whole grains I consumed.

Variety not only keeps down the dose of any one toxic substance, it also means that chemicals in one food may protect you from the harmful effects of chemicals in another. For example, nitrites formed in the digestive tract after eating nitrates naturally present in foods like spinach can detoxify the cyanide in lima beans.

It should be clear by now that *chemicals can be harmful—or harmless—whether natural or synthetic.* "It is naïve to think that . . . purchasing only foods labeled *natural* eliminates poisons from food," notes Martha E. Rhodes, head of the Food Laboratory at the Department of Agriculture and Consumer Services in Tallahassee, Florida. It is even more naïve to think that the word *natural* on a food label somehow confers magical properties.

The Federal Trade Commission proposed in 1978 that "natural" should refer only to foods that are no more than "minimally processed" and that contain no flavor or color additives (natural or artificial) or chemical preservatives or any ingredient that's been synthesized. But as with the term "organic," by mid-1980 there was still no official definition of what could be called natural in food advertising. The Food and Drug Administration's policy on food labeling only prohibits a manufacturer from calling an entire food natural if it contains artificial colors or flavors or any synthetic ingredients. In the face of these loose rules, food producers had a field day with the word *natural,* slapping it on labels of laboratory-concocted foods laced with additives and preservatives that may contain only one truly natural ingredient out of a dozen artificial ones.

Thus, consumers who reached for "a natural" may have gotten one or all of the following:

• "Natural orange flavor" in Tang, which has as its only real ingredient orange oil that is artificially extracted from natural oranges. The rest of Tang is sugar, citric acid (for tartness), malto dextrin (provides body), calcium phosphates (regulates tartness), vitamin C, artificial flavor, cellulose and xanthan gums (provide body), artificial color, vitamin A palmitate, BHA and alpha tocopherol (preservatives).
• "All natural" Colombo peach yogurt, which contains nonfat dry milk solids, sugar syrup, modified food starch, peach flavor and other natural flavors, and annatto extract for color, along with milk, peaches, and yogurt culture. All the ingredients are natural, all right,

but is this highly processed, additive-laden food what people have in mind when they seek to eat "natural"?

• "Natural cheddar cheese" from Kraft. The small type on the label of Kraft's Cracker Barrel cheeses says they contain enzymes, calcium chloride, potassium sorbate as a preservative, and artificial coloring. Manufacturers use the word *natural* to distinguish cheddar and other naturally produced cheeses from process cheese, but does the consumer know that?

• "100% natural flavors" in Welchade Grape Drink, which contains only 10 percent real grape juice. This "natural" ingredient is nearly obscured by the water, sugar, corn sweetener, and additives that form the bulk of the product. Ironically, Welch's Grape Juice, which has nothing but real juice and added vitamin C, makes no claims to being a natural.

• The "natural" beers—Budweiser, Natural Light, Busch, and Michelob—which are not made by traditional brewing processes and do not contain only "natural" ingredients. Tannic acid is used as a preservative and chillproofing agent and carbon dioxide is artificially injected into these Anheuser-Busch beers. They are no more natural than other American commercial beers.

The back-to-nature movement also introduced a "natural" food to the masses that for years had been known only to health food "nuts" —*granola*, a heavy, chewy, dry cereal made from such "healthy" ingredients as whole grains, nuts, seeds, raisins, and honey, and often (though not always) without chemical preservatives. The granola labels proclaim "all natural" and, to their credit, they do contain more protein, fiber, vitamins, and minerals than most popular cereals. But are they an improvement healthwise? Probably not. Their nutritious ingredients are largely offset by lots of fats, especially highly saturated coconut oil, and sugars (honey, after all, is sugar, natural or not), and calories—four to six times as many calories as the same volume of more traditional cereals.

The package label lists the nutritional contents of "a serving," which for cereal is defined as 1 ounce by nearly all manufacturers. But if you read the fine print on a package of granola, you'll see that 1 ounce by weight is only ¼ cup of cereal—just enough to fill the cavities you're likely to get from all that decay-promoting honey! Certainly, ¼ cup is less than what most people put in their cereal bowls. A more likely serving as people actually eat granola is ½ to ¾ cup, which, while giving you more protein, vitamins, and minerals, also gives you a lot more fat, sugar, and calories. But if you eat a 1-ounce serving of Shredded Wheat, you get ¾ cup of cereal at one-fourth of granola's caloric cost for the same volume of cereal. And 1 ounce of Cheerios puts 1¼ cups of high-protein "O's" in your bowl with very little fat, practically no sugar, and one-sixth the calories of 1¼ cups granola.

But the prize for consumer deception on "natural" must go to "natural" potato chips, corn chips, candy, and other junk foods that initially brought the nutrition-conscious consumer's ax down on the heads of the American food industry. Natural or not, junk food is junk food, offering far more calories, fat, sugar, and salt than needed nutrients. If you're really interested in "health foods," skip the snacks regardless of what the labels say.

Magic Foods and False Promises

The American health-food movement actually began 150 years ago when the Reverend Sylvester Graham, with evangelistic oratory, attempted to eradicate spiritual and physical decay with a diet based on bread made from coarse, unrefined flour that is the basis for—you guessed it—the graham cracker. A generation later, Dr. James Caleb Jackson modified Graham's diet by adding "Granula"—baked sheets of graham flour and water, ground into bits, rebaked, and ground again —America's first cold breakfast cereal.

Finally, in Battle Creek, Michigan, in the late 1800s, America's gestating cereal industry was born as a health-food enterprise. Dr. John Harvey Kellogg, who ran a sanitarium with vegetarian Adventists, devised Corn Flakes as a meat substitute for his patients. With his brother W.K., Dr. Kellogg started a flourishing business that swiftly attracted competition. Battle Creek became a boom town as more than forty companies set out to corner the breakfast market with packaged cereals. One company was started by a patient of Dr. Kellogg's, C. W. Post, who became impatient with techniques at the sanitarium and left there to cure himself with foods. In 1895, the same year Dr. Kellogg launched the cereal flake, C. W. Post had introduced Postum, a cereal-based beverage used as a coffee substitute that would make blood "red" and cure "coffee nerves." When Postum sales slacked in the summer heat, Post put out Grape-Nuts, which bore a remarkable resemblance to Dr. Jackson's Granula. The Postum Cereal Company, as he called his business, was netting $1 million a year by 1901 and eventually became the Post division of General Foods.

At about the same time, Henry D. Perky, an inventive genius with dyspepsia, devised little pillow-shaped pads of shredded whole wheat that attracted Dr. Kellogg's interest. But Perky, wary of Kellogg's cleverness, decided to stay clear of Battle Creek and instead set up operations in Niagara Falls, which accounts for the picture of the waterfall on boxes of Nabisco's Shredded Wheat.

With the rebirth of granolas, bran, graham, whole wheat, and other whole grains in the 1970s, you might say that the American cereal industry has come full circle. Had the health-food movement stuck with whole-grain breads and cereals, it might have retained more credibility. Few nutrition specialists today would question the important contribution whole grains can make to nearly everyone's diet. Because they contain both the germ and the bran of the grain, they are a major source of several B vitamins and vitamin E and a good source of protein, calcium, and iron. Rich in dietary fiber, whole grains help to keep your bowels in good working order and fill your stomach before you consume too many calories (see Chapters 5 and 7).

But the native grains were soon exploited to their maximum, and health-food promoters who wanted to make it big had to find other foods to market. And so true believers in a long string of purported health foods, ranging from brewer's yeast and kelp to raw milk, soybean sprouts, and vitamin and mineral supplements, sold an anxious public a host of edible remedies for whatever might ail them. Indeed, many who took the various "food cures" found they worked and soon passed the word to all similarly afflicted friends and acquaintances. Sometimes the remedies worked for the friends and acquaintances as well. Relief of human misery without the cost and inconvenience of a doctor's visit —that's all it takes for nutritional cure-alls to reach the health-food hall of fame.

But if they work, you ask, why knock them? Why, indeed? Because they create false expectations that could lead a few really sick people down the garden path to their graves. The vast majority of ordinary illnesses—colds, flu, aches, pains, and feelings of malaise—are self-limited. They disappear with the mere passage of time, usually leaving no scar on bodily functions. Their disappearance can often be hastened by a time-honored remedy—the placebo, or sugar pill, in which the mind becomes an effective aid to healing the body. (In fact, physicians sometimes prescribe placebos when there is no other specific treatment.) If you believe in a remedy, the chances that it will help you are that much greater. The "remedy" may be a prescription drug, a reassuring talk with the doctor, the hands of a faith healer, or the nostrums in a health-food store. The effectiveness of a placebo depends not on its specific action against the disorder in question (because it has none), but on the recipient's faith in its ability to help.

The danger is that some people turn to health foods and nutritional supplements to cure serious and potentially life-threatening conditions before these people even know (a) what's wrong or (b) whether modern medicine can offer a cure or lasting relief. Others throw good money after bad in a fruitless search for nutritional relief for a malady that can't be touched by diet. Still others reject sound medical advice and go their own health-food way until it's too late.

When health foods are not promoted as cures, they promise to prevent a long list of forbidding ailments and eventualities, from arthritis and cancer to old age. These are false promises indeed. *No one food or nutritional supplement has ever been shown to prevent or cure disease unless the disorder was the result of a specific nutritional deficiency,* such as iron-deficiency anemia. The foods revered by health-food enthusiasts are not all they're cracked up to be, and some can be downright dangerous. We've already talked about the high fat, sugar, and calorie content of granolas. Some other health-food myths worth exploding include the following:

The "nutritious" sweeteners. Disturbed by the emptiness of sugar calories, but unwilling to break their addiction to sweets, millions have abandoned the tiny white crystals of table sugar for raw sugar, honey, or blackstrap molasses. Raw sugar really isn't raw, and, nutritionally speaking, it is no different from white sugar. The calories in honey are only slightly less empty than those in ordinary sugar. Honey is rarely consumed in sufficient quantities to make a meaningful contribution to your diet of anything besides calories. Molasses, the most nutritious of the natural sweeteners, is a good source of iron, but it has no miraculous curative powers (see Chapter 6). The main reason for substituting honey or molasses for white sugar should be taste, not nutrition.

Raw milk. A general dislike for any form of processing and a fear that pasteurization destroys important nutrients in milk has prompted some to reject one of the greatest advances in food sanitation and instead purchase only raw, unpasteurized, unhomogenized milk—straight from the udder to the consumer. It is true that pasteurization destroys some heat-sensitive vitamins in milk—namely, thiamin and vitamin C. But it is also true that milk is not a significant source of these vitamins to begin with. Raw milk, even certified raw milk, can be a

ARE "HEALTH FOODS" NUTRITIONAL WONDERS?

The following table compares products usually carried in health-food stores with those readily available in ordinary food markets. Nutrient comparisons are given for amounts of the products that are nearly equal in calories. As you can see, you don't necessarily get more essential nutrients—or even as many—when you buy health-food products.

Table 26.2 • THE NUTRIENTS IN "HEALTH FOODS" COMPARED TO ORDINARY FOODS

Food	Amount	Calories	Protein (g)	Calcium (mg)	Iron (mg)	Thiamin (mg)	Riboflavin (mg)	Vitamin C (mg)	Vitamin A (IU)*
Brown rice, raw	1 ounce	102	2.1	11.0	.6	.09	.005	0	0
White rice, raw enriched	1 ounce	103	1.9	6.8	.8	.12	.008	0	0
Honey	1 ounce	90	trace	2.0	.2	trace	trace	0	0
Brown sugar	.9 ounce	91	0.0	20.7	.8	.002	.008	0	0
Dried apples	1 ounce	78	0.3	9.0	.5	1.00	.300	trace	—**
Raisins	1 ounce	82	0.7	18.0	1.0	.03	.020	trace	10
Bean sprouts	1 ounce	13	1.7	13.6	.3	.06	—**	4	22
Spinach, raw	2 ounces	15	1.8	55.0	1.8	.06	.110	29	4,592
Pumpkin seeds	1 ounce	180	9.8	11.0	3.3	.13	.040	0	186
Peanuts	1 ounce	167	7.5	20.8	.6	.09	.040	0	—**

Source: Comparisons are made on the basis of data in the U.S. Department of Agriculture Handbook No. 456.
*IU = international units (5 IUs = 1 retinol equivalent).
**—— = no data available.

source of harmful microorganisms, such as those that cause brucellosis (a serious fever-producing infection) and spinal tuberculosis. There's no way to be sure raw milk is safe unless you personally know the cow from which it came (see Chapter 13).

Nuts and seeds. These are good sources of protein, calcium, and B vitamins. As snacks, they are more nutritious than potato chips and pretzels. And they are excellent complements to other vegetable proteins, like beans and grains. But you pay a high caloric price for the nutrients in nuts and seeds because they are also rich in fat, albeit unsaturated vegetable oil. Some 80 percent of the calories in nuts are fat calories, making them no better than meat in terms of the amount of fat. Ten large walnuts add up to 322 calories, 10 peanuts have 105 calories, and 1 ounce of sunflower seeds has 100 calories. Unless you have no problems maintaining a normal body weight, nuts and seeds are best eaten sparingly, not gobbled like popcorn.

Yeast. Fortified nutritional yeast (but not necessarily brewer's yeast) is a reasonable nutritional supplement for persons whose diet is deficient in B vitamins, protein, iron, or phosphorus. But like everything else, it's not a magical cure for whatever ails you, so don't expect anything more from yeast than a little nutritional boost.

Raw and fertile eggs. Eggs do not lose nutritive value when cooked; if anything, they gain it. Raw egg whites contain a substance, avidin, that blocks absorption of the B vitamin biotin. Avidin is destroyed when eggs are cooked. Raw eggs may also carry the food-poisoning bacterium Salmonella. Despite a popular myth, raw eggs have no ability to enhance sexual potency.

Fertile eggs, a purported source of a mysterious force known as "vitalism," are no more nourishing than nonfertile ones. In fact, fertile eggs spoil much more quickly and must be consumed when very fresh to avoid decomposition. While on the subject of eggs, I must point out that the color of the shell is determined by the variety of chicken from which the egg came; white eggs are not more nourishing than brown, or vice versa. Nor does the color of the yolk make a nutritional difference.

Lecithin. This fatty substance is found in egg yolks, soybeans, organ meats, and whole grains. It is used as an emulsifier in processed foods. And it is sold in bulk in health-food stores. While not harmful, it is also not a cure or preventive for arthritis, heart disease, skin disorders, or nervous disorders. It does not lower blood cholesterol. However, recent studies suggest that one of the constituents of naturally occurring lecithin, choline, may counter senile deterioration of the brain. But the lecithin ordinarily sold as a nutritional supplement contains little or no choline.

Bee pollen. People have been eating bee pollen, a rich source of protein, for hundreds of years. But the notion that it has magical powers or bestows athletic prowess is totally without foundation. In a controlled study involving members of the Louisiana State University swimming team, absolutely no difference in performance was noted between those who took 10 pollen tablets a day for six weeks and those who received placebos. At $45 a pound, bee pollen is a very expensive sugar pill!

Vitamins and minerals. See Chapters 8 and 9 for discussions of the benefits (or lack thereof) and hazards from micronutrient megadoses.

The Claims Don't Have to Be True

Some people are under the impression that health-food enthusiasts couldn't legally make the claims they do for various foods and nutritional supplements if these claims weren't proven. This is simply not the case. *The government can only regulate claims made on product labels and in product advertising.* Anyone can publish a book, pamphlet, magazine, newspaper, or leaflet claiming miraculous but totally unproven benefits from one or another food product, and the literature can legally be sold in the same store as the product. This is, in fact, what happens in many health-food establishments. What isn't sold by the label, advertising, or word of mouth is promoted by readily available literature legally printed under the constitutional guarantees of a free press. But even this freedom may be undergoing some voluntary curbs as a result of several lawsuits against health-food writers and publishers for making unsubstantiated claims that led to sickness and death among some who followed the advice. Most notable is a suit against the estate of the late health-food guru Adelle Davis and Signet Books, publishers of her book *Let's Have Healthy Children.* A Florida couple said they followed Ms. Davis's advice and gave their 2-month-old son a large dose of potassium chloride to cure his colic. Four days later the baby died of irreversible abnormalities of the heart rhythm presumably caused by a potassium overdose. An earlier suit, brought by a woman whose son's bone growth was crippled because she followed the same book's advice and gave him massive doses of vitamin A, was settled out of court for $150,000.

The moral of this story is, *don't believe eveything you read, espe-*

cially if it tells you that a particular food or nutrient is your secret to good health. Good nutrition is certainly important, and can help you to look and feel your best. Careless eating habits undoubtedly interfere with proper mental and physical development, good health, achievement, and even personality. But the answer to a careless diet does not lie in a pill, potion, or any "natural" or "organic" edible found in a health-food store, or any combination thereof.

By focusing consumer attention on single sources of nutrients and decrying contamination by various chemical "poisons," the health-food movement distracts people from the far more important connections between nutrition and health that result from distortions in the overall structure of the diet: the overconsumption of sugars, salt, and calories and the overdependence on fat-ridden sources of protein.

It's virtually impossible to convince a true believer in one or another health-food or nutritional supplement that it doesn't work the magic it's purported to possess. But if you're not already hooked, it would be wise to rationally analyze what, if anything, might be wrong with your present diet before leaping to the conclusion that health foods are your salvation from nutritional sins and the panacea and preventive for the world's mental and physical ills.

FOR FURTHER READING

Sidney Margolius, *Health Foods: Facts and Fakes* (New York: Walker, 1973).
Nikki and David Goldbeck, *The Supermarket Handbook* (New York: Signet, 1973).
Ronald M. Deutsch, *The New Nuts among the Berries* (Palo Alto, Calif.: Bull, 1977).
Victor Herbert, M.D., J.D., *Nutrition Cultism* (Philadelphia: George F. Stickley, 1980).
Victor Herbert, M.D., J.D., and Stephen Barrett, M.D., *Vitamins and "Health" Foods: The Great American Hustle* (Philadelphia: George F. Stickley, 1981).

27 ❧ THE LABEL: A TALE PARTLY TOLD

CAROLE wanted to lose the five pounds she'd put on over the holidays, so she bought a box of "diet bars" to eat in place of breakfast and lunch. But not until her third 275-calorie "meal" of these cookielike bars did she notice what was in them. According to the list on the package, fat and sugar were the two main ingredients. Is *that* how to lose weight? Carole wondered. Eating fat and sugar? Aren't those the things to avoid? Carole vowed always to read the label before buying a new product.

Since Robert rarely left enough time for a proper breakfast, he usually relied on an "instant breakfast" drink to hold him until lunch. Still, he would develop a gnawing hunger midway through the morning that interfered with his concentration and made him irritable. Had Robert read the label on his "breakfast," he'd have known the reason why it didn't stick to his ribs. "Sugar, vegetable shortening, water" were the first three ingredients listed. What a way to start the day! For fewer calories, less sugar and fat, and more lasting satisfaction, Robert could have had juice, an egg, toast, and a glass of skim milk.

Since more than half the foods we eat come in packages, learning to read and understand labels is a critically important part of analyzing and improving our diet. It can also help us to determine whether we're getting our money's worth when we choose one product over another. Yet fewer than half of us are regular label readers, and only a quarter of us ever read beyond the ingredients list.

The issue of food labeling is in a state of regulatory and legislative turmoil. A complete overhaul of what the food label says and how it says it is currently under way in federal agencies. Some of the proposals mentioned below may be law by the time you read this book. Others may be revised, abandoned, or deadlocked in controversy. While some changes can be made by regulatory decree, the most significant revisions require new legislation to give more authority to the regulatory agencies involved—the Food and Drug Administration, the U.S. Department of Agriculture, and, to a lesser extent, the Federal Trade Commission.

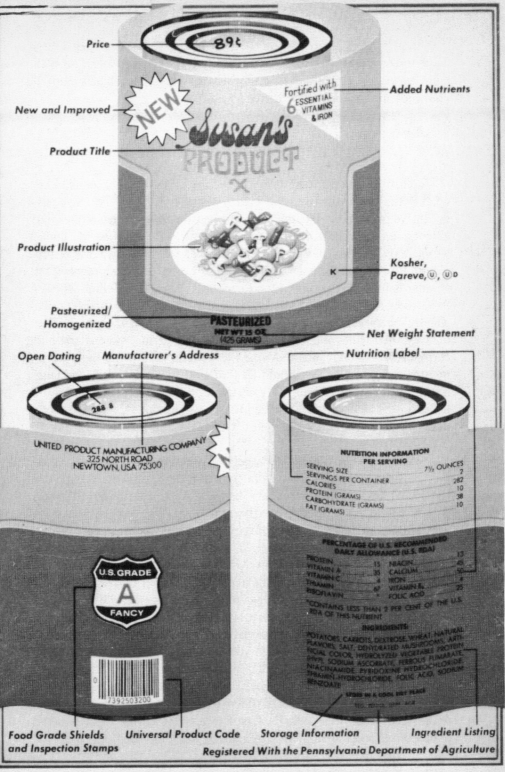

Credit: Allen Wilkis and *Redbook Magazine,* August, 1978.

It will probably be the mid-1990s before fully revamped labels come into widespread use. In the meantime, we have to make do with what we've got. Despite their many shortcomings, food labels can tell you a lot if you know how to read them.

What's the Product Made Of?

Before 1938, manufacturers were not obliged to tell consumers what actually was in the processed foods they bought. To cut costs, expensive ingredients like coffee might be diluted with cheap ones like chicory; an unsuspecting shopper who paid the full price for coffee would have no way of knowing until it was too late. To remedy this situation, a law was passed enabling the FDA to establish ingredients standards for many common food products. The 350 different types of foods covered by these *standards of identity* included bread, milk, cheese, ice cream, macaroni and noodle products, flour, mayonnaise, most canned fruits and vegetables, cocoa, margarine, sweeteners, and certain seafoods. All such foods had to contain everything the government standard said they should. If that's all they contained, the label needn't specify ingredients; only certain optional ingredients had to be listed on the labels of standardized foods. But all other processed foods not covered by a standard of identity had to list all their ingredients on the label.

Today, most manufacturers spell out all ingredients, even for products covered by food standards (although a new law is needed before the FDA can insist upon such a listing). As Carole discovered and Robert might have discovered, the ingredients list can tell you a lot about the contents of the product. *The ingredients must be listed in order of their prominence by weight,* with the main ingredients at the top of the list. In other words, in Carole's diet bars the first item in the ingredients list was vegetable shortening—the main ingredient; it was followed by sugar—the second leading ingredient—all the way down to vitamin B_{12}, the least prominent ingredient in that product.

If a package of breakfast cereal lists sugar (or honey) as the first ingredient, then what's mostly in your bowl are sweet, empty calories. Sometimes, however, several different *sweeteners* are used in a product and listed separately on the label. If sugar is the second ingredient, honey the fourth, and dextrose the sixth, the consumer is in the dark about how prominent sugar is. Chances are, though, if sugar is listed ahead of other major ingredients, such as the grains or flour in cereal, it's a pretty big part of the total product (see pages 132–134).

The ingredients list also tells you something about the *types of fats* used. The most useful label says exactly what the shortening is—for example, corn oil, partially hydrogenated soybean oil, coconut oil, palm oil, butter, etc. If you're trying to avoid saturated fats, don't buy products in which fat is a major ingredient and is a hardened (hydrogenated) vegetable oil, coconut oil, palm oil, or any animal fat, such as butter or lard. Also stay away from those products that just say "vegetable oil" or "vegetable shortening," since it's probably a type you'd best avoid. Sometimes the ingredients list will say something like "vegetable oil (may contain one or more of the following: soybean, coconut, and/or palm oil)." This allows manufacturers to use whichever oil is cheapest at the time of manufacture without having to change the label. The FDA and the USDA have proposed that foods containing more than 10 percent fat on a dry-weight basis be required to state specifically which fats are used. Products with less fat could continue to have the and/or labels.

Food additives must be listed among the ingredients, except for those that are part of the "recipe" for standardized foods, such as artificial coloring for butter. Some manufacturers have voluntarily begun to state the purpose of each additive—for example, "modified food starch (a stabilizer)," "citric acid (for tartness)," "guar gum (a thickener)." If preservatives are used, their purpose *must* be stated.

However, specific *spices, flavors, and colors* do not have to be listed by name. A product may be labeled as containing "artificial flavoring" or "natural flavors" but the manufacturer doesn't have to tell you which ones were used. If any coloring is added, the label must state "artificial coloring" even if the color came from a natural source (such as carotene from carrots), but again you need not be told the name of the coloring agent. Lack of such information can be troublesome to consumers who are allergic to certain spices, colors, or flavors or who wish to avoid foods containing coloring agents of questionable safety (see page 488). New legislation is needed to enable the FDA to require specific flavor, color, and spice names on labels. In contrast, the USDA, which has jurisdiction over labeling of processed meat and poultry products, believes it currently has the authority to require specific listing by name.

The most serious shortcoming of the ingredients list is its failure to indicate how much of each ingredient the product contains. The FDA has proposed new rules requiring label statements to reveal the percent of the characterizing ingredient in a product, such as the amount of shrimp in a shrimp cocktail, or meat in a beef stew. But additional legislation is needed to require quantitative lists of all major ingredients in a given product.

Is It Nutritious?

From a health perspective, even more important than knowing the amount of each ingredient is knowing the total amount in a product of the various nutrients essential to health (like protein and vitamins) and the nutrients that may be detrimental to health (like sugar and sodium). Some of this information can be found under the heading *"Nutrition Information"* on food labels. Under current law, the FDA can require only certain products to provide nutrition information. These are products to which nutrients are added (such as cereals fortified with vitamins), products that make nutritional claims (such as "contains twice as much vitamin C as an apple"), or foods prepared for special dietary uses, such as for feeding infants or for weight reduction. However, many manufacturers voluntarily provide nutrition information, and, as of 1980, nearly half of all packaged foods had such information on the label.

Unfortunately, in its present format, the nutrition label is of limited usefulness to most consumers. Amounts are given in grams and milligrams instead of common kitchen measures or as a percent of total calories. And several important facts, such as cholesterol content, don't have to be listed. But with a little effort and the guidance offered below, you can glean a lot more from the label than you may realize. *All nutrition labels are required to state certain things:* size of a serving; number of servings per container; and, for each serving, number of calories; grams of protein, carbohydrates, and fat; and the percentage of the USRDA for protein, vitamin A, vitamin C, thiamin, riboflavin, niacin, calcium, and iron. In addition, nutrition *labels may contain certain optional information:* per serving, the milligrams of sodium, grams of polyunsaturated and saturated fats, and milligrams of cholesterol, plus the percent of the USRDA (see page 168) for twelve other vitamins and minerals—D, E, B_6, folacin, B_{12}, phosphorus, iodine, magnesium, zinc, copper, biotin, and pantothenic acid. If a food is ordinarily eaten combined with other ingredients, such as cereal with milk or hamburger with "helper," nutrition information may also be listed for the combination.

Finally, a product may optionally list *"carbohydrate information"*

—a breakdown of starches and sugars in grams per serving. This listing, which can now be found on most dry cereal packages, is your clue to total sugar content. But since it is given in grams, you may still be unaware of just how much sugar you're eating. It pays to commit the following to memory: 4 grams of sugar equals 1 teaspoon, 12 grams equals 1 tablespoon, 200 grams equals 1 cup. Thus, when the carbohydrate information on the box of Kellogg's Apple Jacks says 15 grams of sucrose and other sugars per 1-ounce serving, you know you're getting nearly 4 teaspoons of sugar in your morning cereal. Is that how much you would add if you started out with a bowl of unsweetened cereal?

You can also *calculate the percentage of sugar in a serving* and see how well it fits into your nutritional budget. To do this, you have to learn one other fact: 1 gram of sugar (or any carbohydrate) provides 4 calories. Thus, the 15 grams of sugar in a serving of Apple Jacks, multiplied by 4, equals 60 calories worth of sugar per serving. Now check the label for the number of calories in a serving: 110, in the case of Apple Jacks. Divide 60 by 110, multiply the result by 100 and you get 54.5 percent. That's the proportion of sugar calories in a serving of Apple Jacks.

APPLE JACKS

One serving	1 oz.
Calories per serving	110

Carbohydrate Information

Starch and related carbohydrates	11 g
Sucrose and other sugars	15 g
Total carbohydrates	26 g

15 grams of sugar times 4 calories per gram = 60 calories from sugar.
60 sugar calories divided by 110 calories per serving = 0.545.
.545 times 100 = 54.5 percent sugar.

You can make the same calculation for *percent of fat calories* based on the grams of fat per serving listed under nutrition information. But for fat, you have to multiply the number of grams by 9, since each gram of fat provides 9 calories. In Carole's diet bars, each two-bar serving contains 16 grams of fat. Multiplied by 9, that equals 144 fat calories. Divided by the 275 calories per serving and then multiplied by 100, this comes to 52 percent of the calories from fat—far more than the 30 percent fat calories recommended in the Dietary Goals.

Finally, you can use the nutrition information to *calculate whether you're getting your nutritional money's worth*—for example, how much you're paying for protein in various alternatives in the meat group. You may discover that certain products which seem to cost more per pound actually give you a better protein value than those that are cheaper. For instance, if frankfurters cost $1.69 a pound and there are 10 in a 1-pound (16-ounce) package, then each frankfurter costs 17 cents, or 34 cents for a 2-frankfurter (3.2-ounce) serving. If the nutrition information shows that 2 frankfurters contain 12 grams of protein, divide the 34 cents by 12 grams and you get 2.8 cents per gram of protein. Now take a look at the "more expensive" canned ham—$2.19 a pound. Here, there are 16 grams of protein in a 3-ounce serving, which costs 41 cents. Dividing 41 by 16, you see that each gram of protein in the ham costs 2.6 cents, less than the protein in the "cheaper" frankfurters. As a further benefit, the serving of ham has about 100 calories less than the franks, primarily because ham has considerably less fat.

FRANKFURTERS

1-pound package (10 franks) costs $1.69.
$1.69 divided by 10 = $.169 per frank (16.9 cents).
16.9 times 2 franks = 34 cents per serving (3.2 ounces).
Since the label says there are 12 grams of protein per 2-frank serving, divide 34 by 12 = 2.8 cents per gram of protein.

HAM

1-pound package (16 ounces) costs $2.19.
$2.19 divided by 16 = $.136 per ounce (13.6 cents).
13.6 times 3 = 41 cents per 3-ounce serving.
Since the label states there are 16 grams of protein in a 3-ounce serving, divide 41 by 16 = 2.6 cents per gram.

The FDA has proposed a requirement that all foods bearing nutrition information also list the amounts of sodium and potassium and, for foods that contain significant amounts of sugars, the total amount of sugars. But new legislation is needed to require a listing of the amounts of cholesterol and saturated and polyunsaturated fats in foods that do not make claims (such as "lower in cholesterol") about these substances.

A major problem with the current nutrition label is that by listing the USRDA, it emphasizes the amount of protein, vitamins, and minerals in a food. These nutrients are no longer the major nutritional concern in this nation. *What nutritionists, physicians, and consumers worry about today are calories, fats, sugars, sodium, and cholesterol,* since excesses of these nutrients are most closely related to overweight, ill-

How Much Nutrition in a Potato?

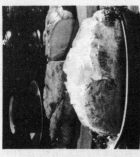

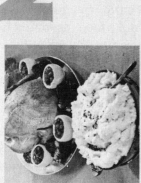

Now we can show you. Because the potato is the first vegetable in the supermarket with a nutrition label. Take a look.

Just one 2½-inch-diameter potato will give you all this nutrition for only 100 calories.

A bigger potato, of course, means much more nutrition for a few extra calories. If you're a potato eater, that's good news. And if you're not, look what you're missing.

The Potato...Something Good That's Good For You.

THE POTATO BOARD

Nutritional information per serving

Serving size	One medium potato (150 grams) about 1/3 pound
Calories	100
Protein	3 grams
Carbohydrate	22 grams
Fat	0 grams

Percentage of U.S. recommended daily allowances (U.S. RDA)

Protein	6	Vitamin B6	20
Vitamin A	*	Folacin (folic acid)	8
Vitamin C	35	Phosphorus	8
Thiamin	4	Magnesium	8
Riboflavin	2	Zinc	4
Niacin	10	Copper	10
Calcium	*	Iodine	15
Iron	10		

*Contains less than 2% of the U.S. RDA of these nutrients.

ness, and death among Americans. When the revisions of food labels are finally completed, they are expected to reflect this new concern about nutritional excesses, perhaps with less emphasis on possible areas of nutritional deficiencies.

A final problem is that even if the law is changed so that all processed foods must bear nutrition information, there are still a lot of foods bought "fresh"—meats, poultry, fish, fruits, vegetables—that have no label and therefore no information of any kind aside from weight, price, and, in some cases, grade (see below). Eventually, this too will probably change, but here again only new legislation will make it happen. However, in 1979, through the determined efforts of the Potato Board (a national association of potato growers), the FDA gave permission for potatoes to have nutritional labeling, making potatoes the first fresh food so labeled. Now, when you shop, you may find a sign or leaflet near the potato bin that looks like the one on page 519.

What Food Grades Mean

Food grades—like "Choice" on beef or "U.S. Grade AA" on eggs —have nothing to do with the food's nutritive value or wholesomeness. Rather, they are *a measure of "quality,"* as defined by the U.S. Department of Agriculture. And a confusing array of ratings they are indeed, with the same grade meaning different things on different foods. Recognizing the confusion, the department in 1980 began to reassess food grades in hopes of making them more intelligible and meaningful to the consumer.

Food grading originated as a means of standardizing food quality and characteristics at the wholesale level. It is entirely voluntary, paid for by whoever packs or processes the food. Unlike food inspection for safety and healthfulness (such as to check on pesticide residues or insect contamination) and honesty in packaging, food grading is not required by law. Even foods that have been graded don't have to be labeled as to their grade.

Critics refer to grading as "a beauty contest" because products are graded mostly on the basis of *how they look.* But other factors, such as *flavor and tenderness,* are considered as well. The foods you're most likely to find labeled with grades are beef, veal, lamb, turkeys, eggs, and butter. Sometimes cheese, instant nonfat dry milk, jams, jellies, frozen concentrated orange juice, and canned, frozen, and fresh fruits and vegetables also carry a USDA grade. Grade labeling currently appears on about 90 percent of turkeys, 75 percent of fresh beef, 40 percent of eggs, and 3 percent of processed fruits and vegetables sold in retail markets. Here is a guide to what the grades mean, according to the standards applied by USDA.

Meat. The three main grades are *Prime, Choice,* and *Good.* In the early 1980s the grades were redefined to permit the use of Prime and Choice on meats of somewhat lower fat content. Prime, the top grade, is the most tender, the most flavorful, and the most expensive. It is usually also the fattiest, since the grade is largely determined by how well marbled the meat is (marbling being streaks of fat among the red muscle of the meat). Choice beef is supposed to be quite tender and juicy, with a good flavor. Good beef is not as juicy or flavorful as Prime or Choice, but still fairly tender and usually containing less fat than the higher grades.

Prime and Choice lamb are tender and can be roasted or broiled; lower-grade lamb is rarely sold retail. Prime and Choice veal is juicier and more flavorful than lower-grade veal. The higher grades can be roasted, but lower grades should be cooked with moist heat for juiciness and flavor.

Poultry. *U.S. Grade A* poultry—the top grade—is meaty and has a better "appearance" than *U.S. Grades B* and *C.* You're not likely to see grade labels on poultry that is not U.S. Grade A.

Dairy Products. For butter, *U.S. Grade AA* is the tops, with a sweet, delicate flavor. *U.S. Grade A* is nearly as good and usually cheaper. The same grades can be used on cheddar cheese, though they rarely are.

On instant nonfat dry milk, a label stating *U.S. Extra Grade* means the milk has a sweet and pleasing flavor and dissolves immediately when mixed with water.

The term *Quality Approved* on products like cottage cheese, pasteurized process cheese, and sour cream means that the product is of good quality and was made in a clean plant under the supervision of a USDA grader.

Eggs. *U.S. Grade AA* is the tops, but *U.S. Grade A* is the one you're most likely to find in markets. Both are considered "attractive" when fried or poached because they don't spread out much in the pan, as do *U.S. Grade B* eggs. The latter are good for cooking and baking.

Fruits and Vegetables. Though most fruits and vegetables that are canned, frozen, or dried are packed according to grade and sold that way wholesale, this information rarely reaches the consumer except in terms of price. There are three grades for processed fruits and vegetables: *U.S. Grade A* is tops, to be used where looks and texture are

especially important; *U.S. Grade B* fruits and vegetables do not have to be as uniform in size and color as Grade A, nor as tender or free from blemishes; *U.S. Grade C* products, though just as nutritious and wholesome, have still lower quality standards and cost less.

Fresh fruits and vegetables bear a different set of grades: *Fancy, U.S. No. 1,* and *U.S. No. 2.* The grade most commonly sold is U.S. No. 1. For apples, there is a different scheme—*U.S. Extra Fancy, Fancy,* and *U.S. No. 1.* The grades are based on color, shape, maturity, and freedom from defects, and the main difference is in appearance and cost.

For further information on how to select food products, you might consult the various booklets in USDA's How to Buy series. Separate booklets on beef roasts; beef steaks; canned and frozen fruits; canned and frozen vegetables; cheese; dairy products; dry beans, peas, and lentils; eggs; fresh fruits; fresh vegetables; lamb; meat for your freezer; potatoes; and poultry can be purchased from the Superintendent of Documents, U.S. Government Printing Office, Washington, D.C. 20402.

What's in the Name?

The name of a product can reveal a lot about its contents, if you know the federal "formulas" for what processed foods can be called. For example, "beef with rice" has more beef than rice; but "rice with beef" has more rice than beef. According to regulations, "beef with gravy" must have more than 50 percent beef, but "gravy with beef" needs to have only 35 percent beef. For "chicken with gravy," the rule says at least 35 percent of the product must be chicken; but for "gravy with chicken," only 15 percent of the product needs to be chicken. If the proposed new rules are put into effect, labels will have to state percentages of such "characterizing" ingredients.

The names of drinks also give clues to their contents. For example, *fruit juice* must contain 100 percent real fruit juice; a *juice drink* can have anywhere from 35 to 69 percent real juice; a *fruit drink* may contain only 10 to 34 percent juice; and a *fruit-flavored drink* has less than 10 percent juice and often no juice at all! What makes up the remaining percentages of these drinks? Water and sugar, flavorings and colorings. And don't be fooled by label claims about added vitamin C, even if it's to the amount naturally present in 100-percent real juice. Real juice has a lot more nutrients than vitamin C, but these other nutrients are not added to the diluted drinks.

The product name can also be a nutritional *dis*service. For example, chocolate milk is whole milk flavored with chocolate, but chocolate drink is made from low-fat milk, making the "drink" nutritionally preferable to the "milk."

Ice cream and ice milk have names that reflect their ingredients. Strawberry ice cream is flavored with real strawberries; strawberry-flavored ice cream has real berries plus artificial flavoring; and artificially flavored strawberry ice cream is 100 percent artificially flavored —it may never have seen the likes of a strawberry.

Some products must be called *"imitation."* These are fabricated foods made to resemble other "natural" foods but, for one reason or another, are not their nutritional equal. Soy steaks might be called "imitation beef" because they resemble beef steaks but do not have quite as much high-quality protein as beef does. However, if the soy steaks are made to equal the percent of the USRDA for protein, vitamins, and minerals in beef, the word *imitation* need not be used and the product can be called by some new name like "soy steak." (The soy product may, however, have less fat and calories than beef without having to be called "imitation.")

The rules on imitation foods are inconsistent and often confusing to consumers. Some foods originally developed to be cheaper imitations of others, and not necessarily their nutritional equals, still do not have to be called "imitation." This is because a standard of identity was established for the new product, specifying what must be in it. Thus, margarine does not have to be called "imitation butter," and salad dressing does not have to be called "imitation mayonnaise." But diet margarine must be called "imitation margarine" because it has less fat per gram than the food standard for margarine allows.

For years, frankfurters, bacon, and other processed meats that had not been cured with sodium nitrite (an additive suspected of causing cancer) had to be called such confusing names as "uncured cooked sausages" for the franks and "pork bellies" or "pork strips" for the bacon. But in 1980, the USDA issued a new rule—over the protests of the meat industry, which took the matter to court—to permit the sale of nitrite-free products under their rightful name as long as they are described as "uncured." As of this writing, the name changes were still being contested.

In 1979, the FDA ruled that foods labeled *"low calorie"* must contain no more than 40 calories per serving, but a food like celery that is naturally low in calories cannot be so labeled. Foods called *"reduced calorie"* must be at least one-third lower in calories than the food for which it substitutes. In addition, a comparison must be made to show what the "reduced calorie" claim is based on. For example, the label might say "Unsweetened applesauce, 50 calories per half-cup serving, 57 percent less than sweetened Mott's Apple Sauce." (But foods called "sugarless" or "sugar-free" do not necessarily qualify for a "low calorie" or "reduced calorie" label. Sausages may be sugar-free, but still high in fat and calories.)

Similar rules have been proposed for foods labeled "low cholesterol," "reduced cholesterol," and "cholesterol-free," as well as "low sodium" and "reduced sodium." The sodium rules were slated to take effect in July, 1986. If a food is labeled "sodium free," it must contain less than 5 milligrams of sodium per serving; if "very low sodium," it can contain 35 milligrams or less per serving; if "low sodium," 140 milligrams, and if "reduced sodium," its sodium content must be reduced by 75 percent or more below what would be in the product it replaces. The words "unsalted," "no salt added," and "without added salt" mean no salt was added in processing to a product that would normally be processed with salt, but these designations do not refer to any limit on sodium. As for claims about fat, processors will have to comply by April, 1987, to these standards: "extra lean" for products with no more than 5 percent fat; "lean" and "low fat" for those with less than 10 percent fat, and "light," "lite," "leaner," and "lower fat" for products with 25 percent less fat than the majority of such products on the market. All products making fat claims will have to disclose the actual fat content on the label.

Canned fruits must state the *kind of liquid* in which they're packed, a nutritionally useful fact for you to note. Fruits packed in water or light syrup have less sugar and fewer calories than fruits packed in heavy syrup. They also cost less, as a rule. Tuna packed in water has 56 percent fewer calories than tuna packed in oil. Even after the oil-packed tuna is thoroughly drained, it has more calories than the water-packed variety.

You can also benefit nutritionally from a statement on the label of certain highly processed foods, such as frozen dinners, breakfast cereals, meal replacements, and pizza. The FDA has established nutritional guidelines (not rules) specifying the minimum amount of protein, vitamins, and minerals that should be in a 100-calorie serving of such products. Products meeting this standard can state: "Provides nutrients in amounts appropriate for this class of food as determined by the U.S. Government."

Unfortunately, current labeling rules do not prevent manufacturers from making true but misleading statements on food packages. For example, a product may claim that it has "more iron than milk" without noting that milk, to begin with, is a poor source of iron. Or a presweetened, highly refined cereal may indicate that it contains the same amount of protein, carbohydrate, fat, and several vitamins and minerals as a whole-wheat cereal without saying that, unlike whole wheat, its carbohydrate is mostly sugar and that it is missing other micronutrients found in whole wheat.

Another word of nutritional significance you're likely to find on some products is *"enriched."* Enrichment of flour and grain products refers to the addition of certain nutrients that are lost during refining and processing. But not all the missing nutrients are replaced in the enriched product. Whole-grain products always contain more. Nonetheless, enriched white flour, rice, or pasta is more nutritious than refined, *un*enriched flour, rice, or pasta.

Some foods are *"fortified"* with vitamins and minerals that are not naturally present in those products. For example, vitamin D is usually added to milk, helping to ensure an adequate supply of the vitamin, especially for growing children during the winter months. Breakfast cereals, too, may be fortified with various vitamins and minerals—particularly iron—to enhance the cereals' nutritional value.

If a food has been fortified with 50 percent or more of the USRDA for any nutrient (protein, vitamin, or mineral), it must be called a *diet supplement.* Thus, General Mills' Total—wheat flakes fortified with 100 percent of the USRDA for ten vitamins and minerals—cannot be called a cereal at all! The same for Kellogg's Most, which earned its label as a diet supplement and the right to its product name by being fortified with 100 percent of the USRDA for *eleven* different vitamins and minerals.

Fortification

As you probably guessed by now, "fortification" is one of the food industry's most popular gimmicks, designed to exploit consumer interest in vitamins and minerals. It's hardly surprising that companies try to make the numbers look good. But is fortification good for the consumer? Usually not, for the following reasons:

It's misleading. A product heavily dosed with added vitamins and minerals creates the impression that it's a healthful food. But fortification provides no indication of what else the product may contain—such as saturated fats or lots of added sugar—or what may be missing from the product—such as the rest of the essential micronutrients. We cannot live by the USRDA alone: no amount of vitamins or minerals added to Kellogg's Most negates the fact that 29 percent of the calories in a serving are sugar calories—the equivalent of 2 teaspoons of sugar in ¾ cup of cereal. Yet, compared to Most, Shredded Wheat—which has no sugar, just natural whole wheat—looks like a nutritional weakling, because none of its USRDA percentages is above 10. Yet which do you think is the better food?

The potential for making "junk" foods appear nutritious through fortification is worrisome to many nutritional specialists. If potato chips were fortified with all the required micronutrients, they'd still contain too much fat and salt to be good for you. The Nestlé Company developed a candy bar called Go Ahead and stuffed it with 10 percent of the USRDA for all nineteen of the vitamins and minerals that can be listed on the label. Yet Go Ahead is still candy, too high in sugar to be healthful. In fact, under current law, as the Center for Science in the Public Interest points out, you could fortify cardboard with all the nutrients in wheat cereal and not even have to call it "imitation."

It's unnecessary. Why should you consume 100 percent of your day's allotment for any nutrient all in one meal? Or in one part of a meal, since the 100-percent level doesn't count the milk you add to your cereal, or the juice, toast, or anything else you may eat with it? By the time the day is out, you will have consumed several times the recommended amount of several of the vitamins and minerals in such overfortified products. Yet, there's no evidence that this is desirable. Indeed for some nutrients, such as vitamins A and D, it may even be harmful.

It's expensive. You pay a lot more for heavily fortified products than the company spends giving you the added nutrients. The Center for Science in the Public Interest, which filed a complaint with the Federal Trade Commission claiming that the ads for Total are misleading, says that General Mills has "overcharged" the public $40 million since Total was introduced in 1973. The center based this conclusion on a comparison with another General Mills cereal, Wheaties, which is nearly identical to Total except that it is not nearly so heavily fortified. "It costs General Mills only about two cents to add the extra nutrients to a 12-ounce box of Total, yet the retail price of Total is about 30 cents higher than the price of Wheaties," the center stated in its publication, *Nutrition Action.* In my supermarket in April, 1986, an 18-ounce box of Wheaties cost $2.09, whereas the same size box of Total sold for $3.03—94 cents more for 3 cents' worth of vitamins which you don't even need in the first place!

To be fair, fortification is not always undesirable. If a certain nutrient, such as iron, is found to be chronically in short supply in the diet of a large segment of the population, fortification of a common food, such as bread, with that nutrient might be highly beneficial (just as fortification of milk with vitamin D has practically eliminated rickets in American children). It's just that fortification has gotten out of hand. Federal regulations are needed that spell out which foods can be fortified with which nutrients and to what levels. There should also be rules as to what claims companies can make about fortified products and what consumers must be told to prevent deception.

Other Label Information

Though less directly concerned with nutrition, there are many other items on food labels that may be of potential use to consumers who want to know what they're buying and whether it's worth the price. Among them are:

Weight statement. *"Net weight"* (or volume), given in common weights and measures, refers to the weight of the entire product minus the package it comes in, including the liquid of canned fruits and vegetables. If you want to know how much "real food" you're getting, you'd have to know the *"drained weight"* (the product minus the liquid) or the *"filled weight"* (how much of the product actually went into the package), but currently such information is rarely provided. For dry foods, net weight would be the same as filled weight.

Date. All processed foods that are packaged in a factory are dated, but usually the date is in a code that only the manufacturer and perhaps the market manager can interpret. Certain perishable foods are required by law in some states to have an "open date"—that is, a date that consumers can readily understand. Currently, four kinds of open dates are used:

"Packed on"	The date the food was packed. It is really only useful if you know how long the food remains fresh. In general, frozen foods are best used within a few months of the "pack" date and canned foods within a year.
"Sell by"	The last date the product should be sold. These "pull" dates are often found on breads, dairy products, cold cuts, and fresh fruit juices. Some bakery products can be sold at a reduced price after this date.
"Best if used by"	The date by which you should use the product if you want it to be top quality. It doesn't mean,

however, that you can't use the product after this "quality assurance" or "freshness" date has passed. It might be found on cheeses.

"Expiration (EXP)" The date after which the product should not be used. Yeast, baby formula, and milk may have expiration dates.

Product illustration. If a picture of a product appears on the label, it must represent what the consumer would find inside the package or what the food would look like if prepared according to directions.

Storage information. Some food labels tell you to store the product in a cool, dry place (always best for any packaged foods, including canned goods) or to refrigerate it after purchase or after opening. You'll get the best quality and least waste if you follow these instructions.

Universal product code. These are bunches of parallel blue or black lines of various widths with a long serial number beneath them. They are designed for computerized inventories and check-out that provides you with a sales slip showing an abbreviated description of the product and its manufacturer. The computer is programmed with the product's price, so few mistakes are made by the check-out clerk.

Product guarantee. This is a voluntary statement that some companies offer on their products to assure consumer satisfaction. If you are in any way displeased with the product, send a note to the company with the reason for your dissatisfaction (see instructions on the label); you will probably get your money back.

Manufacturer. All food products must carry the name and address of the manufacturer, packer, or distributor. Write to them (attention: customer service) if you want more information about a product—such as the amount of sodium or cholesterol it contains—or if you wish to register a complaint.

What the Label Cannot Say

The federal government does not allow any manufacturer to make health claims on food labels or in advertisements for food products. *No one can say the following:*

• The presence of a particular nutrient (or lack of it) makes the food useful for the prevention, treatment, or cure of any disease.
• A food has dietary properties that are of no significant value in

human nutrition. This prohibits claims about "nonvitamins" like rutin or inositol and other quasinutrients in food and vitamin preparations.

• A natural vitamin is better than one that has been added to a food.

• An adequate amount of nutrients cannot be obtained from a normal balanced diet.

• The soil in which a food is grown has made it nutritionally inadequate or deficient in quality. This prohibits claims of superiority for "organically grown" foods unless these claims are supported by scientific data.

• The processing or handling of a product has made it inadequate or deficient. This prohibits claims that certain foods, such as those prepared without additives, are more nutritious than others unless supported by scientific data that show these products to be nutritionally superior to competing products.

INDEX

abortions, spontaneous, 336
accidents:
alcohol and, 261, 262, 274
overweight and, 287
acid controllers, as additives, 471
acidophilus milk, 252, 254, 335
acne, 401–2
additives, food, 463–91
acid controllers as, 471
amounts allowed by FDA of, 475
benefits of, 464–66, 470–72
cancer and, 468, 469, 470, 473, 476, 478–85
coloring agents as, 469, 474, 477–78, 486–88, 515
description of, 466–68
federal legislation on, 473–75
flavorings as, 468–69, 474, 486–88, 515
as food industry name for chemicals, 464
functions of, by type of substance, 468–72
GRAS substances as, 473–76, 483
in "health foods," 492–93
human vs. laboratory animals reactions to, 474–75
hyperactive children and, 486–88
initials used for, 464
interaction of substances and, 476, 481
label identification of, 514–15
leavenings as, 471
minerals as, 471–72
"natural" labeling and, 490
natural substances as, 466
preservatives as, 469–71
in "prior sanctioned" status, 473
problems with, 465, 471, 486–88
rational approach to, 489–90
safety of, 7, 8, 468–69, 472–86, 488–89, 526–27
salt as, 467, 468, 489, 490
spices as, 515
sweeteners as, 467, 468, 483–86, 489, 490
synthetic copies of natural substances as, 466

testing of, 472, 473–76
texture agents as, 471
unintentional, 466
vitamins as, 468, 471–72
wholly synthetic chemicals as, 466
yearly individual consumption of, 467, 468
see also labels, labeling
adolescents, 389–403
acne and, 401–2
appetite of, 389
boys, 389–90, 394, 400–401, 450
calcium needs of, 394
calorie needs of, 389–90
consumption patterns of, 392–93
crash diets and, 401, 402–3
eating at home by, 399–400
fast foods and, 395–99
girls, 389–90, 394, 400–401, 402–3, 426
growth spurt in, 389
iron needs of, 394, 450
milk for, 394
nutrition needs of, 389–403
overweight, 400–401
snacking by, 399–400
underweight, 401
vegetarian diets of, 400, 449
vitamin-mineral deficiencies in, 390
vitamin-mineral needs of (table), 391
see also children
aflatoxin, 502
Agriculture Department, U.S., 9, 11, 13, 131, 204, 396, 482, 494
grading standards of, 520–23
How to Buy series of, 423
Human Nutrition Center of, 11
labeling and, 512, 515, 524
meal plans of, 23, 26–29
nutrient information published by, 49
school breakfast programs and, 373
school lunch program of, 382–83
alcoholic beverages, 15, 258–74
athletics and, 423, 424
benefits of, 258, 259–60
calories and, 266, 267
congeners in, 269

ABOUT THE AUTHOR

A native of New York City, JANE E. BRODY studied biochemistry at the New York State College of Agriculture and Life Sciences at Cornell University, receiving a B.S. degree in 1962, and studied science writing at the University of Wisconsin School of Journalism, receiving an M.S. degree in 1963. She has been a science and medical writer for the *New York Times* since 1965 and has been writing the Personal Health column for the *Times* since 1976. Other books she wrote are *Secrets of Good Health* (with Richard Engquist), *You Can Fight Cancer and Win* (with Dr. Arthur I. Holleb as consultant), *Jane Brody's The New York Times Guide to Personal Health,* and *Jane Brody's Good Food Book.* An inveterate jogger, cyclist, tennis player, swimmer, skater, walker, gardener, and cook, she lives with her husband and twin sons in Brooklyn, New York.